Fundamentals of Aquatic Veterinary Medicine

Fundamentals of Aquatic Veterinary Medicine

Edited by

Laura Urdes
University of Agricultural Sciences and Veterinary Medicine
Bucharest, Romania

Chris Walster
The Island Veterinary Associates
Stafford, UK

Julius Tepper
Long Island Fish Hospital
Manorville, NY, USA

WILEY Blackwell

This edition first published 2022

Registered Offices
John Wiley & Sons, Inc., 111 River Street, Hoboken, NJ 07030, USA
John Wiley & Sons Ltd, The Atrium, Southern Gate, Chichester, West Sussex, PO19 8SQ, UK

Editorial Office
9600 Garsington Road, Oxford, OX4 2DQ, UK

For details of our global editorial offices, customer services, and more information about Wiley products visit us at www.wiley.com.

Wiley also publishes its books in a variety of electronic formats and by print-on-demand. Some content that appears in standard print versions of this book may not be available in other formats.

Library of Congress Cataloging-in-Publication Data

Names: Urdes, Laura, editor. | Walster, Chris, editor. | Tepper, Julius, editor.
Title: Fundamentals of aquatic veterinary medicine / edited by Laura Urdes, Chris Walster, Julius Tepper.
Description: First edition. | Hoboken, NJ : Wiley-Blackwell, 2022. | Includes bibliographical references and index.
Identifiers: LCCN 2021036619 (print) | LCCN 2021036620 (ebook) | ISBN 9781119612704 (paperback) | ISBN 9781119612711 (Adobe PDF) | ISBN 9781119612728 (epub)
Subjects: MESH: Veterinary Medicine | Aquatic Organisms | Animal Diseases | Fishes | Amphibians | Invertebrates
Classification: LCC SF997.5.A65 (print) | LCC SF997.5.A65 (ebook) | NLM SF 997.5.A65 | DDC 636.089–dc23
LC record available at https://lccn.loc.gov/2021036619
LC ebook record available at https://lccn.loc.gov/2021036620

Cover Design: Wiley
Cover Images: courtesy of Wes Baumgartner, Chris Walster, Julius Tepper, Laura Urdes

Set in 9.5/12.5pt STIXTwoText by Straive, Pondicherry, India

10 9 8 7 6 5 4 3 2 1

Contents

Preface

Of the various subspecialties of veterinary medicine, aquatic veterinary medicine is unique in that it encompasses the knowledge, skills and experience needed to care for multiple classes of organisms living in an aquatic environment very different from our own. Although many of the practice techniques and drugs are familiar to the clinician, the aquatic environment poses additional problems that are not encountered in a terrestrial setting. Despite these requirements for advanced knowledge, many veterinary school curricula have limited or no formal studies of aquatic veterinary medicine, even though this has been recommended by the World Organisation for Animal Health (OIE).

This book is intended for veterinary students looking to acquire day-one competency, as defined by the OIE, and are advised to use this book in the order of presentation, as each chapter builds on the previous one. It is also suitable for veterinary schools wishing to establish a course covering the nine core areas of aquatic veterinary medicine. For veterinarians interested in practicing aquatic veterinary medicine, and aquatic veterinarians looking to become certified through the CertAqV program of the World Aquatic Veterinary Medical Association, it provides a valuable resource to obtain necessary skills and technical understanding.

There is a significant amount of information contributed by dozens of authors from around the world on the nine core areas of the CertAqV certification program, so a companion website has been created with access to supplementary data. Each chapter in the book has links to the companion website, where additional text, figures, and further reading and resources can be found.

The diseases presented in this printed version of the text are those that are considered to have worldwide importance. Diseases found primarily in one locality or isolated to only one or a few species can be found in the online text. With respect to exploratory surgery in aquatic birds, mammals, amphibians and reptiles, it should be considered that the procedures and techniques are similar to their terrestrial counterparts except where noted throughout the book.

List of Contributors

Olanike K. Adeyemo
Fish and Wildlife Unit, Department of Veterinary Public Health and Preventive Medicine, University of Ibadan
Ibadan, Nigeria

Acacia Alcivar-Warren
ONE HEALTH Epigenomics Educational Initiative, Environmental Genomics Inc.
Southborough, MA, USA
Fundación para la Conservación de la Biodiversidad (FUCOBI)
Quito, Ecuador

Kelly Bateman
Crustacean Health Theme Lead, OIE Collaborating Centre for Emerging Aquatic Animal Diseases, Cefas
Dorset, UK

Wes Baumgartner
University of Illinois
Urbana, IL, USA

Trista Becker
US Fish and Wildlife Service, Fish Health Program Lead, Southwestern Fish Health Unit
Dexter, New Mexico, USA

James E. Bogan, Jr.
The Critter Fixer of Central Florida
Oviedo, Florida, USA

Morag Clinton
University of Alaska, Fairbanks
Fairbanks, AK, USA

Erdem Danyer
Veterinary Control Central Research Institute, Wildlife Department
Ankara, Turkey

Pádraig Duignan
The Marine Mammal Center
Sausalito, California, USA

Mansour El-Matbouli
University of Veterinary Medicine
Vienna, Austria

María J. Forzán
College of Veterinary Medicine, Long Island University
Brookville, New York

Leo Foyle
College of Public Health, Medical and Veterinary Sciences, Division of Tropical Health and Medicine, James Cook University
Townsville, Queensland, Australia

Farah Gonul Aydin
Department of Pharmacology and Toxicology, Ankara University Faculty of Veterinary Medicine
Ankara, Turkey

Soliman Hatem
University of Veterinary Medicine
Vienna, Austria
Faculty of Veterinary Medicine, Assiut University
Assiut, Egypt

Sherry Kasper
The Animal Hospital &
Pet Resort at Southwood
Tallahassee, FL, USA

Myron Kebus
Department of Agriculture, Trade and Consumer Protection
Madison, WI, USA

Jack Kottwitz
College of Veterinary Medicine, Auburn University
Auburn, AL, USA

Gregory Lewbart
College of Veterinary Medicine, North Carolina State University
Raleigh, NC, USA

Richmond Loh
The Fish Vet
Perth, Australia

Matt Longshaw
Q2 Lab Solutions
Livingston, Scotland, UK

Adolf Maas
ZooVet Consulting, PLLC
Toledo, Ohio, USA

Nicole Marie Nemeth
Southeastern Cooperative Wildlife Disease Study, Department of Pathology, University of Georgia
Athens, Georgia, USA

Nicholas Saint-Erne
Arizona Exotic Animal Hospital
Phoenix, Arizona, USA

Mona Saleh
University of Veterinary Medicine
Vienna, Austria

David Scarfe
Faculty of Veterinary Sciences, University of Pretoria
Onderstepoort, South Africa
Aquatic Veterinary Associates International
Bartlett, IL, USA

Julius Tepper
Long Island Fish Hospital
Manorville, NY, USA

Laura Urdes
University of Agricultural Sciences and Veterinary Medicine
Bucharest, Romania

Vasile Vulpe
University of Agricultural Sciences and Veterinary Medicine
Iasi, Romania

Chris Walster
The Island Veterinary Associates
Stafford, UK

Acknowledgement

Special thanks to Dr. Craig Harms for the input on exploratory surgery in fish in chapter 6.

About the Companion Website

Don't forget to visit the companion web site for this book:

www.wiley.com/go/urdes/aquatic-veterinary-medicine

There you will find valuable materials, including:

- Further supplementary materials for each chapter, additional references, and further readings

Scan this QR code to visit the companion website

1

Aquatic Environment and Life Support Systems

Sherry Kasper, Olanike K. Adeyemo, Trista Becker, David Scarfe, Julius Tepper, and Wes Baumgartner

Learning Objectives
Students should demonstrate knowledge of the elements of life support systems and water found within these systems.

1.1 Introduction

For veterinarians to adequately evaluate the health or disease problems of aquatic animals, it is imperative that they understand the impact of, and assess the conditions in which the animal lives. Like terrestrial animals, the health of aquatic species is impacted by their environment. Suboptimal conditions can result in non-infectious diseases or create situations favorable for opportunistic pathogens, which can lead to decreased growth, increased morbidity and clinical disease. It is therefore imperative to include an assessment of water quality and a history of any changes in the environment as part of a clinical evaluation of any health problem.

Fish health management is a term used in aquaculture to describe management practices designed to prevent fish disease. Once fish get sick it can be difficult to salvage them. Successful fish health management begins with prevention of disease rather than treatment, accomplished through, among other considerations, good water quality management. Without this foundation it is impossible to prevent outbreaks of opportunistic diseases. Fish are constantly bathed in potential pathogens, including bacteria, fungi, and parasites. Suboptimal water quality generally associated with stressful conditions allows potential pathogens to cause disease.

The biotic integrity of an ecological system is often reflected by the health of organisms that reside in that system. Proper management of the aquatic environment therefore offers optimum environmental conditions for the growth and better health of the cultivated fish. It also strengthens the defense mechanism of the body to fight against invading disease-producing organisms. Eradicating any predatory or invasive fish species, disinfecting the pond, selecting quality and healthy seed for stocking, maintaining proper species ratios and stocking density, regulating water quality, as well as feeding and handling fish properly, are the various steps of these management measures.

Fundamentals of Aquatic Veterinary Medicine, First Edition. Edited by Laura Urdes, Chris Walster, and Julius Tepper.

Companion website: www.wiley.com/go/urdes/aquatic-veterinary-medicine

With a very large number of cultured aquatic species, and hence different water systems in which they may live, the task of evaluating optimal conditions for every species may seem daunting. However, if considered on an ecosystem level for those that thrive naturally in freshwater, brackish or marine aquatic ecosystems, and evaluating these as life-support systems for different taxa, the task is simplified. Furthermore, many biotic and abiotic physicochemical features of fresh, brackish or marine water bodies are similar, even for very different taxa.

This chapter provides general information about basic features of aquatic environments and life-support systems important to the health of finfish, amphibians, mollusks, crustaceans and invertebrates that veterinarians might encounter. As aquatic mammals, birds and other homeothermic species are generally covered in veterinary curricula, they are not addressed here.

1.2 The Life-Support System in Aquaculture and Ornamental Fish Care

Aquaculture is the farming of aquatic organisms including fish, mollusks, crustaceans and aquatic plants, with some sort of intervention in the rearing process to enhance production, such as regular stocking, feeding, and protection from predators. Farming also implies individual or corporate ownership of the stock being cultivated. Aquatic ecosystems provide the basis for aquatic production. The worldwide practice of aquaculture runs the gamut from low-technology extensive methods to highly intensive systems. Although used for housing and maintaining ornamental fish, similar aquasystems are found in large public aquaria and private homes and are discussed in this chapter. The term 'life-support system' is understood as a complete system that satisfies the physiological needs of an aquatic organism in question. Diagrams and photographs of examples of life-support systems can be found in Chapter 3.

Managed ecosystems form the basis for aquaculture production, which has been widely offered as a means of complementing and ultimately supplementing traditional fisheries. Here, unlike fisheries, inputs, production processes and quality of output can be at least partially controlled, and ownership, care and environmental responsibility might be more easily established. By removing natural constraints to survival and productivity, and by husbandry and management, production need be limited only by availability of simple inputs such as land, water, seed (hatchling, spawn, fry or fingerling), fertilizers and feeds. The design of a life-support system is dependent on the type of aquatic system in question, being either a flow-through system or a closed system. In a flow-through system, the main elements include a spigot or waterfall that is adjustable for the amount of water flow necessary, a drain that is usually positioned at the opposite end of the system, potential for increased aeration, and, possibly, temperature controls.

A closed system may be a pond, tank or aquarium. In a pond, the most important elements are circulation and aeration, and it may also include a filtration system. Tanks and aquaria usually require a filtration system, aeration, and often temperature control. The source of the water is important when deciding on the type of aquatic system and the type of life-support system. A large well, river or lake is necessary for a flow-through system because of the high volume of water that is needed to maintain proper water quality. If city water is being used in a system, it is important to have a reservoir to dechlorinate any new water entering the system. In recirculating systems, water circulation and purification is accomplished with the use of powered pumps and filtration systems. The type of equipment used will depend on the type of fish, number of fish and the expected growth rate of those fish.

In aquaculture, high-intensity growth of fish leads to higher ammonia levels and waste production. The output of the pump should allow for a flow of the full volume of water in the system to pass through the filter every two to three hours. This is referred to as the "turnover time". It is calculated by dividing the water volume in the system by the volume per time rating of the circulation, measured at the return (the volume/time is variously described in gallons/minute or hour as GPM, GPH or metric m^3/hour). In tanks and ponds, flow rates are very variable, from less than five minutes in the smallest aquaria to more than 10 hours in larger ponds. Submersible pumps with low maintenance sealed impellors may be used in small ponds and aquaria, but larger aquasystems typically use external pumps. The filtration system should contain biological media with an appropriate surface area to allow for detoxification of ammonia based on the number of fish. On average, 1 m^2 of active surface area can process 1 gram of ammonia every 24 hours (Wildgoose, 2001).

Monitoring of the system may be fully automated or may be performed by individuals. The benefits of automated monitoring equipment include the ability to set alarms for power outages, changes in dissolved oxygen and large changes in ammonia. Some systems are able to calculate flow rates and water usage, which is beneficial for production calculations. Monitoring should include ammonia, nitrite, nitrate, dissolved oxygen, temperature, total alkalinity and pH to assure proper water quality parameters.

1.2.1 Extensive Culture System

The extensive culture system is characterized by low to no inputs (food, fertilizer, etc.) and low stocking densities. Extensive aquaculture is practiced in lakes, reservoirs, lagoons, ponds and tanks.

1.2.1.1 Ponds

The most common production system in use is the earthen pond. Earthen ponds are extremely popular among fish growers due in part to ease of construction, low maintenance, relatively small area requirements and ability to grow a wide variety of species. Additionally, because earthen ponds mimic nature, they may produce fish of an overall healthier appearance than other techniques. A natural supply of food is often available in earthen ponds, which may lead to better fish health. Pond culture can vary, from all life stages naturally occurring in a single pond to elaborate systems with discrete ponds for holding broodstock, spawning, rearing, growing and catch-out or harvest.

1.2.1.2 Tanks

Tanks essentially act as ponds but are generally constructed of concrete or fiberglass. Wood can also be used but must first be treated to prevent rotting. Concrete tanks have the advantage of being less expensive, easily constructed and formed into various shapes.

- Plastic, fiberglass or glass tanks are ordinary tanks which are either designed and constructed for rearing fish or used for storing water. They can be moved from one place to another.
- Wooden troughs are constructed with planks. They vary in size and depth. After construction, the tank is lined with nylon to prevent leakage. It can be moved from one place to other.

1.2.2 Semi-Intensive Culture System

The semi-intensive culture system is distinguished by increased stocking rates and the requirement for some level of input, such as food, fertilizer, chemicals, etc.

- Cage culture uses existing water resources (i.e. lakes or ponds) but encloses the fish in a cage or basket, which allows water to pass freely between the fish and the pond or lake. One of the main advantages is the ease of harvesting.

- Fish pens are enclosures installed in open waters that are not too deep for raising fish. The fish have access to the water bottom, unlike in cages.
- Rafts/trays or long lines are mostly used for oyster culture.
- Some improvised containers such as bathroom tubs, big plastic containers, abandoned plank canoe, earthen pots are used to culture fish where the farmer cannot afford the conventional rearing facilities. Some fish farmers in Lagos use these containers for breeding. Apart from breeding purposes, this type of rearing facility is not suitable for commercial fish farming.

1.2.3 Intensive Culture System

Intensive culture system is where animals are maintained in systems such as ponds, tanks and raceways, where the support parameters are carefully controlled and dependence on the natural environment is minimal. Such systems require a high degree of management and usually involve substantial investment and operating costs, resulting in high yields per unit area. They typically feature recirculating systems, which filter and reuse all or a portion of their water. Currently, this technique is in limited use due to its high start-up and maintenance costs. It has several advantages, however, in that this system is highly desirable in areas where a constant water supply may be questionable or a discharge is not appropriate. Other advantages of this type of system include the ability to incorporate the growth of a second product through hydroponics and the use of settled material as fertilizer. As the technology evolves and water withdrawal and discharge requirements become more stringent, this technique is bound to see an increase in use. Ponds are also very popular for housing ornamental fish, such as koi or goldfish. Typically lined with EPDM rubber, these can be fairly simple in having only a recirculating system and waterfall or extremely complex, with sophisticated filtration and water conditioning systems.

1.3 Physical Features of Life-Support Systems

Multiple designs from simple box filters to multistage proprietary units can be found in use for home aquaria. For freshwater systems, these typically include a mechanical filter to remove particulate and a biofilter placed afterwards in the return water flow. Often an ultraviolet (UV) light unit is installed to control planktonic algae. In saltwater systems, a protein skimmer is also used to remove dissolved organic matter. Adequate gas exchange is generally assured by the simple water turnover provided by the filter system, although additional aeration is often provided with the use of air pumps and air stones. Ponds will usually have the same components as freshwater aquaria, scaled up to meet the needs of larger fish. The most modern designs will typically feature a prefilter, mechanical filter, biofilter and UV light. Water is returned to the pond via a spillway or waterfall, which assures adequate gas exchange. Designs for these components vary, with some rudimentary systems having only a biofilter and waterfall. As this system relies on in-pond sedimentation, regular depopulation and cleanout is needed. Public aquaria differ only by size and scale from home aquarium systems. However, some large-scale water purification equipment is described below. Some examples of aquaculture open and closed husbandry systems (raceways, recirculating, ponds, net pens) are given in Chapter 3. Different systems for different life stages are described in Chapter 10.

1.3.1 Mechanical, Chemical and Other Types of Filtration

Recirculating systems can vary in complexity and design. Depending on the water source, varying types of water purification may be required or recommended to prevent pathogens at the point of entry as well as within the system itself. Mechanical filters are often used to improve water quality and reduce pathogen loads by removing particulate matter in the system. Recirculating systems that are considered self-cleaning remove waste solids and provide some water purification prior to system reentry. Mechanical filter design based on water flow direction can be described as "downflow", where the water to be processed passes by gravity or under pressure down through the media or "upflow", where it is forced under pressure up through the media. The advantage of this upflow design is to allow sediment to fall away from the media, making it somewhat self-cleaning (Tepper, 2000). Media used may be sand, polypropylene or fiberglass mesh or polypropylene brushes in downflow systems and polypropylene beads in upflow systems.

Prefilters can be used to separate settleable solids by rotating the water in an upflow direction. This strips off the heavier particulate, enabling more efficient water processing before entering the mechanical filter.

Industrial aquaculture facilities may use self-cleaning tanks in recirculating systems to remove waste solids and provide some water purification using large rotating drum filters. Also, water sources with high total solids prior to system entry may also require large screen filtration to remove solids. Other large facilities may employ pressurized canisters of upflow design for this purpose (floating bead filters). These canisters are also often seen in home pond filtration, although downflow box filters with filter mesh for particulate removal are also used, where they are the most common type of filter for small aquasystems like freshwater and marine home aquaria. Sand canister filters are sometimes used due to their high efficiency at removing solids and low cost. They have the disadvantage of being hard to maintain over time due to "caking" of the sand media.

1.3.1.1 Ultrasonic Cavitation

Life stages of larger organisms such as the salmon louse may be effectively removed from discharge water with ultrasonic cavitation (Svendsen *et al.*, 2017). Anecdotally, some hatcheries have seen reduction in levels of other parasites with the installation of some types of low-head oxygenators, perhaps through a similar mechanism such as microbubbles.

1.3.1.2 Ultraviolet Filtration

Pathogens can be removed effectively from water by UV filtration. These filters cause DNA damage to microorganisms by radiating with light in the UV-C spectrum. The dose required to inactivate an organism varies, with some organisms proving more difficult and thus requiring a higher dose than others. Published values for specific pathogens can be found and may vary with the system used, the source of water, species being reared, and the potential pathogens of concern. These doses are calculated under ideal laboratory conditions and, in reality, the effective dose required may be much higher in a system with poor water quality. UV filters consist of a light source (bulbs) contained within a vessel that permits water to be passed through at varying rates. The amount of time the water is in contact with the light and the wattage of the bulb determines the dose. These systems are subject to impacts from turbidity of the water and require regular maintenance to remain effective. The glass must be cleaned of debris and silt and most manufacturers recommend bulb replacement at a minimum of once a year. Water with a high organic load will reflect the UV radiation and cause a decline in the effective dose. Systems with high total solid loads or otherwise high in organics may require prefiltration to assure reliable UV effectiveness. Flows must be monitored and not increased to exceed the capabilities of the UV filter.

Other factors that may impact the dose requirements for pathogen inactivation in a system are the bacterial repair mechanisms – photoreactivation and dark repair – that may allow bacteria to resist being killed by repairing the UV damage. Preventing exposure of the water to natural light will help to inhibit photoreactivation of bacteria in the system, as will increasing the UV dose in the system beyond the standard published doses. Preventing reduction of lamp intensity, which can occur with poor water quality or increased flow, will also help to reduce photoreactivation in the system. In cold-water aquaculture with short water retention times, photoreactivation is more likely to become a problem than dark repair. Likewise, in recirculating systems that have long water retention times (many cycles of the same water or a high reuse percentage with very few additions of new water) dark repair may be more of a concern. UV filtration at lower doses is often employed in aquasystems for planktonic algae control (using a UV light unit).

1.3.1.3 Ozone Filtration

Another type of water treatment that can be used is ozone. This effective oxidizer is produced in an onsite system and requires a high voltage generation unit. It is usually reserved for larger industrial aquasystems and public aquaria. A large source of purified oxygen is required to produce the ozone, which can be linked to a low head oxygenator or other oxygen feed systems that may already be in use to increase production capacity of a facility. Ozone oxidizes cell membranes, making it effective at killing bacteria, but fish and humans should not be directly exposed to it. As with UV, contact time in the water is important, with considerations for an initial killing dose followed by a residual dose to meet the required contact time. The residual dose can be reached inside a residual holding tank, allowing for longer contact time. The ozone must be transferred to the water by some method of injection system and inactivated before reaching the fish holding tanks, as fish are highly sensitive to residual ozone. When used in seawater systems, additional byproducts may need to be managed.

1.3.1.4 Biological Filtration

The conversion of ammonia to nitrite and nitrate is critically important in aquasystems where new water exchange is minimal. These systems must be treated with care to ensure that adequate levels of beneficial bacteria are maintained to perform this conversion. In cases of high recirculating water reuse systems that recirculate water in the 90% range, a dedicated biofilter is used before the water reenters the main system. In the biofilter, the conversion is accomplished through the use of specialized media designed to maximize bacterial performance.

Features of a biofilter that impact its capacity to convert ammonia through to nitrate in any aquasystem are the type of media used and the surface area per unit volume for bacterial growth, as well as the water flow pattern, degree of oxygen exchange and adequacy of sediment removal. Most biofilters use plastic composite material, although older systems may employ lava rock. Sand can also be used in upflow-designed tanks, called fluidized bed bioreactors, after the water has been cleared of settleable solids. Many types of biological filters that use varying technologies are already in use in recirculating aquaculture. This field is rapidly growing and expanding. With increasing popularity and utility of recirculating systems, the capabilities of these units continue to improve and it is important that a system is designed to allow for upgrades and improvements. While biofiltration conserves water and increases production capacities, these filters require substantial floor space and add a high cost to initial system installation. In selecting this type of system, the long-term benefits such as water usage savings, increases in production capacity, and decreased effluent discharge should be weighed against the initial cost. The details of biofilters are complex. Additional information can be found in specialized texts such as *Recirculating Aquaculture* by Timmons *et al.* (2018). Further study is recommended prior to working with these types of complex systems.

1.3.2 Aquasystem Water

1.3.2.1 Abiotic (Chemical and Physical) Properties

Oceans, rivers, lakes, and even ponds, are various types of aquatic ecosystems. The abiotic components of aquatic ecosystems are the physical and/or chemical factors characteristic of the environment that act on the living organisms during any part of their life. These abiotic factors are also called ecological factors. They vary from ecosystem to ecosystem; for example, the abiotic factors in the marine biome differ from those of fresh water in terms of chemistry, light, current and temperature.

Some of the chemicophysical parameters of water have a direct influence on fish health. Any abrupt and wider than normal fluctuations of such values cause a state of stress in fish, sometimes resulting in widespread disease outbreaks. Dissolved oxygen content, pH, turbidity, temperature, introduction of some chemicals, detergents, pesticides and naturally produced toxic products like hydrogen sulfide, ammonia, dinoflagellate toxins are potential stress-related parameters.

1.3.2.2 Temperature

Fish are ectotherms, which means that they do not regulate their body temperature internally so it fluctuates with external environmental changes. Sudden change often causes stress and sometimes even death in extreme situations. Temperature affects the development and growth of fish more than any other single factor and also influences other variables. Metabolic rate either increases or decreases two-fold for every 8°C. Each species has an optimal temperature range for growth and reproduction. Cultured species should be selected according to the prevailing water temperature in each locality. This is because the temperature range at which an organism can survive depends on their temperature adaptation pattern over time.

Water temperature greatly influences water quality, because the growth and metabolism of phytoplankton, bacteria and other microorganisms increases with increasing temperature. Moreover, water holds less oxygen at higher temperatures. Dissolved oxygen depletion is much more likely to occur during hot weather than during cooler periods. Rates of chemical processes such as ionization, mineral dissolution, adsorption and ion exchange also increase in response to higher water temperature. The onset of potentially harmful water quality events is faster in warmer weather. A deep pond can also be subject to thermal stratification, with large temperature fluctuations among layers of the water column.

- Warm-water species grow best above 21°C
- Cold-water species grow best below 21°C
- Cool-water species grow best at mid-range from 21°C to 28°C
- Sudden temperature changes cause stress and even death.

1.3.2.3 pH

The term "pH" is a mathematical transformation of the hydrogen ion (H^+) concentration; it conveniently expresses the acidity or basicity of water. The lowercase letter "p" refers to "power" or exponent, and pH is defined as the negative logarithm of the hydrogen ion concentration. Each change of one pH unit represents a 10-fold change in hydrogen ion concentration. The pH scale is usually represented as ranging from 0 to 14, where lower number reflects higher acidity and the higher number reflects higher alkalinity. Water with a pH of 4.5 or lower has no measurable alkalinity. Water with a pH of 8.3 or higher has no measurable acidity. At 25°C, a pH value of 7 is neutral; this describes the neutral point of water at which the concentrations of hydrogen and hydroxyl ions (OH^-) are equal (each at 10–7 moles/l). The pH of freshwater ecosystems can fluctuate considerably within daily and seasonal timeframes, and most freshwater animals have evolved to tolerate a relatively wide environmental pH range. Animals can, however, become stressed or die when exposed to pH extremes or when pH changes rapidly, even if the change occurs within a pH range that is normally tolerated. The pH of water in ponds often increases during the day and decreases at night. Fish and other vertebrates have an average blood pH of 7.4. Recommended pH range for cultured fish is 6.5–9.0. Acid death point is around 4; alkaline death point is around 11. The hydrogen ion concentration affects aqueous equilibria involving ammonia, hydrogen sulfide, chlorine and dissolved metals. Interactions of pH with these variables are often more important than the direct effects of pH on aquatic animals. For example, the toxicity of ammonia to fish increases with an increase in pH. Chemical interactions among carbon dioxide, hydrogen ions and the anions that produce alkalinity buffer the pH of most natural waters in a range of about 6–8.5.

1.3.2.4 Dissolved Oxygen

Dissolved oxygen monitoring is critical in aquaculture. Temperature, salinity and elevation affect dissolved oxygen. As these three factors increase, dissolved oxygen at saturation decreases. For example, the cold temperature of the Antarctic results in higher dissolved oxygen concentrations compared with warmer tropical waters. Freshwater at sea level holds 9.2 ppm at 20°C and 7.6 ppm at 30°C. Fish become more active and increase their metabolic oxygen needs as temperature increases. As temperature rises, fish also need more dissolved oxygen to grow muscle tissue. Minimum tolerable dissolved oxygen levels increase with a rise in temperature.

In general, most fish species will grow and thrive within a dissolved oxygen range of 5–12 mg/l (parts per million). However, if levels drop below 4 mg/l they may stop feeding, become stressed and begin to die. Dissolved oxygen ranges for cultured fish are as follows:

- 0–2 ppm – small fish may survive a short exposure, but lethal if exposure is prolonged. This range is lethal to larger fish.
- 2–5 ppm – most fish survive, but growth is slower if prolonged; may be stressful; aeration devices are often used below 3 ppm.
- 5 ppm to saturation – the desirable range for all.
- With rainbow trout, the minimum lethal limit is 1.6 ppm at lower temperatures and 2.5 ppm at higher temperatures.

Oxygen and pH are best measured in situ (with probes) or as soon as possible after collection (preferably before leaving the site) as, in most situations, levels will change during storage and transport.

Biological oxygen demand is a measure of the oxygen used by all organisms in an aquasystem.

1.3.2.5 Carbon Dioxide

Carbon dioxide (CO_2) is consumed during photosynthesis by plants and expired during respiration by animals, plants (at night) and bacteria in an aquasystem. When added to pond water by respiration or diffusion, it forms a weak acid (carbonic acid), which lowers the pH. Dissolved oxygen and pH cycles follow the same daily peaks and troughs. Carbon dioxide levels of below 10 mg/l are thought to be well tolerated by fish. While levels greater than 20 ppm often harm fish, especially if dissolved oxygen levels are low, sensitivity to CO_2 varies between species. The level of CO_2 in source water varies greatly, and is further affected by the respiratory and photosynthetic activity of animals and plants, and the level of decomposition of organic material in that water (a very significant contributor to CO_2 levels in some nutrient-rich waters). CO_2 can build up to significantly high levels in systems with large numbers of animals and relatively slow water turnover.

The effect of increased CO_2 in water is to reduce the rate at which CO_2 from the animal's own metabolism can be released from the blood through the gills. As a result, CO_2 in the blood also increases (known as hypercapnia), resulting in a drop in the blood pH and acidosis. At the same time, the oxygen-carrying ability of the hemoglobin in the blood is reduced. The animal can counteract the effect by balancing the acidosis with an exchange of ions, such as increasing the uptake of bicarbonate and losing hydrogen and phosphate ions and little harm is done. In the long term, this balancing act can have a more profound effect on the health of the animal. Carbon dioxide causes problems in recirculating aquaculture systems without aeration or degassing.

1.3.2.6 Nitrogen

The nitrogen (N_2) biogeochemistry of aquaculture ponds is dominated by biological transformations of nitrogen added to ponds in the form of inorganic or organic fertilizers and formulated feeds. Nitrogen application in excess of pond assimilatory capacity can lead to the deterioration of water quality through the accumulation of nitrogenous compounds (e.g., ammonia and nitrite) toxic to the fauna. Principal sources of nitrogen include animal excretion and sediment flux derived from the mineralization of organic matter and molecular diffusion from reduced sediment, although cyanobacterial nitrogen fixation and atmospheric deposition are occasionally important.

1.3.2.7 Hydrogen Sulfide

Hydrogen Sulfide (H_2S) is a poisonous gas with a "rotten egg" smell, produced by anaerobic decomposition of organics. Sulfur is an essential element for plants, animals and bacteria. H_2S is present in natural waters and in aquaculture systems, mainly as the sulfate ion. Sulfide can occur in water because it is a metabolite of Desulfovibrio species and certain other bacteria found in anaerobic zones, usually in sediment. These bacteria use oxygen from sulfate as an alternative to molecular oxygen in respiration. There are three forms of sulfide (H_2S, HS^- and S_2^-), and they exist in a pH and temperature-dependent equilibrium. As pH increases, the proportion of H_2S declines, and that of HS^- rises until the two forms have roughly equal proportions at pH 7. At greater pH, HS^- is the dominant form, and there is no S_2^- until the pH is above 11. Hydrogen sulfide is toxic to aquatic animals because it interferes with reoxidation of cytochrome a3 in respiration. This effect is caused almost entirely by H_2S, while HS^- is essentially non-toxic. Even if it is toxic, S_2^- is not an issue, because it does not occur at pH values found in aquaculture systems.

1.3.2.8 Chlorine

Chlorine is harmful/toxic to fish at values greater than 0.03 ppm. Tap water may range from 4.0 to 8.0 ppm. Sodium thiosulfate can be used to neutralize the chlorine. Chlorine may be used to disinfect equipment, tanks, countertops, and nets at 10 ppm for 24 hours or 200 ppm for 30–60 minutes. Effectiveness is reduced by organic material such as mud, slime and plant material. Sodium hypochlorite is available at concentrations of 15%, 50%, or 65% active.

1.3.2.9 Alkalinity

Alkalinity is the ability of the water to accept hydrogen ions and neutralize them and offers a buffering system to reduce pH swings. It is measured by the amount of acid (hydrogen ion) that water can absorb (buffer) before achieving a designated pH. Total alkalinity is expressed as milligrams per liter or parts per million calcium carbonate (mg/l or ppm $CaCO_3$). It consists of negatively charged bases – carbonates, bicarbonates, and hydroxides. Alkalinity is expressed in equivalent concentrations of calcium carbonate.

Carbonates and bicarbonates are sources of carbon for plants, which is used in photosynthesis to make carbohydrates. Carbonates and bicarbonates are the most common and most important components of alkalinity. A desirable range of total alkalinity for fish culture is $CaCO_3$ 75–200 mg/l. Carbonate–bicarbonate alkalinity (and hardness) in surface and well waters is produced primarily through the interactions of CO_2, water and limestone. Rainwater is acidic because of exposure to atmospheric carbon dioxide and sulfuric acid (H_2SO_4).

1.3.2.10 Hardness

Hardness refers to the concentration of divalent cations (calcium, magnesium, and sodium). Water hardness is important to fish culture and is a commonly reported aspect of water quality. It is also expressed as the calcium carbonate equivalent concentration. The same carbonate rocks responsible for most of the alkalinity are the main sources of calcium and magnesium cations for hardness. Hardness may be an index of potential pond productivity. The minimum hardness for fish is 20 ppm and optimum hardness is around 100 ppm.

Hardness is traditionally measured by chemical titration. The hardness of a water sample is reported in milligrams per liter as calcium carbonate (mg/l $CaCO_3$). Calcium carbonate hardness is a general term which indicates the total quantity of divalent salts present and does not specifically identify whether calcium, magnesium and/or some other divalent salt is causing water hardness. If limestone is responsible for both hardness and alkalinity, the concentrations will be similar, if not identical. However, where sodium bicarbonate ($NaHCO_3$) is responsible for alkalinity, it is possible to have low hardness and high alkalinity.

1.3.2.11 Conductivity, Salinity, Total Dissolved Solids

Conductivity is a measure of water's capability to pass an electrical current. This ability is directly related to the concentration of ions in the water (US Environmental Protection Agency, 2016). These conductive ions come from dissolved salts and inorganic materials such as alkalis, chlorides, sulfides and carbonate compounds (Miller *et al.*, 1988). Compounds that dissolve into ions are also known as electrolytes (Sommer and Spitzer, 2004). The more ions that are present, the higher the conductivity of water. Likewise, the fewer ions that are in the water, the less conductive it is. A sudden increase in pond conductivity can indicate pollution. Agricultural runoff or a sewage leak will increase conductivity due to the additional chloride, phosphate, and nitrate ions.

Salinity is a measure of the total concentration of dissolved solids, usually in parts per thousand (ppt). Anions (negatively charged) are chloride, sulfate, bicarbonate and bromide. Cations (positively charged) are sodium, magnesium, calcium, potassium, and strontium. Sodium and chloride are the major solids. Because the electrolytes form ionic particles as they dissolve, each with a positive and negative charge, salinity is a strong contributor to conductivity. The concentration of water is as follows:

- Freshwater: less than 2 ppt
- Brackish water: 2–16 ppt
- Saltwater: 35 ppt.

Most aquatic organisms can only tolerate a specific salinity range (Clean Water Team, 2002). The physiological adaptation of each species is determined by the salinity of its surrounding environment. Salinity tolerances depend on the osmotic processes within an organism. Fish and other aquatic life that live in fresh water (low salinity) are hyperosmotic (cells have a high ability to eliminate water and retain ions). On the other side of the spectrum, saltwater (high salinity) organisms are hypo-osmotic and maintain a lower internal ionic concentration than seawater. Most species of fish are stenohaline, exclusively freshwater, or exclusively saltwater (Myers, 1949). However, there are a few organisms that can adapt to a range of salinities. These euryhaline organisms can be anadromous, catadromous or true euryhaline. Anadromous organisms live in saltwater but spawn in freshwater. Catadromous species are the opposite – they live in freshwater and migrate to saltwater to spawn (Myers, 1949). True euryhaline species can be found in saltwater or freshwater at any point in their life cycle (Myers, 1949). Estuarine organisms are true euryhaline.

The sum of all ion particles that are smaller than 2 microns (0.0002 cm) is the total dissolved solids. This includes all the disassociated electrolytes that make up salinity concentrations, as well as other compounds such as dissolved organic matter. Freshwater aquasystems should have less than 2000 mg/l of total dissolved solids and most water sources should have much less than that (American Public Health Association *et al.*, 2017).

1.3.2.12 Light, Color, Vibration and Noise

Aquasystem water color influences microplankton growth, which can affect the stability of the water chemistry. Water clarity can affect fish. If fish that prefer turbid waters (e.g., bullhead, catfish, walleye) are cultured in relatively clear water they will experience stress; survival and growth will be adversely affected. Intensive aquaculture systems, particularly recirculating systems, utilize equipment such as aerators, air and water pumps, blowers, and filtration systems that inadvertently increase vibration and noise levels in fish culture tanks (see also vibration and noise in Chapter 10). Field and laboratory studies have shown that fish behavior and physiology can be negatively impacted by intense sound. Chronic exposure to aquaculture production noise could therefore cause increased stress, reduced growth rates, and cold feed conversion efficiency, and decreased survival. In the wild, geological and geophysical exploration, pile driving, drilling, dredging, and vessel traffic all produce manmade noise and vibrations, which may have negative effects on native fauna, which may range from physiological and behavioral effects to physical damage.

1.3.2.13 Greenhouse Gases and Climate Change

Elevation of carbon dioxide in the atmosphere leads to acidification of our water. This change affects all aquatic life. Millions of dollars are lost each year on decreased growth and increased mortality due to large fluctuations in the pH and temperatures of the water. Elevation in the CO_2 levels of the atmosphere push the chemical reaction:

$$HCO_3 \rightarrow H^+ + CO_3^{\,2}$$

to move more toward a disassociation of water molecules and increase the HCO_3^-. In the ocean, this fluctuation is well buffered by salt water, but in coastal areas and rivers the addition of runoff increases the nitrogen, carbon and Ca_2^+, creating large fluctuations in the pH. Climate change has resulted in an increase of the ocean temperatures, changes in mixing and increased intensity of storms globally. These changes, together with large fluctuations in pH, result in large hypoxic zones and the inability of fish to acclimate to them.

Fish in estuaries and coastal areas are affected the most by acidification due to the increased fluctuation of the pH. This fluctuation is exaggerated by nutrient runoff, coastal upwelling, and atmospheric pollution. Fish have been shown to be able to regulate their pH within days, but they rely on the ability to move the CO_2 into the lower partial pressure of carbon dioxide (pCO_2) of the aquatic environment. As atmospheric CO_2 increases, fish can compensate metabolically and regulate their pH but still show elevated levels of the CO_2 in their extracellular fluids. Studies have shown that this elevated level of CO_2 can cause problems with osmoregulation. In addition, studies have shown this increased level of CO_2 can result in increased otolith size in clownfish, Atlantic cod and pollock (Heuer and Grosell, 2014).

The increased CO_2 in the plasma has been shown to affect the metabolic rate and the formation of $CaCO_3^+$. This occurs when HCO_3^- is secreted into the intestinal lumen. This secretion stimulates the secretion of CO_2. This combination precipitates the $Ca2^+$ from the seawater that has been ingested. These then combine to form $CaCO_3^+$. The higher PCO_2 in the plasma has been proven to increase these secretions in midshipmen and toadfish. $CaCO_3^+$ is important for osmoregulation in fish by influencing the osmotic pressure in the luminal cavity. Changes in the amount of $CaCO_3^+$ has the potential to decrease the osmotic balance (Heuer and Grosell, 2014).

Elevations in atmospheric CO_2 have been shown to decrease calcification rates in the carbonate equation:

$$Ca\,CO_3 + CO_2 + H_2O \rightarrow Ca_2^{\;+} + CO_3^{\;2-} + CO_2 \rightarrow Ca2^+ + 2HCO_3^{\;-}$$

Decreases in calcification rates affect coral reefs, planktonic microalgae, coccolithophores, phytoplankton, and all shellfish. Coral reef growth has been shown to decline due to the decrease of calcification, with a predicted decrease of 21–40% over the period of 1880–2065 (Turley *et al.*, 2006). This decline is also dependent on the temperature of the water and other available nutrients. Oysters and abalone have been the focus of many studies in regards to acidification. These organisms have been shown to have a decreased rate of survival at the larval stage due to lack of calcification of the shell and decreased ability to ingest nutrients. The shell of mollusks is produced throughout all its life stages. During the larval stages, the shell is made from deposition of amorphous calcium carbonate, which then forms into a crystalline aragonite. Both these stages of shell development are more soluble in a low pH. Studies have shown that certain levels of pH will cause holes to form in the shells (Wessel *et al.*, 2018).

Acidification of our oceans has a great effect on the ecosystem of the ocean. It is leading to changes in the phytoplankton that are available for ingestion by fish and cultivation. It is predicted to decrease the available fish population of our reefs, which will damage the animal protein consumption of many developing nations. The high fluctuations of pH in the estuaries and coastal areas have the potential to greatly affect fisheries. Mitigation of these fluctuations should include consistent monitoring of the water to enable fisheries to add buffering if necessary (Clements and Chopin, 2017). Options for buffering may include:

- Crushed shell hash in the sediment
- Sodium bicarbonate
- Movement of fish pends away from river mouths.

Further mitigation strategies should include breeding plants and animals that have a high tolerance for low pH. Integration of a multitrophic aquaculture system can help to mitigate pH fluctuations and other stress caused by run-off and increased population. An integrated system should include three levels of nutrient absorption (Clements and Chopin, 2017):

- Shell fish: small organic particle suspension extractive.
- Seaweed: dissolved nutrients suspension extractive.
- Invertebrates: large organic particle deposit extractive.

While acidification of natural aquasystems can only be mitigated by global reduction of atmospheric carbon dioxide, further research is necessary to fully understand the impacts of global climate change and the acidification of our oceans.

1.3.2.14 Ammonia, Nitrite and Nitrate

Ammonia is a colorless, odorless substance which can accumulate in aquasystems and cause direct mortality, a decrease in production and increased incidence of many diseases. In water, ammonia occurs in two forms, which together are called the total ammonia nitrogen. Ammonia gas is usually released from the gills or from decomposing organics dissolved in the water. Some reacts with the water to produce ammonia ions. The remainder is present as un-ionized, which is acutely toxic to aquatic life. Chemically, these two forms are represented as NH_4^+ and NH_3. NH_4^+ is called ionized ammonia because it has a positive electrical charge, and NH_3 is called un-ionized ammonia (UIA), since it has no charge. This is important to know, since NH_3, UIA is the form that is toxic to fish. The percentage of UIA in solution depends on the pH and temperature of the water; as both go higher, so does the toxicity.

A typical aquasystem has bacteria, which in the presence of dissolved oxygen converts (oxidizes) ammonia to the intermediate form of nitrite and then to nitrate. Ammonia is converted into nitrite (NO_2^-) due to the influence of *Nitrosomonas* bacteria. Nitrite (NO_2^-) is converted into nitrate (NO_3^-) due to the influence of *Nitrobacter* bacteria. Most test kits measure total ammonia nitrogen, so the aquarist must determine what percentage of the total is toxic.

Nitrite is an intermediate in the oxidation of ammonium to nitrate. Nitrite is less toxic to fish than ammonia. An elevated ambient nitrite concentration is a potential problem for freshwater fish since nitrite is actively taken up across the gills in competition with chloride. Nitrite is a well-known toxicant for fish, as well as a disrupter of multiple physiological functions including ion regulatory, respiratory, cardiovascular, endocrine and excretory processes. One critical consequence of nitrite accumulation is the oxidation of hemoglobin to methemoglobin, compromising blood oxygen transport (Kroupova *et al.*, 2005). Nitrite toxicity to fish varies considerably and depends on many external and internal factors. Among the most important ones are water quality (e.g. pH, temperature, cation, anion and oxygen concentration), length of exposure, fish species, fish size and age, and individual fish susceptibility.

Nitrate is relatively non-toxic; however, high concentrations reduce animal growth and can decrease survival. For example, concentrations over about 400 mg NO_3^-N/l have been shown to depress the growth rate and survival of marine shrimp (*Litopenaeus vannamei*). In intensive biofloc aquaculture systems used for shrimp culture, concentrations of 400 mg NO_3^-N/l have been observed after using water for roughly three culture cycles. Salinity influences the toxicity of nitrate, as it does with ammonia and nitrite. At higher salinities, these compounds are less toxic to aquatic animals. Several options exist for dealing with nitrate, including water exchange, phytoremediation, denitrification, and heterotrophic assimilation (Svobodova and Kolarova, 2004; Svobodova *et al.*, 2005; Tepper, 2000).

It is recommended that un-ionized ammonia should be less than 0.02 ppm to prevent stress and reduced growth. Ammonia has been reported to be lethal to catfish at about 0.4 ppm (Jensen, 2003). Ammonia, nitrite and nitrate are labile ions and must be analyzed rapidly or samples frozen as soon as possible after filtration. Samples that cannot be submitted within a few hours should be filtered (0.45 mm) then frozen to reduce the loss of ammonia and changes in nitrite/nitrate concentrations. Plain blood collection tubes are suitable containers for freezing. Two 10-ml tubes will provide enough samples for all three tests. Do not fill completely; leave space for expansion during freezing.

1.3.2.15 The Nitrogen Cycle

In aquaculture, the nitrogen cycle eliminates ammonia from the water column by bioconversion to nitrite and then nitrate. Nitrate is used by plants, including algae, as a nutrient. This constant change from ammonia to nitrite to nitrate is called the nitrogen cycle (Figure 1.1). In ponds, this

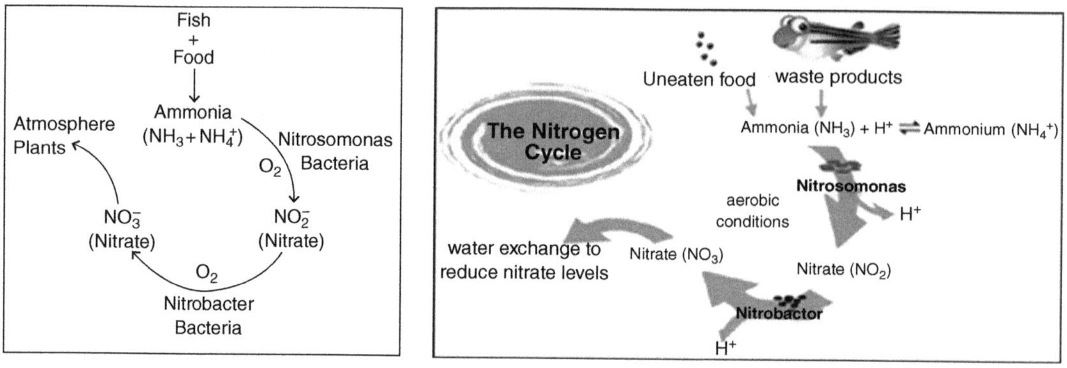

Figure 1.1 The nitrogen cycle (Francis-Floyd, 2003). *Source:* image on the right courtesy of Gillian Taylor.

process takes place in the surface layers of the mud, but in tanks or aquaria, a special place is provided for the bacteria to live and flourish. This is called a biological filter, or biofilter. One important point to mention about the nitrogen cycle is that both groups of nitrifying bacteria need oxygen to function. If oxygen levels are insufficient, the process can slow down and the levels of ammonia and nitrite will rise in the system.

1.3.2.16 Interaction of Chemical and Physical Properties of Water that Affect Aquatic Animal Health

Some chemicophysical parameters of water have a direct influence upon fish health. Any abrupt or large fluctuations of these parameters often cause a state of stress in fish, sometimes resulting in widespread disease outbreaks. Dissolved oxygen content, pH, turbidity, temperature, introduction of some chemicals, detergents, pesticides and naturally produced toxic compounds like hydrogen sulfide, ammonia, and dinoflagellate toxins are potential stress-related parameters. Carbon dioxide concentration up to 20–30 mg/l can be tolerated by fish provided that oxygen is near saturation. At lower levels of dissolved oxygen, the toxicity of carbon dioxide increases. The optimum pH range is between 6.7 and 8.6; liming agents may be applied to correct a low pH.

Ammonia concentration above 1 mg/l can indicates organic pollution. Hydrogen sulfide toxicity increases with decreasing pH and it is harmful even at a concentration of 1 mg/l. Making the aquasystem environment more congenial and hygienic reduces stress and promotes fish health. For example, excessive application of inorganic fertilizers and accumulation of organic matter in older aquasystems may cause an over production of phytoplankton, and the appearance of algal and bacterial blooms, leading to dissolved oxygen depletion to lethal levels. For health and optimum growth, the dissolved oxygen level should not drop below 2–5 mg/l. Carbon dioxide concentration up to 20–30 mg/l can be tolerated by fish provided oxygen is near saturation. Nephrocalcinosis in salmonids has long been recognized as a pathological entity related to high dissolved CO_2, eventually leading to the formation of large mineralized deposits within the excretory tissue of the kidney and associated kidney pathology. The condition can result in poor condition and performance and occasional fish loss, particularly if other stressors are present.

At lower levels of dissolved oxygen, the toxicity of carbon dioxide increases. The optimum pH range is between 6.7 and 8.6; liming agents may be applied to correct low pH. Problems with high pH are common in fry nursery ponds and in ponds used to grow freshwater prawns (*Macrobrachium rosenbergii*). This is because fertilization practices used to prepare ponds for stocking are designed to promote fast-growing phytoplankton blooms that rapidly take up carbon dioxide. Unfortunately, the early life stages of fish and crustaceans are particularly susceptible to pH toxicity and juveniles are less able than older animals to avoid areas of pH shift by moving to areas of stable pH in the pond (such as deeper waters).

Ammonia concentration above 1 mg/l indicates organic pollution. Ammonia is very important in intensive systems; in small amounts, ammonia causes stress and gill damage. Fish exposed to low levels of ammonia over time are more susceptible to bacterial infections, have poor growth and will not tolerate routine handling. Deformities and significant behavioral changes associated with chronic exposure to nitrates have been documented in rainbow trout (*Oncorhynchus mykiss*) raised in recirculating aquaculture systems with nitrate concentrations at levels less than one-tenth the recommended maximum nitrate nitrogen level of 1000 mg/l.

Hydrogen sulfide toxicity increases with decreasing pH and it is harmful even at 1 mg/l concentration level. Proper and timely management of soil and water by manipulating feeding, fertilization, liming, addition of water and aeration eliminates most of the environmental stressors and provides better and healthier environments for the growth of fish. Hydrogen sulfide has been referred to as a silent killer of shrimp, causing tissue corrosiveness by irritating soft tissues in the gills, gut, stomach walls and hepatopancreas. H_2S stresses shrimp, lowering their resistance to infection. A safe level for H_2S in giant tiger shrimp (*Penaeus monodon*) ponds has been reported as 0.033 ppm while white shrimp (*P. vannamei*) post larvae has been said to tolerate up to 0.0087 ppm and juveniles up to 0.0185 ppm (Panakorn, 2016).

1.3.3 Biotic Factors of Water

1.3.3.1 Biological Oxygen Demand

The biological oxygen demand is a measure of the oxygen used by all organisms in the aquasystem. Microbes (bacteria and fungi) use oxygen to decompose organics (may use 1–3 ppm dissolved oxygen in 24 hours). Phytoplankton respire at night to use oxygen (may use 5–15 ppm dissolved oxygen nightly). Fish respire day and night (may use 2-6 ppm dissolved oxygen in 24 hours). Dissolved oxygen levels fall at night, since all organisms are respiring, and rise during the day, since plants photosynthesize to use carbon dioxide and eliminate oxygen (may gain 5–20 ppm dissolved oxygen daily). Diffusion and wave/wind action add oxygen (may add 1–5 ppm dissolved oxygen).

The measurement of biological oxygen demand is a chemical procedure which determines the amount of dissolved oxygen needed by aerobic organisms in a body of water to break down organic material present in a given water sample at a certain temperature over a specific time period. It is not a precise quantitative test, although it is widely used as an indication of the organic quality of water. It is most commonly expressed in milligrams of oxygen consumed per liter of sample for five days of incubation at 20°C and is often used as a robust surrogate of the degree of organic pollution of water. Sources of biological oxygen demand include topsoil, leaves and woody debris; animal manure; effluents from pulp and paper mills, wastewater treatment plants, feedlots, and food-processing plants; failing septic systems; and urban rainwater runoff.

1.3.3.2 Plants and Algae

The type and amount of vegetation in an aquatic environment can have a positive or negative effect on the health of the aquasystem. Vegetation can improve the growth of fish by allowing for shade, shelter, and removal of nitrates and phosphates from the water. At night, excessive vegetation can also decrease the oxygen available to the fish, since plants will use oxygen for respiration and may impede movement of the fish and decrease their ability to catch prey or avoid predation. Studies performed on bass, sunfish and brill have shown that different species of fish react differently to vegetation levels. In one study, the size and life stages of fish also affect the amount of vegetation that is most appropriate. In this study, bass were less tolerant of the plants filling the water column than brill or sunfish. Larger bass were negatively affected when 30% of the water column was filled with plants, while smaller bass were negatively affected when 50% of the water column was filled. These studies express the importance of knowing the species of plant and the species of fish for which the veterinarian is caring.

Floating beds of vegetation are a good answer to nitrate and phosphate removal. Studies performed on rye grass in floating beds has shown that it effectively removes a significant amount of the NO_3 (Bartucca *et al.*, 2016). By creating floating beds of vegetation, the nitrate and phosphate levels can be reduced without encumbering the water column. It is important to monitor the oxygen, nitrogen, and phosphorous levels to decide the best density of planting.

1.3.3.3 Algal Bloom

Overabundance of nutrients like phosphorus, particularly when the water is warm and the weather is calm, can lead to excessive growth of algae. According to the World Health Organization standard, when the population of algal cells exceeds 100 000 cells/ ml, the condition is termed an algal bloom. Excessive algal growth can lead to nocturnal hypoxic conditions where fish may start to gasp on the water surface, and mass mortality events may occur. Phytoplankton blooms can also cause large diurnal fluctuations in other water quality variables (e.g. very high pH due to excessive use of free CO_2 for photosynthesis) in mid-afternoon. Such conditions are stressful to fish. Blue-green algae can also produce toxic substances that are lethal to some fish (see also Harmful Algal Bloom below). They can also produce compounds that impart a strong off-flavor to fish. In addition, dead algae can accumulate at the pond bottom and create toxic gases from decomposition.

The best approach to controlling algae is to regulate nutrient inputs by moderate stocking and feeding rates. Phosphorus is one of the major factors responsible for increased levels of phytoplankton in an aquasystem. It is possible to precipitate phosphorus from pond water by applying sources of iron, aluminum, or calcium ions. These ions precipitate phosphorus as insoluble iron, aluminum or calcium phosphates. The use of alum (aluminum sulfate) 20–30 mg/l or gypsum (calcium sulfate) 100–200 mg/l to precipitate excessive concentrations of phosphorus may also be feasible. Alum is acidic and more suitable for use in waters of 500 mg/l total alkalinity and above. Gypsum is better for use in low alkalinity waters.

1.3.3.4 Larger Aquatic Plants

Larger aquatic plants or macrophytes include pondweed and milfoil. These plants are undesirable in aquasystems because they interfere with fish management (feeding and harvesting), compete with plankton for nutrients, provide shelter for undesirable fish, contribute to oxygen depletion and high ammonia levels when they decompose and contribute to water loss through transpiration. Drying and desilting of aquasystems every one or two years will keep the growth of aquatic plants in check.

1.3.3.5 Pests and Predators

Pests and predators are unwanted animals or plants that destroy fish or hinder the production of target fish species. Birds, fish, reptiles, amphibians, mammals and even certain invertebrates are known predators of cultured fish. Bird predation is the major source of fish loss at aquaculture facilities. Tadpoles feed on aquatic plants and animals, while frogs can eat fish fry. They lay eggs on the surface of ponds, which interferes with surface oxygenation, thereby restricting fish growth if not checked. Sea anemones can grow on boards, sluice gates and grooves, and on concrete dikes in high-salinity, brackish water areas, and are poisonous to fish.

Fish predators can be used in controlling an overpopulation of fish in ponds. Wild fish are one of the potential sources of fish pathogenic organisms. Some of these wild species are predatory in nature and prey upon the young of cultivated species. They can rapidly multiply and compete for food with the cultivated fish. Control of nuisance fish can be done by poisoning or dewatering the pond. Piscicides of plant origin are preferred over common chemical insecticides used in agriculture due to the long-lasting toxicity and residual effect of the latter. Moreover, fish killed by insecticides become unfit for human and animal consumption. Piscicides derived from plants such as mahua oil cake are most commonly used as their toxicity lasts for about two weeks and the fish killed are fit for human consumption. Mahua oil is applied at 200–250 ppm. However, the poisoning process kills only the unwanted fish species of the pond without affecting the pathogenic organisms they may carry. Disinfection of water is an effective means of disease control in fish culture by reducing the numbers of pathogens to minimum levels.

1.4 Monitoring and Regulation of Life-Support Systems

Proper and timely management of soil and water by manipulating feeding, fertilization, liming, addition of water, aeration, bottom raking, and so on, eliminates most of the environmental stressors and provides better, healthy environments for the production of fish and other aquatic animals. Proper management also increases the immune response against pathogens. Eradication of predatory and nuisance fish, disinfecting the pond, selection of quality and healthy seed for stocking, maintaining proper species ratio and stocking density, water quality regulation, proper feeding and proper handling are the important steps of this management exercise. Water quality parameters that are commonly monitored in the aquaculture industry include temperature, dissolved oxygen, pH, alkalinity, hardness, ammonia, nitrites and nitrates. Depending on the culture system, carbon dioxide, chlorides, and salinity may also be monitored. Some parameters such as alkalinity and hardness are fairly stable, but others like dissolved oxygen and pH can fluctuate daily. Most of these parameters are measured with physical reagents or meters. However, there are several classical methods of water analysis which are still used today. Atomic absorption analysis provides the atomization of a sample in flame or electrothermal plasma. Liquid sample is turned into an atomic gas through desolvation, evaporation, and volatilization. Electrochemical methods are based on an analysis of the processes occurring at the electrodes and in the inter-electrode space followed by the measurement of the potential and/or current in an electrochemical cell containing the analyte. Gravimetric analysis involves determining the amount of analyte through the measurement of mass (Table 1.1).

Relative concentration changes for dissolved oxygen, carbon dioxide and pH in ponds over 24 hours are shown in Table 1.2. Biological oxygen demand measurement requires taking two measurements. One is measured immediately for dissolved oxygen (initial), and the second is incubated in the laboratory for five days and then tested for dissolved oxygen remaining (final). This represents the amount of oxygen consumed by microorganisms to break down the organic matter present in the sample during the incubation period.

In ponds with moderate to high alkalinity (good buffering capacity) and similar hardness levels, pH is neutral or slightly basic (7.0–8.3) and does not fluctuate widely. Higher amounts of CO_2 (i.e. carbonic acid) or other acids are required to lower pH because more base is available to neutralize or buffer the acidity. The relationship of alkalinity, pH and CO_2 is shown in Table 1.3. The number (factor) found in the table which corresponds to the measured pH and water temperature is multiplied by the measured alkalinity value (mg/l as $CaCO_3$). The product of these numbers estimates CO_2 concentration (mg/l).

Table 1.1 Water quality factors, commonly used monitoring procedures, and preferred ranges for fish culture. Details for specific test procedures can be obtained from a commercial supplier or appropriate text (e.g. APHA 1989).

Water quality factor	Test procedure	Preferred ranges for fish culture
Temperature	Thermometer, telethermister	Species dependent
Dissolved oxygen	Titrimetric (modified Winkler) polarographic meter, calorimetric kits	> 4–5 ppm for most species
Total ammonia-nitrogen (ionized and un-ionized)	Calorimetric kits, (Nesslerization or salicylate), ion specific probes	NH < 0.02 ppm
Nitrite	Calorimetric kits (diazotization), ion specific probes	< 1 ppm; 0.1 ppm in soft water
pH	Electronic meter, calorimetric kits,	6–8 ppm
Alkalinity	Titrimetric with pH meter, titrimetric with chemical indicator	50–300 ppm calcium carbonate
Hardness	Titrimetric kit	> 50 ppm, preferably > 100 ppm calcium carbonate
Carbon dioxide	Titrimetric kit	< 10 ppm
Salinity	Conductivity meter	species dependent typically < 0.5–1.0 ppt for freshwater fish)
Hydrogen sulfide	Calorimetric kit	No detectable level
Clarity	Secchi disk, turbidimeter	Species dependent

Table 1.2 Relative concentration changes for dissolved oxygen, carbon dioxide, and pH in ponds over 24 hours (Tucker 1984).

	Change		
Time	Dissolved oxygen	Carbon dioxide	pH
Daylight	Increases	Decreases	Increases
Night	Decreases	Increases	Decreases

Since most test kits measure total ammonia nitrogen, it is important to determine what percentage of the total is toxic. In healthy ponds and tanks, ammonia levels should always be zero. Since the toxicity of UIA begins as low as 0.05 mg/l, a positive total ammonia nitrogen test needs to be followed by a test to find the actual concentration of UIA. Once the pH and temperature are known, the fraction of UIA present can be determined (Table 1.4), as presented in Table 1.5. Samples that cannot be submitted within a few hours should be filtered (0.45 mm) then frozen to reduce the loss of ammonia and changes in nitrate/nitrite concentrations.

Salinity is usually not measured directly, but is instead derived from the conductivity measurement (Wagner *et al.*, 2006). This is known as practical salinity. These derivations compare the specific conductance of the sample to a salinity standard such as seawater. Salinity measurements based on conductivity values are unitless but are often followed by the notation of practical salinity units (Nelson and Siegel, 2014).

Table 1.3 Factors for calculating carbon dioxide concentrations in water with known pH, temperature and alkalinity measurements.[a]

	Temperatures (°C)						
pH	5	10	15	20	25	30	35
6.0	2.915	2.539	2.315	2.112	1.970	1.882	1.839
6.2	1.839	1.602	1.460	1.333	1.244	1.187	1.160
6.4	1.160	1.010	0.921	0.841	0.784	0.749	0.732
6.6	0.732	0.637	0.582	0.531	0.495	0.473	0.462
6.8	0.462	0.402	0.367	0.335	0.313	0.298	0.291
7.0	0.291	0.254	0.232	0.211	0.197	0.188	0.184
7.2	0.184	0.160	0.146	0.133	0.124	0.119	0.116
7.4	0.116	0.101	0.092	0.084	0.078	0.075	0.073
7.6	0.073	0.064	0.058	0.053	0.050	0.047	0.046
7.8	0.046	0.040	0.037	0.034	0.031	0.030	0.030
8.0	0.029	0.025	0.023	0.021	0.020	0.019	0.018
8.2	0.018	0.016	0.015	0.013	0.012	0.012	0.011
8.4	0.012	0.010	0.009	0.008	0.008	0.008	0.007

Source: Tucker, 1984.
[a] Factors should be multiplied by total alkalinity (mg/l) to get carbon dioxide (mg/l). For practical purposes, CO_2 concentrations are negligible above pH 8.4.

Total dissolved solids are reported in mg/l and can be measured by gravimetry or calculated by multiplying a conductivity value by an empirical factor; standard methods for the examination of water and wastewater accepts a total dissolved solids constant of 0.55–0.7 mg/l, although if the water source is known to be high in calcium or sulfate ions, a constant of 0.8 mg/l may be used (American Public Health Association *et al.*, 2017). Depending on the ionic properties, excessive total dissolved solids can produce toxic effects on fish and fish eggs. Salmonids exposed to higher than average levels of $CaSO_4$ at various life stages experienced reduced survival and reproductive rates. When total dissolved solids ranged above 2200–3600 mg/l, salmonids, perch and pike all showed reduced hatching and egg survival rates (Scannel and Jacob, 2001).

It is important for the clinician to be familiar with the types of life-support system monitoring reports used in modern aquatic facilities. Each facility will have its own template or digital form tailored to the specific monitoring procedures.

1.5 Maintaining Optimal Conditions

Various processes, both natural and artificial, as well as varied physical components, are all involved with creating an aquasystem that provides the healthiest environment for maintaining its inhabitants.

Table 1.4 Fraction of un-ionized ammonia in aqueous solution at different pH values and temperatures. *Source:* calculated from data in Emmerson *et al.* (1975).

pH	Fraction at temperature													
(°F)	42.0	46.4	50.0	53.6	57.2	60.8	64.4	68.9	71.6	75.2	78.8	82.4	86.0	89.6
(°C)	6	8	10	12	14	16	18	20	22	24	26	28	30	32
7.0	0.0013	0.0016	0.0018	0.0022	0.0025	0.0029	0.0034	0.0039	0.0046	0.0052	0.0060	0.0069	0.0080	0.0093
7.2	0.0021	0.0025	0.0029	0.0034	0.0040	0.0046	0.0054	0.0062	0.0072	0.0083	0.0096	0.0110	0.0126	0.0150
7.4	0.0034	0.0040	0.0046	0.0054	0.0063	0.0073	0.0085	0.0096	0.0114	0.0131	0.0150	0.0173	0.0198	0.0236
7.6	0.0053	0.0063	0.0073	0.0086	0.0100	0.0116	0.0134	0.0155	0.0179	0.0206	0.0236	0.0271	0.0310	0.0369
7.8	0.0084	0.0099	0.0116	0.0135	0.0157	0.0182	0.0211	0.0244	0.0281	0.0322	0.0370	0.0423	0.0482	0.0572
8.0	0.0133	0.0156	0.0182	0.0212	0.0247	0.0286	0.0330	0.0381	0.0438	0.0502	0.0574	0.0654	0.0743	0.0877
8.2	0.0210	0.0245	0.0286	0.0332	0.0385	0.0445	0.0514	0.0590	0.0676	0.0772	0.0880	0.0998	0.1129	0.1322
8.4	0.0328	0.0383	0.0445	0.0517	0.0597	0.0688	0.0790	0.0904	0.1031	0.1171	0.1326	0.1495	0.1678	0.1948
8.6	0.0510	0.0593	0.0688	0.0795	0.0914	0.1048	0.1197	0.1361	0.1541	0.1737	0.1950	0.2178	0.2422	0.2768
8.8	0.0785	0.0909	0.1048	0.1204	0.1376	0.1566	0.1773	0.1998	0.2241	0.2500	0.2774	0.3062	0.3362	0.3776
9.0	0.1190	0.1368	0.1565	0.1782	0.2018	0.2273	0.2546	0.2836	0.3140	0.3456	0.3783	0.4116	0.4453	0.4902
9.2	0.1763	0.2006	0.2273	0.2558	0.2861	0.3180	0.3512	0.3855	0.4204	0.4557	0.4909	0.5258	0.5599	0.6038
9.4	0.2533	0.2847	0.3180	0.3526	0.3884	0.4249	0.4618	0.1985	0.5348	0.5702	0.6045	0.6373	0.6685	0.7072
9.6	0.3496	0.3868	0.4249	0.4633	0.5016	0.5394	0.5762	0.6117	0.6456	0.6777	0.7078	0.7358	0.7617	0.7929
9.8	0.4600	0.5000	0.5394	0.5778	0.6147	0.6499	0.6831	0.7140	0.7428	0.7692	0.7933	0.8153	0.8351	0.8585
10.0	0.5745	0.6131	0.6496	0.6844	0.7166	0.7463	0.7735	0.7963	0.8207	0.8408	0.8588	0.8749	0.8892	0.9058
10.2	0.6815	0.7152	0.7463	0.7446	0.8003	0.8234	0.8441	0.8625	0.8788	0.8933	0.9060	0.9173	0.9271	0.9389

Table 1.5 Stepwise determination of un-ionized ammonia.

STEP	ACTIVITY
1	Measure pond TAN with commercial test kit
2	Measure Pond temperature
3	Measure Pond pH
4	Find the multiplication actor in Table 1.1 using the pond temperature and pH
5	Multiply TAN and factor from step 4 to determine un-ionized ammonia nitrogen

TAN, total ammonia nitrogen.

1.5.1 Biofilms

Millions of bacteria and viruses are found in every milliliter of water in a healthy aquasystem and on every surface, and they comprise very complex ecosystems called biofilms. The relationship between beneficial and pathogenic organisms is very complex. Culturing bacteria only identifies less than 1% of the bacteria in water. Current technologies such as quantitative polymerase chain reaction are demonstrating a vastly diverse microbial ecosystem. A managed system demonstrated over 890 genera and over 2500 species of bacteria which only accounted for 69% of the bacterial DNA; the rest were unidentified (Stamper, 2015).

Aquatic microorganisms occur in two realms: planktonic and sessile. The planktonic state is fairly straightforward, whereas the sessile biofilm ecology is extremely complex. Biofilms include organisms beyond bacteria and comprise fungi, algae, protozoans and metazoans. An intricate ecological process occurs as various environmental parameters change. These organisms secrete an assortment of chemicals known as extracellular polymeric substances, which add to the total organic carbon within the water column and are critical to the health of the organisms and water environment (Stamper, 2015; Tepper, 2019).

An important consideration in any aquatic system is the potential for pathogenic bacteria to create a biofilm that will allow it to persist in a tank or other culture system. Biofilm formation and disinfection can be especially problematic in recirculating aquaculture systems. Once a highly pathogenic organism is introduced, it can persist in the system indefinitely and continue to cause recurrent disease outbreaks.

Secreting a protective coating can allow bacteria to survive desiccation and standard cleaning techniques. If recurrent bacterial disease becomes an issue in cultured species, additional disinfection of the system may be indicated. This may require depopulation while strong disinfectants are used, following a period of dewatering and drying of the system. Physical methods such as heat and pressure washing can be used and a combination of physical and chemical treatment techniques may increase the effectiveness of the disinfection.

1.5.2 Chemical Flocculation and Bioflocculation

As urban populations grow and the science surrounding water quality improves, regulatory changes in discharge limits for large-scale aquaculture operations have led to a need for more intense handling of solids. One sophisticated and large-scale method of processing biological solid wastes uses the theory of biological flocculation or “bioflocculation”. While the veterinarian may not typically be called upon to manage such systems, it is important to understand that these systems might be in use, how they operate at a basic level, and how they may impact animal health. Perhaps the most common concern for aquatic veterinarians is how chemicals used for disease treatment in a system may impact the function of these solids treatment systems.

Flocculation involves the clumping of suspended particles together into a settleable "floc". Chemical flocculation is used in wastewater treatment plants to remove solids from water on a large scale, where surfactant chemicals such as alum or ferric chloride are used. More recently, polyacrylamide has also been used.

Large-scale aquaculture systems with large biological loads (and thus a high volume of fecal wastes) may use this chemical flocculation method. Home aquaria are also often treated with chemical flocculants to clear cloudy water.

Another method that may be used in small-scale aquaculture systems is bioflocculation, where microorganisms cause particles to clump together when natural chemicals such as polysaccharides are secreted as a result of their normal biological functions. This naturally occurring process is important for the proper functioning of all filter systems. Small-scale aquaculture facilities may employ an enhanced system of bioflocculation. While fine suspended organic particles from animal wastes will settle out on their own in a stagnant tank or pond over time, organic particles such as phosphorus never quite settle out. Microorganism activity speeds up the process and leads to a more effective solids removal by clumping particles together into a floc which can be removed from the water. This type of system can be used to treat wastewater and reduces the total dissolved solids and phosphorus following prefiltration to remove larger particles. The intensity of the wastewater treatment required will depend on many factors, and the discharge of such chemicals as nitrogen and phosphorus may be limited by a water jurisdiction agency to reduce eutrophication impacts on the environment. Flocculation is commonly used in combination with coagulation, which creates microflocs by decreasing the negative charges that repel particles and cause them to remain in suspension.

The budget, amount of land area available for this application, biological load in the system, and the regulatory limits of the discharge permit will determine the type and size of system used. Typically these systems require a long time to "turn over" and are limited in volume. These methods are well suited to a settling basin or belt filter.

As with a biological filter, the type and amount of chemicals or microorganisms present in the system will impact the speed and effectiveness of this water treatment method. Treatment chemical residues in the wastewater may interact with chemical flocculants. High concentrations of toxic chemicals containing formaldehyde or chlorine used to treat diseases in fish may negatively impact the microorganism population of the system and treatment may need to be altered to a lower concentration over a longer period to reduce the lethal dose in the water treatment system. In some cases, bypassing the settling basin or belt filter may be considered.

The principle of bioflocculation has other applications and is currently a growing area of research for aquatic animal feeds, pathogen reduction, and biofuel production.

1.5.2.1 Effect of Therapeutants and Disinfectants on Biofilters

Certain therapeutants and disinfectants, such as iodine and ozonation can have a detrimental effect on the functioning of active biofilters. Always consult product information before using these products in an aquasystem.

1.5.3 Environmental Toxins and Pollutants

1.5.3.1 Heavy Metals

Heavy metals occur naturally in the environment due to geologic weathering but can also occur from human use. It is important to survey the immediate environment as well as the areas upstream to the water source used in an aquasystem. Atmospheric pollution from coal combustion is a major cause of many heavy metals being found in source water. Residential and agricultural use of pesticides and fertilizer may contribute to several types of heavy metals in groundwater, well water, lakes, ponds and estuaries. Other types of industrial waste to consider are leather tanneries, textile industry, battery storage or production, plastic production, metal finishing, mining, and pigment production.

There are essential and non-essential heavy metals. Essential metals include copper, zinc, chromium, nickel, cobalt, molybdenum and iron. Nonessential metals include cadmium, mercury, tin and lead (Sfakianiakis *et al.*, 2015).

Essential metals can cause disease if they are deficient and if the levels are too concentrated. The most bioavailable form of these metals is the dissolved ionic form. These metals help during larval development of the neurologic and gastrointestinal systems (Sfakianakis *et al.*, 2015; Authman *et al.*, 2015).

Essential and nonessential heavy metals can cause damage at high concentrations. Knowing that there is potential for heavy metal in the water source is an important part of diagnosing decreased reproductive health, slow growth, and acute mortalities. The periods during which fish are most susceptible to heavy metal toxicity are the embryonic and larval stages. They can cause lordosis, increased mortality, hatching delays and other anomalies. According to Sfankianakis *et al.* (2015), morphological deformities are commonly used as a biomarker to study the effects of contamination.

Fish are susceptible to heavy metals through their gills, gastrointestinal tract and through skin absorption. These metals will accumulate in the liver, kidney, and gills. Arsenic has also been found to accumulate in the retina and cadmium has been found in the heart muscle (Authman, 2015).

Although there are differences in the mechanism of action, most heavy metals cause damage to the liver, gills, reproductive, immune, and neurologic systems. They cause damage to the gills through hyperplasia and necrosis. Aluminum causes lamellar fusion which leads to necrosis. Iron accumulates in the gills as a precipitate causing vascular occlusion. At chronic doses, many heavy metals negatively affect leukocytes, erythrocytes, and antibodies. They can also affect the endocrine system, decreasing reproductive health. Iron can precipitate on eggs causing a reduction of oxygen reaching the larvae. Other heavy metals decrease growth through increased biological stress, disruption of osmotic balance, and developmental changes. Many heavy metals cause neurologic damage, including mercury, which causes behavior changes, cognitive changes, ataxia, and convulsions (Kennedy, 2002).

Studies on cadmium show that it is primarily absorbed via the gastrointestinal system and the gills. It interrupts the absorption of calcium, which can cause problems with reproduction, growth, and development. It can also cause acute death from hypocalcemia. Cadmium levels as low as 0.001 ppm affect the hatching and larval survival of many species of fish.

Studies have been performed showing that excessive copper can affect the gills, gastrointestinal system, and the sensory system. These studies showed that zebra fish larvae had difficulty orienting in the water column, reduced hatching and impairment of growth (Authman, 2015).

1.5.3.2 Insecticides

Insecticides may be used in the local environment for the control of agricultural pests or insects that cause vector borne diseases. These compounds can affect fish through runoff and atmospheric accumulation on pond surfaces. There are many types of insecticides on the market. Most insecticides affect the neurologic system using different mechanisms of action. They may affect acetylcholinesterase activity, block sodium channels, bind nicotinic receptors, affect the peripheral nervous system and directly degrade neurotransmitters in several other ways. They can also cause chromosomal aberrations, decrease protein levels, affect the immune system, and mimic or block reproductive hormones (Sabra and Mehana, 2015). Compared with insects, they differ in their specificity for vertebrates, their toxicity, their bioaccumulation, and their environmental persistence.

Organochlorines have been banned in most countries due to their highly toxic nature. They are toxic to most animals, have a high level of bioaccumulation, and persist in the environment for long periods of time (Fulton *et al.*, 2013).

Organophosphates have a lower level of bioaccumulation and a shorter half-life in the environment. They may be used as a treatment for several fish parasites, but can be easily overdosed. Some fish are more sensitive to organophosphates than others. If using organophosphates for treatment of disease, always determine the species sensitivity.

Carbamates are frequently used for agriculture and residential insect control. They also have minimal bioaccumulation and environmental persistence. They are less toxic to fish than organophosphates, but still can cause chronic toxicity if overused around an aquasystem (Fulton *et al.*, 2013).

Pyrethroids and nicotinoids are also commonly used in the environment. Nicotinoids cause irreversible block of the post synaptic nicotinoid receptors. Pyrethroids cause damage to the sodium channel in the neurons leading to hyperexcitability, tremors, ataxia and paralysis (Sabra and Mehana, 2015).

There are many other types of insecticides to consider. Although most will not persist in the environment more than one or two weeks, if used consistently, they may lead to chronic disease. This may appear as decreased growth, low reproduction, and slow increase in mortality.

1.5.3.3 Herbicides

There are many different classes of herbicides. Most herbicides do not directly affect fish; however, different species of fish respond to varied levels and classes of herbicides. Studies performed on forestry herbicides in regard to fish development showed no evidence of toxicity in zebra fish to picloram, clopyralid, imazapic, glyphosate, imazapyr, and triclopyr (Stehr *et al.*, 2009). However, studies evaluating *Cyprinus carpio* and rohu showed an increased mortality and histologic changes in the kidney, liver, and gills when exposed to glyphosate at 86 mg/l. This same study showed increased mortality in response to the use of the salt formulation of 2, 4-D at 100 mg/l and paraquat at 26 mg/l.

Atrazine has been shown to affect the hypothalamus–pituitary–gonadal axis in vertebrates. One study has shown that this herbicide negatively affects the egg production of fathead minnows (Tillitt, 2010).

Pretilachlor is frequently used in rice fields. Studies performed on *Clarias batrachus* exposed to this herbicide had significant behavioral changes, including decreased feeding and increased buccal activity (Soni, 2018).

At high levels, triazine has been shown to cause acute toxicity in fish. This herbicide can also cause negative affects regarding reproduction and reproductive development (Hostovsky *et al.*, 2014).

When diagnosing possible toxic exposure in a fish population, herbicides should be considered if they have been used in the water or in the area nearby due to potential runoff. When developing a farm management program that includes herbicides, it is important to consider the following:

- The sensitivity of the species you are working with.
- The potential exposure to wild fish in the area and their sensitivity.
- The bioaccumulation of the herbicide directly into the water or in the runoff.
- The half-life of the chemical if it is used in an unpopulated pond.

1.5.3.4 Harmful Algal Blooms

Micro- and macroalgae have been implicated in millions of dollars of loss in aquaculture over the past decade (Hallegraeff *et al.*, 2017) and large numbers of deaths of aquatic animals in the wild and in aquariums. These harmful algal blooms have recently increased in our environment due to increased migration, climate change, CO_2 levels, and nutrients in the water. Harmful algal blooms are caused by microalgae species including diatoms, cyanobacteria, raphidophytes, prymnesiophytes, pelagophytes, and silicoflagellates (Landsberg, 2002). The most common freshwater algal blooms are caused by cyanobacteria.

Increased water traffic has allowed for migration of algal blooms from continent to continent, allowing the microalgae to find the most conducive environment for growth. Changes in water temperature, pH, and nutrient upwelling have allowed many of these microalgae species to bloom in new areas where animals are not adapted to their presence (Anderson *et al.*, 2012). Climate change has also affected the percentage of toxic compared with nontoxic strains such as *Microcystis* and a decreased overwintering period as seen in *Cylindrospermopsis* (Wood *et al.*, 2015).

The effects of harmful algal blooms are very difficult to anticipate due to the variety of microalgae, the toxins that each species contain, and the sensitivity of aquatic animals to those toxins. Each species of microalgae has a different environmental niche. Some are benthic and require limited sunlight. Others must remain near the surface. There are some microalgae that can adjust their buoyancy to move to the most effective area where both photosynthesis and nutrient absorption are greatest. Many adaptations of microalgae allow for them to have an advantage over other algae. These adaptations also tend to give the nontoxic forms of the species less of an advantage over the toxic forms.

The toxins of algal blooms include hepatotoxins, neurotoxins, and dermatotoxins. Each bloom may occur without the presence of toxins in the water and the toxins may only be found in the water before the mortality is detected. This adds to the difficulty in the diagnosis of algal bloom toxicity. The Centers for Disease Control and Prevention list the majority of toxins that are known at this time (Roberts *et al.*, 2020). A more complete explanation of the individual events that have shown proven effects of the toxins in aquatic animals can be found in Jan Landsberg's (2002) article "The effects of harmful algal blooms on aquatic organisms".

Cyanobacteria can cause fresh water algal blooms. They are found in ponds, lakes and estuaries. When fresh water incursion occurs and nutrient levels are high, these blooms can reach marine life on the coast. Cyanobacteria most commonly produce microcystins, anatoxins, and cylindrospermopsin. Most aquatic species appear to be resistant to anatoxins and cylindrospermopsin. There have been bird deaths with anatoxin-a(s) and a possible alligator mortality with cylindrospermopsin. Microcystins have been shown to cause both acute disease and chronic disease. The route of uptake is through the gastrointestinal tract, gills, and skin. There have been many field observations and laboratory experiments with fish regarding microcystin-LR. These studies have shown that microcystins affect the leukocytes, liver enzymes, growth rate, and ionic stability. The histopathological changes are dose dependent and include degenerative changes to the kidney, liver, and gills (Malbrouck, 2009).

Fish appear to be more resistant than mammals to many neurotoxins, such as brevetoxins, domoic acid, and saxitoxins. These toxins bioaccumulate in fish and cause high mortality rates in birds and marine mammals. Saxitoxins cause paralytic shellfish poisoning (PSP) in mammals due to sodium channel blockage. There are 21 derivatives of saxitoxins involved with PSP. Recent studies show a direct effect on mollusks causing increased mortality and poor growth. Herring exposed to *Alexandrium tamarense* show increased mortality due to asphyxiation (Landsberg, 2002). Brevetoxins include nine types of neurotoxins, several of which are found in sea spray and act as a respiratory irritant. The neurotoxins alter membrane properties in the neurologic cells. Manatee deaths caused by brevetoxins is postulated to be caused by the ingestion of tunicates found on the surface of sea grass and through inhalation when traveling through large blooms (Landsberg, 2002).

Domoic acid is an excitatory neurotransmitter binding glutamate receptors. There are some copepods that are very sensitive to domoic acid, others are less sensitive and act as a vector. Domoic acid has not been identified in fish mortality events, but it has caused mortalities in brown pelicans after ingestion of anchovies (Lansberg, 2002).

Harmful algal blooms can also cause a reduction in the available oxygen during respiration, exaggerating the toxic effects. Many of the species involved in these blooms are more tolerant to the low oxygen levels and will thrive on the nutrients created by the increased mortality of other organisms. Harmful algal blooms also contain superoxide radicals, phycotoxins and fatty acids that have been acknowledged to play a role in aquatic species mortality through gill damage (Dorantes-Aranda, 2015; Hallegraeff *et al.*, 2017). Studies performed by Hallegraeff show that reactive oxygen species do not cause damage to fish independently, but when free fatty acids are present they work in synergy to increase the potency of the fatty acid. This results in damage to the gills and to osmoregulation. Microalgal blooms such as barbed diatoms can also cause damage to the gills through mechanical stress by lodging in fish gills (Hallegraeff *et al.*, 2017).

There is no effective treatment for the toxicity that occurs due to harmful algal blooms. Avoidance of the blooms is best achieved by decreasing runoff of high nutrient materials, planting grasses and other plants near waterways to help reduce nutrient runoff and use the nutrients in the water, and careful monitoring. If a large bloom occurs in an aquaculture facility, there are several considerations that need to be made before action is taken:

- Is the toxin present a danger to humans, aquatic species, or both?
- Is an early harvest an option?
- Will killing the algae cause more toxin to be suddenly released?

With blooms that are specifically ichthyotoxic due to fatty acids and reactive oxygen species, the fish may still be safe for harvest. If so, it is important to prevent histamine build-up by keeping the fish alive long enough to allow the system to be flushed. This can be accomplished by airlift upwelling and targeted clay applications to remove the ichthyotoxins (such as bentonite clay at 0.05–0.25 g/l for *Prymnesium*, *Karenia*, *Karlodinium*, *Chattonella*, *Heterosigma*, and *Alexandrium*). The last three listed have a lower removal percentage then the first three (Hallegraeff *et al.*, 2017). If an early harvest is not an option, then means for movement of the fish and decreased nutrient load should be considered. The feed should be stopped to decrease nutrient levels. Cages can be moved to unaffected areas if possible. To reduce concentration, surrounding the fish with perimeter skirts and increased aeration or airlift upwelling can be used. Clay flocculation should be carefully considered based on the area the fish are in and the type of algal blooms present. Most clays can cause damage to benthic fauna present, especially mollusks (Hallegraeff *et al.*, 2017)

1.6 Diseases Associated with Suboptimal Water Quality

Many diseases or conditions have been wholly, or in part, associated with suboptimal water quality. Examples may be found in Chapter 4.

Supplementary materials available online

- Bibliographic references.
- Further Resources.

References

American Public Health Association, American Water Works Association, Water Environment Federation. (2017). *Standard Methods for the Examination of Water and Wastewater*, 23e. Baltimore, MD: American Public Health Association, American Water Works Association, Water Environment Federation.

Anderson, D.M., Cembella, A.D. and Hallegraeff, G.M. (2012). Progress in understanding harmful algal blooms: paradigm shifts and new technologies for research, monitoring, and management. *Annual Review of Marine Science* 4: 143–176.

Authman, M.M. (2015). Use of fish as bio-indicator of the effects of heavy metals pollution. *Journal of Aquaculture Research and Development* 6(4). doi:10.4172/2155-9546.1000328.

Bartucca, M., Mimmo, T., Cesco, S. et al. (2016). Nitrate removal from polluted water by using vegetated floating system. *Science of the Total Environment* 542: 803–808.

Clean Water Team. (2002). *Electrical Conductivity/Salinity Fact Sheet.* Fact Sheet 3.1.3.0. Clean Water Team Guidance Compendium for Watershed Monitoring and Assessment State Water Resources Control Board, Version 2.0. Sacramento, CA: California State Water Resources Control Board.

Clements, J.C. and Chopin, T. (2017). Ocean acidification and marine aquaculture in North America: potential impacts and mitigation strategies. *Reviews in Aquaculture* 9: 326–341.

Dorantes-Aranda, J.J., Seger, A., Mardones, J.I. et al. (2015). Progress in understanding algal bloom-mediated fish kills: the role of superoxide radicals, phycotoxins and fatty acids. *PLOS One* 10(7): e0133549.

Francis-Floyd, R. (2003). *Sanitation Practices for Aquaculture Facilities.* VM87. Gainsville, FL: Florida Cooperative Extension Service, IFAS, University of Florida.

Fulton, M., Key, P., and Delorenzo, M. (2013). Insecticide toxicity in fish. *Fish Physiology* 33: 309–368.

Hallegraeff, G., Dorantes Aranda, J.J., Mardones, J. *et al.* (2017). Review of progress in our understanding of fish-killing microalgae: implications for management and mitigation. In: *Marine and Fresh-Water Harmful Algae. Proceedings of the 17th International Conference on Harmful Algae. International Society for the Study of Harmful Algae and Intergovernmental Oceanographic Commission of UNESCO 2017.* (ed. L.A.O. Proença and G.M. Hallegraeff), 148–153. ISBN 9788799082766 (2017) (eds). Helsinki: International Society for the Study of Harmful Algae.

Heuer, R.M., and Grosell, M. (2014). Physiological impacts of elevated carbon dioxide and ocean acidification on fish. *American Journal of Physiology-Regulatory, Integrative and Comparative Physiology* 307: R1061–R1084.

Hostovsky, M., Blahova, J., Plhalova, L. et al. (2014). Effects of the exposure of fish to triazine herbicides. *Neuro Endocrinology Letters* 35(Suppl 2): 3–25.

Jensen, F.B. (2003). Nitrite disrupts multiple physiological functions in aquatic animals. *Comparative Biochemistry and Physiology Part A Molecular and Integrative Physiology* 135: 9–24.

Kennedy, C. (2011). The toxicology of metals in fishes. In: *Encyclopedia of Fish Physiology: From gemone to environment.* (ed. A.P. Farrell), 2061–2068. London: Academic Press.

Kroupova, H., Machova, J. and Svobodova, Z. (2005). Nitrite influence on fish: a review. *Veterinarni Medicina – UZPI (Czech Republic)* 50: 461–471.

Landsberg, J.H. (2002). The effects of harmful algal blooms on aquatic organisms, *Reviews in Fisheries Science* 10: 113–390.

Malbrouck, C. and Kestemont, P. (2006). Effects of microcystins on fish. *Environmental Toxicology and Chemistry* 25: 72–86.

Miller, R.L., Bradford, W.L. and Peters, N.E. (1988). *Specific Conductance: Theoretical considerations and application to analytical quality control.* US Geological Survey Water-Supply Paper 2311. Denver, CO: United States Government Printing Office.

Myers, G.S. (1949). *Salt-tolerance of Fresh-water Fish Groups in Relation to Zoogeographical Problems.* Early Classics in Biogeography, Distribution and Diversity Studies to 1950. http://people.wku.edu/charles.smith/biogeog/MYER1949.htm (accessed 14 June 2021).

Nelson, N. and Siegel, D. (2014). Chromophoric dissolved organic matter (CDOM) in the global ocean. [Presentation]. http://www.ioccg.org/training/SLS-2014/Siegel_CDOM_Nelson.pdf (Accessed 19 April 2021).

Panakorn, S. (2016). H2S toxicity: the silent killer, *Aquaculture-Asia Pacific*, 12(2): 14.

Roberts, V.A., Vigar, M., Backer, L. *et al.* (2020). Surveillance for harmful algal bloom events and associated human and animal illnesses: one health harmful algal bloom system, United States, 2016–2018. *MMWR Morb Mortal Wkly Rep 2020*; 69: 1889–1894.

Sabra, F. and Mehana, S.D. (2015). Pesticides toxicity in fish with particular reference to insecticides. *Asian Journal of Agriculture and Food Sciences.* 3: 40–60.

Scannell, P.W. and Jacobs, L.L. (2001). *Effects of Total Dissolved Solids on Aquatic Organisms: A literature review.* Alaska Department of Fish and Game, Division of Habitat and Restoration. Technical Report 01-06.

Sfakianakis, D., Renieri, E., Kentouri, M. *et al.* (2015). Effect of heavy metals on fish larvae deformities: a review. *Environmental Research* 137: 246–255.

Sommer, K., and Spitzer, P. (2004). Session H: Ocean Salinity. Plenary lecture presented at the WMO-BIPM WS Geneva 30 March–1 April.

Soni, R. and Verma, S.K. (2018). Acute toxicity and behavioral responses in *Clarias batrachus* (Linnaeus) exposed to herbicide pretilachlor. *Heliyon*, 4(12): e01090.

Stamper, M.A. (2015). Microbes and the Aquarium. Proceedings of the International Association for Aquatic Animal Medicine Conference, April 6–11, 2015, Chicago, IL.

Stehr, C.M., Linbo, T.L., Baldwin, D.H. *et al.* (2009). Evaluating the effects of forestry herbicides on fish development using rapid phenotypic screens. *North American Journal of Fisheries Management* 29: 975–984.

Svendsen, E., Dahle, S.W., Hagemann, A. *et al.* (2017). Effect of ultrasonic cavitation on small and large organisms for water disinfection during fish transport. *Aquaculture Research* 49: 1166–1175.

Svobodova, Z. and Kolarova, J. (2004). A review of the diseases and contaminant related mortalities of tench (*Tinca tinca* L.). *Veterinarni Medicina* 49: 19–34.

Svobodova, Z., Machova, J., Poleszczuk, G. *et al.* (2005). Nitrite poisoning of fish in aquaculture facilities with water-recirculating systems: three case studies. *Acta Veterinaria Brno* 74: 129–137.

Tepper, J.M. (2000). A phytoremedial device for koi ponds. IAAAM 2000: Proceedings of the International Association for Aquatic Animal Medicine Conference, Spring 2000, New Orleans, LA. https://www.vin.com/apputil/content/defaultadv1.aspx?pId=11125&meta=generic&id=3980412 (accessed 19 April 2021).

Tepper, J.M. (2019). Water biology for healthy freshwater aquasystems. Proceedings of the World Small Animal Veterinary Association Congress Proceedings, 2019 July 16–19, 2019, Toronto, Canada. https://www.vin.com/apputil/content/defaultadv1.aspx?pId=24437&catId=137405&id=9382753&ind=301&objTypeID=17 (accessed 19 April 2021).

Tillitt, D.E., Papoulias, D M., Whyte, J.J. *et al.* (2014). *Atrazine Reduces Reproduction in Fathead Minnow* (Pimephales promelas)*: Raw data report*. Data Series 805. Reston, VA: US Geological Survey.

Timmons, M.B., Guerdat, T. and Vinci, B.J. (2018). *Recirculating Aquaculture*. 4e. New York, NY: Ithaca Publishing Company.

Tucker, C.S. (1984). Carbon dioxide. *For Fish Farmers. Mississippi Cooperative Extension Service Newsletter* 84(2).

Turley C., Blackford J.C., Widdicombe, W. *et al.* (2006). Reviewing the impact of increased atmospheric CO_2 on oceanic pH and the marine ecosystem. In: *Avoiding Dangerous Climate Change*. (ed. H.J. Schellnhuber, W. Cramer, N. Nakicenovic *et al.*), 65–69. Cambridge University Press.

US Environmental Protection Agency. (2012). 5.9 Conductivity. In Water: Monitoring and Assessment. https://www.epa.gov/national-aquatic-resource-surveys/indicators-conductivity (accessed 14 June 2021).

Wagner, R.J., Boulger, Jr., R.W., Oblinger, C.J. *et al.* (2006). *Guidelines and Standard Procedures for Continuous Water-Quality Monitors: Station operation, record computation, and data reporting*. Techniques and Methods 1-D3. Reston, VA: US Geological Survey.

Wessel, N., Martin, S., Badou, A. *et al.* (2018). Effect of CO_2-induced ocean acidification on the early development and shell mineralization of the European abalone (*Haliotis tuberculata*). *Journal of Experimental Marine Biology and Ecology* 508: 52–63.

Wildgoose, W. (ed.) (2001). *BSAVA Manual of Ornamental Fish*, 2e. Chichester, UK: Wiley.

Wood, S.A., Puddick, J., Borges, H. et al. (2015). Potential effects of climate change on cyanobacterial toxin production. In: *Climate Change and Marine and Freshwater Toxins* (ed. L.M. Botana, C. Louzao and N. Vilariño), pp. 155–180. Berlin: De Gruyter.

2

Taxonomy, Anatomy, and Physiology

Matt Longshaw, Acacia Alcivar-Warren, Wes Baumgartner, Trista Becker, James E. Bogan, Jr., Erdem Danyer, Sherry Kasper, Nicole Marie Nemeth, and Adolf Maas

Learning Objectives
Students should demonstrate knowledge of basic anatomy and physiology of the major aquatic animal taxa.

2.1 Introduction

It is an unstated but important truism that to treat an animal one must be able to place the animal within a recognized taxonomic framework and to acknowledge that differences in anatomy and physiology of these animals can differ markedly between and within those taxa. This should not be seen as a need to learn a whole new set of skills, as it is natural for humans to try to classify their surroundings and the flora and fauna within it. The binomial system created by Carl Linnaeus, which relies predominately on morphological similarities and differences between organisms, has been universally adopted and continues to be used to this day. A move toward DNA barcoding has been seen as potentially leading to the death of classical taxonomy and as a stimulus for new species discovery. Indeed, the combination of morphological and molecular techniques is now considered the norm and has led to the identification of a number of cryptic species, even in the absence of clear morphological differences, across a wide range of taxa. Although taxonomy will continue to develop with shifts in the systematic classification of animals and plants, the overarching view is that the higher taxonomy of most living species is well established and is unlikely to change fundamentally.

In most cases, the underlying principle of taxonomy is to identify similarities and differences in taxa. These criteria extend to the anatomical features and to physiological responses. It follows that it is highly likely that the responses and reactions to any treatment, infection or insult will be similar for taxonomically related animals and therefore, with some limited exceptions, analogous therapies can be applied across related taxa.

Further exploration of the effect of this taxonomic diversity is concluded through the comparative analysis of the anatomy and physiology of animals that live in the aquatic environment for all

Fundamentals of Aquatic Veterinary Medicine, First Edition. Edited by Laura Urdes, Chris Walster, and Julius Tepper.

Companion website: www.wiley.com/go/urdes/aquatic-veterinary-medicine

or part of their life cycle. It is recognized that due to space limitations, not all aquatic and semi-aquatic animals are covered within this chapter but the text provides the fundamental knowledge required to recognize the major variations likely to be encountered and highlights the need to be mindful of these differences.

Taxonomy provides a concise review of the major aquatic animal taxa. There are seven main classifications: kingdom, phylum, class, order, family, genus, and species. Each of these classifications may be further subdivided. The list comprises vertebrates (i.e., fish including teleosts and elasmobranchs), amphibians, reptiles, birds and mammals, and invertebrates such as mollusks and crustaceans. An understanding of these taxa and their relationships is critical in recognizing the diverse range of aquatic and semi-aquatic species likely to be encountered and the potential impact of this diversity on the anatomy and physiology and on the responses of the hosts to infection. Be aware that classifications are continuously being revised and may differ from those cited in the book.

Anatomy and physiology provide a comparative review of the major aquatic animal taxa of economic importance. Differences across (and within) taxa are commonplace; it is imperative to be able to recognize the similarities and differences between the taxa to ensure that appropriate treatment is administered. For example, respiration in lower invertebrates and some amphibians can be via cutaneous respiration/diffusion; in higher invertebrates and fish, respiration is typically via gills in direct contact with water, compared with mammals and birds that respire using lungs that do not come into contact with the aquatic medium. Other examples of differences include swim bladders, unique to bony fish, which can vary markedly in structure, and major differences in the structure of the integument (e.g. scales in fish, pelage in mammals, feathers in birds).

The taxonomy of Mollusca and oysters is available in the website materials accompanying this text.

2.2 Invertebrates

2.2.1 Crustacea

The large subphylum Crustacea contains a large variety of arthropods, including mobile species such as crabs and lobsters, sessile forms such as barnacles, and parasitic and commensal species such as parasitic copepods and branchiurans (e.g., *Argulus* spp.). More than 30,000 crustacean species have been described, with the majority occurring in marine and freshwater habitats, although terrestrial species are known (e.g., woodlice, some terrestrial crabs). Crustacea are extensively exploited, with many species being cultivated, kept in captivity, or fished worldwide. While some members of the class Maxillopoda (e.g., copepods) can be cultured as live animal feed, the main class exploited and/or kept in captivity is the class Malacostraca, which contains around 40,000 species occurring in a broad range of aquatic ecosystems. Representative examples in the order Decapoda are available in the website materials accompanying this text for those species that are commercially exploited or maintained under captive situations (including aquaculture).

The taxonomy chart is available in the website materials accompanying this text.

2.2.1.1 Superfamily Penaeidae

Most crustaceans are aquatic. A large proportion of them are marine species. Among other organisms, the crustaceans group includes shrimps, crayfish, lobsters, crabs and copepods (Myers, 2020; National

Center for Biotechnology Information, 2020; WoRMS, 2020). "Lobsters, crayfish, barnacles, and crabs are important to human economies. Others, such as krill, are at the base of extremely important marine food chains. Still others are crucial in recycling nutrients trapped in the bodies of dead organisms"(Myers, 2020).

Many crustacean species are free living, with just a few being sessile or parasitic species. The body of a crustacean is mainly composed of head, thorax, and abdomen. The head has paired antennae, paired compound eyes, paired mandibles and maxillae. Each body segment has a pair of appendages primitively branched (biramous). All crustaceans have a hard, flexible exoskeleton. Crustaceans respire via gills and use their maxillae and mandibles to ingest food. With the help of their walking legs and the specialized chelipeds they are able to capture prey. Some crustaceans filter plankton and bacteria from the water, scavenge nutrients from detritus, or act as effective predators.

Most crustaceans are dioecious (distinct male and female individuals). The fertilization mechanisms in crustaceans vary greatly. The young stages of some crustaceans are like miniature adults, whereas others, such as shrimp, go through a larval stage called a nauplius.

There are five classes of Crustacea: Remipedia, Cephalocarida, Branchiopoda (fairy shrimp, water fleas, others), Maxillopoda (ostracods, copepods, barnacles) and Malacostraca (isopods, amphipods, krill, crabs, shrimp, etc.; Myers, 2020; Holthius, 1980; National Center for Biotechnology Information, 2020; WoRMS, 2020).

The morphology and biology of Penaeus shrimps are available in the website materials accompanying this text.

2.3 Vertebrates

2.3.1 Fish and Elasmobranchs

The Classification of fish is available in the website materials accompanying this text.

Class Pisces (fish) comprises three groups:

1) Agnatha – jawless fish
2) Chondrichthyes – cartilaginous fish
3) Osteichthyes (Teleost) – bony fish

For further information, refer to the taxonomy of fish in Fish Base and the *Catalog of Fishes* (Fricke *et al.*, 2021).

Depending on the author cited, the number of species vary. There are about 50 Agnatha species, over 1000 species of Chondrichthyes and 30 000 species of Osteichthyes in the world. Most bony fish species belong to the ray-finned group. There are about 70 fish orders found in the world, including sharks and rays; sturgeon and gars; herring-like fish; trout and salmon; eels, minnows, suckers, and catfish; flying fish and relatives; cod-like fish; flatfish; seahorses and relatives; mullets and silverside.

2.3.1.1 Agnatha

Agnatha represents an ancient vertebrate lineage. *Gnathos* is Greek for "jaw" and the prefix "a" means "without"– Agnatha fish lack jaws. They have an elongate body and persistent notochord throughout life. A notochord is a flexible rod-like cord of cells that provides the main support for the body during its embryonic stage. There are two extant lineages (hagfish and lamprey), which are often grouped together on account of their similar body form. There are 70 living species of agnathans (42 lampreys and 28 hagfish species).

- Hagfish are primitive eel-like fish, classified as Myxini, which lack a vertebral column. The skeleton of a hagfish is composed of cartilage, which includes a cartilaginous notochord that runs the length of the body and provides support to the hagfish's body. Unlike true vertebrates, hagfish do not replace the notochord with a vertebral column during development.
- Lampreys are classified as Petromyzontidae. They are morphologically similar to hagfish and also lack paired appendages. However, lampreys develop some vertebral elements as an adult. Their notochord is surrounded by cartilaginous structures called arcualia, which may resemble an evolutionarily early form of the vertebral column.

2.3.1.2 Chondrichthyes

Chondrichthyes, also referred to as gnathostomes (jawed vertebrates), are vertebrates that possess jaws. The class Chondrichthyes comprises the cartilaginous fish, which encompasses skates, sharks, rays, and chimaeras. The class contains 12 orders divided between two monophyletic subclasses, the Elasmobranchii (sharks, rays and skates) and Holocephali (chimaeras). With the Holocephali, now represented by only around 40 living species of chimaera in the single order Chimaeriformes, the vast majority of extant chondrichthyans are elasmobranchs.

- Elasmobranchii (Elasmobranch): There are over 1000 species in the class Elasmobranchii, including the southern stingray, whale shark, basking shark, and shortfin mako shark. The classification of elasmobranchs has undergone revision. Recent molecular studies have found that skates and rays are different enough from all of the sharks that they should be in their own group under elasmobranchs. Sharks swim by moving their tail fin from side to side, while a skate or ray may swim by flapping their large pectoral fins like wings. Rays are adapted for feeding on the ocean floor. Sharks are well known and feared for their ability to kill by biting and tearing. Sawfish, now endangered, have a long snout with protruding teeth that looks like a chainsaw blade, used for slashing and impaling fish and prowling in mud. Electric rays can generate an electric current to stun their prey and for defense. Stingrays have one or more barbed stingers with venom which they use for self-defense.
- Holocephali: Chimaera or ghost sharks, like other sharks and rays, have cartilaginous skeletons but have a single external gill opening. Chimaeras are tapered fish with large pectoral and pelvic fins, large eyes, and two dorsal fins, the first preceded by a sharp spine. They have slender tails, from which the name ratfish, applied to some, has been derived. There are about 47 species of chimaeras, ranging in length from about 24 to 80 inches (60–200 cm) and in color from silvery to blackish. The species are placed in three families: Chimaeridae (including the species called rabbit fish), characterized by a rounded or cone-shaped snout; Callorhinchidae (elephant fish), with an unusual, hoe-shaped, flexible snout; and Rhinochimaeridae (long-nosed chimaeras) with an extended, pointed snout.

2.3.1.3 Osteichthyes (Teleost)

The main characteristics of bony fish are that bone replaces cartilage developmentally, opercula cover the gills, and the swim bladder maintains buoyancy. They have specialized jaw musculature and skeletal elements. Bony fish are made up of the classes Sarcopterygii (lobe-finned fish) and Actinopterygii (ray-finned fish). The vast majority of fish are members of Osteichthyes, which is an extremely diverse and abundant group consisting of 45 orders, over 435 families and 28 000 species. The scientific name Pisces has also been used to identify these groups of fish.

- Actinopterygii, or ray-finned fish: constitute a class or subclass of the bony fish. The ray-finned fish are so called because they possess lepidotrichia or "fin rays", their fins being webs of skin supported by bony or horny spines ("rays").
- Sarcopterygii or lobe-finned fish: The living sarcopterygians are the coelacanths, lungfish, and the tetrapods. Early lobe-finned fish had fleshy, lobed, paired fins joined to the body by a single bone. Their fins differ from those of all other fish in that each is borne on a fleshy, lobe-like, scaly stalk extending from the body. Pectoral and pelvic fins have articulations resembling those of tetrapod limbs.

2.3.1.3.1 Morphology and Physiology of Teleost Fish

The anatomy of bony fish has been the subject of numerous studies and books over the past 200 years. In place of a comprehensive description in this chapter, there will be a focus on prototypical species, especially zebrafish (*Danio rerio*), as a starting point. In a general sense, fish anatomy is similar across species and, where pertinent, variations that may be of particular interest to clinicians will be mentioned.

Body Fish are composed of a head, trunk, and tail. The head encloses the brain, eyes, mouth, and gills, with plate-like gill coverings called opercula (sing. operculum). The trunk extends from the head to the caudal extent of the abdominal (pleuroperitoneal, coelomic) cavity, which is generally at the anus. The abdomen of a fish is, relatively speaking, much smaller relative to the trunk as compared with that of mammals. Caudal to this is the caudal peduncle. Fish have several sets of fins; the paired pectoral fins just caudal to the gills, the paired pelvic fins associated with the anus, the unpaired dorsal fin, and smaller unpaired caudal dorsal fin, the unpaired anal fin, and the caudal fin, or tail. Some species may lack any variety of fins (Roberts and Ellis, 2012).

Integument The skin of a fish is the largest mucosal surface of the animal; it is continuous with the mouth, gills, nose, digestive, and urogenital organ systems. The skin serves not only as a barrier to the environment, but as a means of communication, immune function, ion regulation, and even respiration. In general, fish skin is similar to mammalian skin, but there are significant differences. Fish epithelium is stratified (Figure 2.1) but keratinization occurs only in specific areas (nuptial

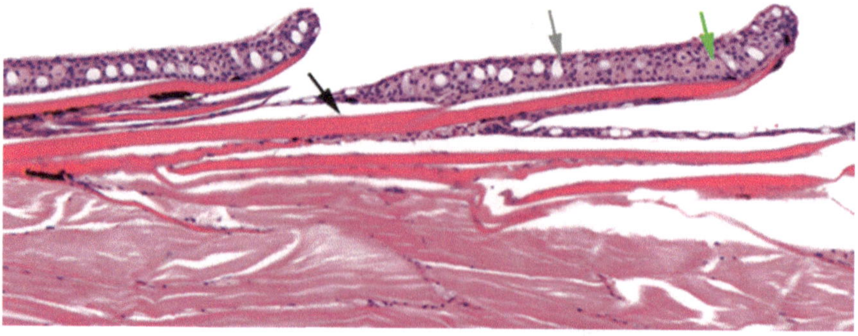

Figure 2.1 Zebrafish skin. Black arrow indicates the scale, green arrow indicates the club cell (alarm substance), and grey arrow the goblet cells. Wes Baumgartner hematoxylin and eosin stain.

tubercles) and in certain species. It is highly permeable and highly susceptible to chemical injury. For the most part, fish skin is protected by a mucus layer (cuticle) that is produced by the epidermis; it is in continuous production and cleanses the skin surface and also contains lysozyme and immunoglobulins. Fish skin has several types of mucus/gland cells (goblet cells, club cells, others), which function to produce mucus and aid the immune response. The maintenance of the mucus layer is of vital importance to the fish, and care must be taken when handling them. A primary indicator of disease in a fish will be a change in mucus production, especially hypersecretion. Since fish live in water, even relatively small areas of skin injury can have significant consequences to health, not only in terms of microbial infection, but in terms of osmolar shifts between the fish and the water.

Fish skin heals rapidly; epithelium can cover defects within hours. In such cases, areas of skin injury will assume a change in color (often pallor/milky) as a result of epidermal necrosis, hyperplasia, and edema. They can also regenerate fin tissue. The stages of skin wound healing are similar in fish and mammals.

Scales are mineralized skeletal elements that occur in most species of fish, and there are various types described. The scales reside in the dermis just beneath the epidermis, and can be easily rubbed off or lost. Fish lose scales at least once in their lifetime, and can readily regenerate them. Scales serve as a primary calcium/mineral reservoir in times of need, although calcium is generally not a limiting metabolite since it is abundant in water. Scales develop in very fine scale "pockets" in the dermis; they enlarge by the addition of outer rings, much like tree rings.

The color of fish skin is partially determined by the pigment cells (chromatophores) in the dermis and subcutis. Melanophores (melanocytes) and other pigment cells (erythrophores, iridophores, leucophores, xanthophores, etc.) have been described.

Bone Fish have an axial and appendicular skeleton of a nature similar to mammals (Figure 2.2); it comprises an endoskeleton and exoskeleton. The former includes the bone and cartilage elements that are commonly thought of as the 'skeleton' in mammals. The exoskeleton is of mesodermal origin (Shimada *et al.*, 2013), and is composed of teeth, dermal bone, scales/scutes, spines, and fin rays. Fish grow continuously throughout life, and the skeleton is continually remodeled in response to diet, environmental cues, light, and temperature; adaptation can occur over the animal's lifetime in response to mechanical loads, diet, etc. Changes also occur in some species with migration and spawning.

Fish have a complex skull and simple vertebral column. The skull houses the gills within the oropharynx. The vertebrae are block-like with prominent spines (neural and hemal) that protect the dorsal spinal cord and ventral artery/vein. Vertebrae are biconcave with intervening disks composed of notochord-derived tissue. In lateral radiographs, vertebrae appear as an X shape, being formed by the conical ends of the bone.

In contrast to mammals, fish lack hematopoietic tissue in the bones. Instead, marrow elements are preserved in the kidneys.

The regulation of calcium in bony fish is primarily accomplished by the gill and intestine. Kidneys maintain calcium levels through excretion. Calcium deficiency is uncommon; however, phosphorus is a limiting nutrient, and uptake is vitamin D dependent.

Muscle The majority of fish muscle is present in the trunk to provide locomotion. Interlocking folded muscular units (myomeres) occupy quadrants of the body when viewed in transverse section; they work in unison and are white anaerobic fiber-type (*muscularis lateralis profundus*). Red aerobic fibers are present just beneath the skin (*muscularis lateralis superficialis*), especially

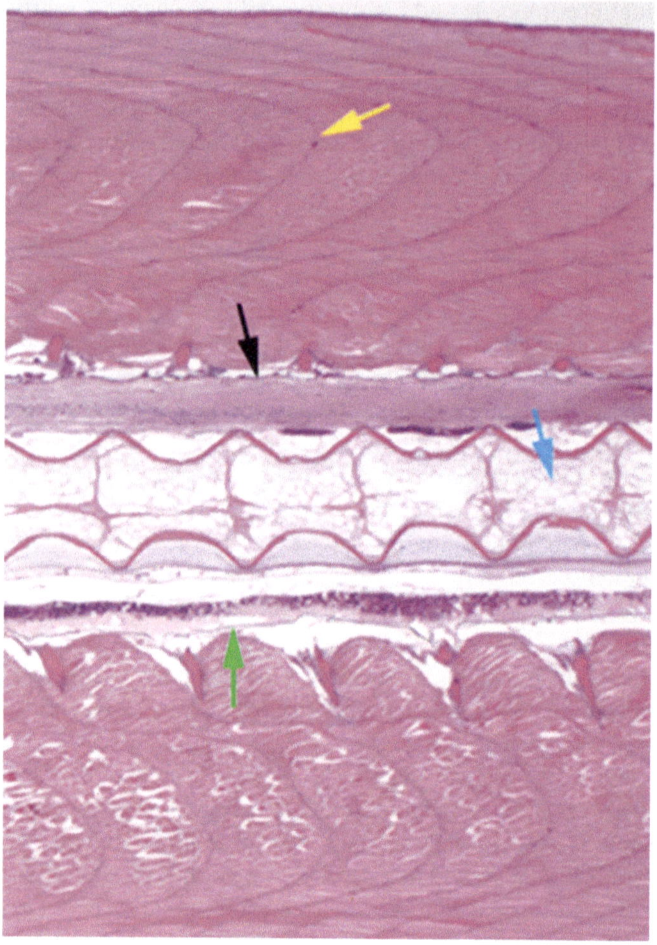

Figure 2.2 Channel catfish fry; sagittal section of the tail. Black arrow indicates the spinal cord, green arrow indicates the ventral hemal canal, blue arrow the vertebrae (still developing), and yellow arrow the muscle myomere junctions. Wes Baumgartner hematoxylin and eosin stain.

along the lateral aspect of the trunk; these function for sustained slow swimming. Drug injections in the red muscle will have different pharmaco-kinetics compared to white muscle (Roberts and Ellis, 2012).

Adipose Fat physiology and anatomy is similar to that in mammals. Fish have only white fat. Adipose accumulates in the mesentery, viscera (especially liver), muscle, and subcutis at the base of the fins. Laboratory and pet fish often suffer from nutritional imbalance and can have excessive adipose tissue in the liver.

Circulatory System The fish circulatory system is relatively simple and is similar to that in mammals, although blood pressure is much lower. From the heart, poorly oxygenated blood is circulated through the gills, where gas exchange occurs. Blood then courses through the dorsal aorta to supply the tissues, with return of fluids through veins, lymphatics, and the secondary vascular system.

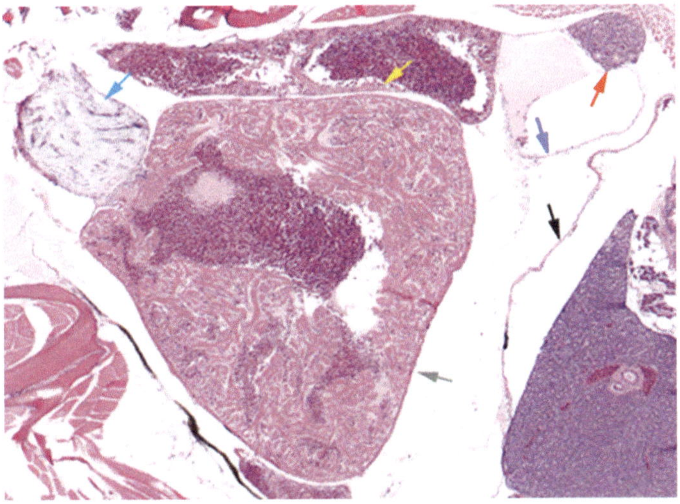

Figure 2.3 Zebrafish heart. The black arrow denotes the septum transversum, the dark blue arrow is the sinus venosus, the yellow arrow the atrium, the gray arrow the ventricle, the light blue arrow the bulbus arteriosus, and the red arrow the ultimobranchial body. Wes Baumgartner hematoxylin and eosin stain.

The heart is positioned between the gills, within a rigid pericardial cavity that is separated from the liver by a transverse septum. It has four chambers in series; a thin-walled sinus venosus that receives blood from the cardinal veins and liver, a thicker atrium that empties through one valve into the thick-walled ventricle, and finally a bulbus arteriosus, which is elastic and is separated from the ventricle by a valve. Fish electrocardiograms are similar to other vertebrates, with a QRS wave. Systolic pressures of 30–70 mmHg and diastolic pressures of 10–30mmHg are reported. Heart rates can vary markedly, depending on the temperature (Figure 2.3).

Most fish have a renal portal system, where venous blood (partially or totally) from the tail and flank pass through the kidney. In all species, the kidneys are supplied by blood from the flank (segmental veins), but segmental venous blood may also go directly to the liver or heart. Venous blood from the tail (caudal vein) bypasses the viscera and goes directly to the heart in some species (salmonids, tuna, perch). This renal portal system can have significant effects on pharmacodynamics, depending on where drugs are administered (Roberts and Ellis, 2012).

Study of the fish lymphatic system is controversial. Fish have lymphatics to supply viscera (with the possible exception of the intestine), but also have a secondary vascular system that serves the skin, gills, fins, peritoneum, and oral mucosa. The secondary vascular system is composed of narrow bore vessels that connect to the blood vessels, but restrict erythrocyte access. The volume in the secondary vascular system can be up to twice that in the primary circulation; it may function in osmotic buffering and nutrition in the skin, but this is poorly understood.

Gills/Pseudobranch The gills are the primary respiratory organs of fish; they reside within the oral cavity on either side of the pharynx, behind the opercula. Gills also serve as the primary site for osmoregulation, acid-base balance, nitrogenous waste excretion, and hormone metabolism. They are highly adaptive and delicate structures. Fish gills are arranged in arches, typically four on each side; they are bow-like when viewed laterally and are composed of bony tissues that support the

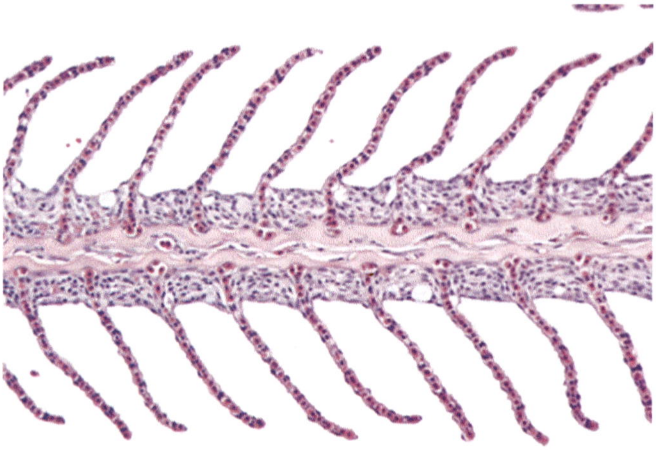

Figure 2.4 Channel catfish gills. The filament runs horizontal, and many lamellae arise perpendicularly. Pillar cells form spaces for erythrocytes to travel. Wes Baumgartner hematoxylin and eosin stain.

vascular filaments (primary lamellae). On each arch are two rows of filaments, like teeth on a comb. Each filament is covered on both sides by plate-like (secondary) lamellae which are oriented with the flow of water (Figure 2.4); it is in these lamellae where gas exchange occurs between the water and the erythrocytes. The lamellae are an envelope of thin epithelial cells that are separated by pillar cells, which also delimit the capillary-sized lumen of the vascular channels. Blood flow in the gills is such that a countercurrent exchange system occurs, where oxygen loading is maximized (Roberts and Ellis, 2012).

In addition, fish have pseudobranchs, which are not respiratory organs. They arise from the first gill arch and are embedded in the anterior wall of the opercular cavities; they receive oxygenated blood to supply the ocular retia.

Digestive System The pharynx of teleost fish includes the teeth or beak, tongue and oral cavity. They vary widely, depending on the species. Some fish have no teeth. Fish can have oral teeth along the jaws, lingual teeth, or pad-like arrangements deep in the pharynx. Fish can continuously grow and shed teeth, and the frequency of shedding depends partly on the diet. Zebrafish have only pharyngeal teeth, with a keratinized pharyngeal grinding pad as in other cyprinids. Some eels have a secondary jaw within the mouth.

In some species, the start of digestion occurs through mastication. In other species, a majority of the food is swallowed in its entirety. Fish lack salivary glands and a tongue may or may not be present. The gastrointestinal tract is composed of a mucosa, submucosa, muscularis, and serosa similar to that in mammals.

The size and function of the stomach varies between species. The definition of a true stomach is a dilation of the gastrointestinal system that contains glands which produce digestive enzymes and acids. The amount of digestion that occurs in this area depends on the species, and some fish (approximately 20%) lack true stomachs in this regard (like zebrafish and other cyprinids). The fundus and pylorus are the main areas of the stomach found in fish. It may be J, Y, U, I-shaped, or a straight tube, when present. In some species (gizzard shad), a muscular grinding stomach is present.

The intestines include the duodenum, small intestines, and colon; the zebrafish has only an intestine and no demarcations are found. The length of each portion typically varies by what the animal is eating and how much digestion and absorption still needs to occur posterior to the stomach. Some fish have digestive systems that are larger than 50% of their body while others have digestive systems that are only 10% of their body. True herbivores tend to have a longer digestive tract than omnivores and carnivores. Much of the digestion occurs in the duodenum either due to glands in the duodenum or through ducts that allow bile and enzymes to flow into the duodenum from the pancreas and liver. Fish intestinal mucosa in all but a few species lack villi, but have many irregular folds.

In many species of fish (salmonids, cod, trout) there are fingerlike pyloric ceca at the junction of the pylorus and the intestines. They may be free floating or condensed, appearing as a mass. Their function is likely in absorption.

The intestines are the main area for digestion and absorption. In herbivorous fish, the ratio of body length to intestinal length may be as long as a 30 : 1 ratio. In carnivorous fish, the ratio may be as close as 1 : 1. The pancreas and the gall bladder have ducts that empty into the first part of the intestine to help with digestion. The fish intestine can be divided into three functional segments; the anterior segment is the longest and absorbs lipids, while the second shorter segment absorbs protein. The third, shortest segment absorbs water and electrolytes. Carnivorous fish may not tolerate plant substances/proteins in their diet, which can lead to severe enteritis, hepatitis, and death. Bony fish lack cloacas; gut, urinary, and genital tracts empty into separate openings at the vent.

The liver and biliary system in fish is comparable to that of mammals (Figure 2.5); hepatocytes are arranged in cords but lobular organization is clearly appreciated. The liver functions in processing carbohydrates, proteins, fats, vitamins, and xenobiotics. Also, fish produce vitellogenin for eggs. In some species, the liver can be highly pigmented, which is usually due to the presence of

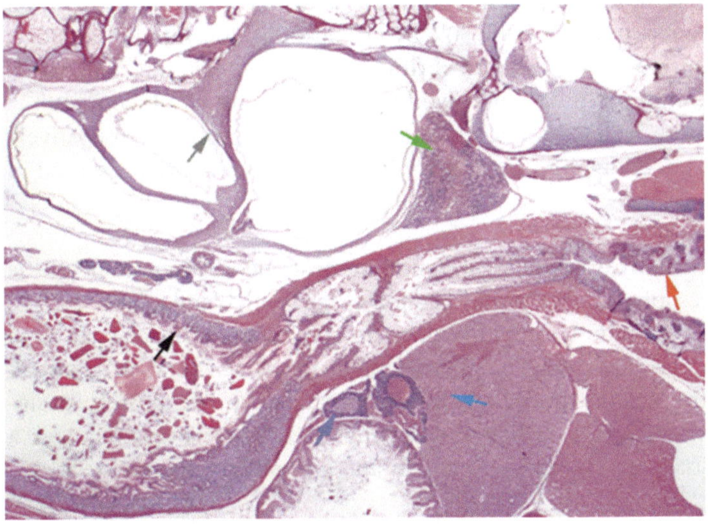

Figure 2.5 Channel catfish fry, abdominal viscera; the spine is along the top, and the ventrum is the bottom of the photomicrograph. Black arrow indicates the stomach, green arrow indicates the pronephros, red arrow the mouth/teeth, dark blue arrow the pancreas with endocrine islet, light blue arrow the liver, and gray arrow the swim bladder. Wes Baumgartner hematoxylin and eosin stain.

melanomacrophage centers (collections of reactive macrophages). Liver swelling and pale/yellow discoloration are common in housed fish, which is often due to excess lipid or glycogen; this is a consequence of excessive nutrition or malnutrition. In situations of cyclical starvation, livers may accumulate ceroid and become tan/bronze.

The exocrine pancreas is highly variable and is often diffusely distributed into the mesentery, liver, and even spleen. Endocrine pancreas tissues are also distributed in this area, and may form rather distinctive nodules in the mesentery. Exocrine function is similar to mammals.

When discussing the anatomy of the gastrointestinal tract, it is also important to equally consider the roles that digestion and absorption of nutrients play in the growth and maintenance of normal functions in animals. A widely accepted model organism for laboratory studies of fish is the zebrafish (*Danio rerio*). Considerable research has contributed extensive knowledge to the understanding of nutrition in other important aquaculture fish – namely food fish, such as salmonids and catfish. Advances in the understanding of nutrition and growth in aquaculture have been made with the use of the zebrafish model for nutritional genomics (nutrigenetics and nutrigenomics) studies on the impacts of individual and population genetics on growth in production as well as the impacts of nutrition on phenotypic expression of growth traits (Ulloa *et al.*, 2013). However, little is known of the exact nutritional requirements of zebrafish, probably due to their versatility in husbandry and feeding conditions.

Gastrointestinal transit time will increase or decrease with a respective change in water temperature, as will feed intake and metabolic rate. The type of diet, wet or dry, has also been shown to change transit time. Studies on several species of fish have shown that a higher water content will slow transit time (Le *et al.*, 2019). General nutrient requirements can be used for fats, protein, carbohydrates, vitamins, and minerals. Fish cannot synthesize polyunsaturated fatty acids and thus must obtain them from the diet. Coldwater fish like salmonids have high omega 3 fatty acids requirements (linolenic acid, 18 : 3) and warm water fish have higher omega 6 fatty acid requirements (linoleic acid, 18 : 2). Not only are lipids an important energy source, but they provide building blocks for pheromones, hormones, and cell membranes. Inadequate levels of these essential fatty acids can affect growth and reproduction (especially fertilization rates). Protein requirements vary from 30% to over 50% by species and developmental stage, with 10 essential amino acid requirements of fish and shrimp – threonine, leucine, isoleucine, methionine, lysine, arginine, valine, tryptophan, histidine, phenylalanine (Tacon, 1987). Carbohydrate requirements are less well understood, and inadequate levels may negatively affect growth. The basics of feeds, feeding, and husbandry in aquatic species are presented in more detail in Chapter 3.

Swim Bladder The swim bladder is a hydrostatic organ found in most teleosts. The tissue of the swim bladder originates from the esophagus. The main function of the swim bladder is to regulate buoyancy but it also plays a role in respiration, sound reception and production. One classification of fish is by the type of swim bladder they have. The physostomous fish (like zebrafish) retain at least one connection with the gastrointestinal tract called the pneumatic duct. The main physostomous fish include cyprinids, salmonids, eels, catfish and herring. The physoclistous fish lack a connection with the gastrointestinal tract. Many benthic fish and elasmobranchs tend to lack a swim bladder.

The tissue of the swim bladder is made up of two layers: an internal tunic composed of transitional or simple epithelium (some authors further subdivide this layer into mucosa, submucosa, muscularis) and an external tunic composed of connective tissue. The mucosa is made of cuboidal epithelium. The muscular tissue is of smooth muscle type (Demski *et al.*, 1973). The submucosa and the external layers are made of fibroblasts and collagen. The healthy swim bladder has a shiny white serosal surface.

The size and shape of the swim bladder is dependent on species. Typically, the swim bladder is found at the dorsal surface of the coelomic cavity. The average size of the swim bladder is approximately 30% of the coelomic cavity. It may be as small as 3% of the coelomic cavity or as large as 50% as seen in some fish of the phylum Acanthomorpha. In physostomous fish, there can be one or several connections with the gastrointestinal system. The swim bladder may be U-shaped, tube like, or oval, with one or more compartments. In some fish, such as in freshwater butterflyfish, the bladder infiltrates the vertebrae. Physoclistous fish have a gas gland to produce gas and an oval gland to absorb it.

Some species of fish have swim bladder horns that connect with the otic capsule or the supracleithral lateral line canal. The *Chaetodon* species have several different types of connection of the swim bladder to the supracleithral lateral line. The function of this connection is to enhance the detection of sound. The effectiveness of this sound enhancement is dependent on the size of the swim bladder and the type of connection that is present. There are six main types of connections of the anterior swim bladder horns and the supracleithral lateral line. These are separated into direct or indirect connections. The direct connections have a direct tissue attachment between the soft tissue in the medial opening of the supracleithrum with a tympanic separation between the fluid-filled lateral line canal and the air of the swim bladder. This is further separated with some species having mucoid connective tissue present at this layer. The indirect connections are separated into four categories based on length of horns, presence of one or two chambers and the presence of mucoid connective tissue.

The swim bladder is innervated by the sympathetic and autonomic nervous system. A study of zebrafish has shown that there are many types of receptors present, including serotonin, neuropeptide Y, tyrosine hydroxyls, and choline acetyltransferase-immunoreactive somata. Both the sympathetic and autonomic nervous system effect the diffusion of gas into and out of the swim bladder.

The nervous system input, the glands of the swim bladder, and the permeability of the swim bladder wall contribute to the physiology of gas retention and release. Fish need to maintain a percentage of their size as gas volume to maintain the appropriate buoyancy. The volume of the gas needed in the swim bladder is affected by the water salinity, water temperature, and the depth the fish prefers to inhabit. Most fish maintain 5% of their body weight in gas volumes. The gas present is composed of oxygen, carbon dioxide and nitrogen. The percentage of each is dependent on the species. Salmonids, for example, have a high nitrogen level.

Boyle's law explains that atmospheric pressure and volume of air are inversely related. Therefore, the deeper the fish goes in the water column, the more compressed the gas will be, effectively decreasing the volume present. A physostomous fish will gulp air at the surface which will enter the swim bladder through the physostomous duct. As this fish swims deeper in the water column the air will compress and there will be no air to add via the pneumatic duct. Some physostomous fish, such as goldfish and koi, adapt to this condition by also having a *rete mirabile*. The *rete mirabile* is found in physostomous fish as their primary source of gas into the swim bladder. Physostomous fish have an anteroventral secretory region which contains the gas gland and the *rete mirabile*. The gas gland secretes lactic acid into the countercurrent capillary loop, the *rete mirabile*, which acidifies the region. The low pH causes both the Bohr and Root effects. The Bohr effect is that hemoglobin will decrease its affinity for oxygen at a low pH. The Root effect is a change in the structure of the hemoglobin that allows for the release of oxygen. This drives oxygen into the blood, which is diffused from the blood via the gas gland. The "salting-out effect" causes small bubbles of oxygen to form, also driving the oxygen from the blood. Since the oxygen coming into the *rete* is bound to hemoglobin, the countercurrent of the *rete mirabile* effectively keeps the oxygen in the *rete* because the oxygen moves down the gradient and the blood leaving the rete will be higher in dissolved oxygen that is not attached to hemoglobin.

Fish move air out of the swim bladder either by the pneumatic duct or the oval. The oval is an area developed from the degenerating pneumatic duct. It is a capillary bed separated from the swim bladder by a muscular ring. The muscles contract to expose the oval and release air. Both these areas may be blocked by tumors, swelling from infection, or foreign bodies, effectively preventing air escape.

Osmoregulation Osmoregulation in aquatic animals will vary with the environment and is a highly active process triggered by chloride levels in the body. Animals in marine or otherwise saline habitats have adaptations for acquisition and retention of H_2O, while freshwater animals have adaptations for excretion of H_2O and retention of sodium and other minerals. Regardless of being adapted to a marine or freshwater lifestyle, fish face a challenge maintaining body salinity concentrations vastly different from that of their environment. The respiratory, gastrointestinal, and urogenital systems have important osmoregulatory functions in fish, and may be highly specialized in some.

Fish in freshwater face a water overload and must take up as well as retain sodium and chloride, while constantly getting rid of excess water. Marine fish are perpetually dehydrating and have a salt overload to manage. Marine fish must drink saltwater and then continually remove those excess salts, while trying to balance osmotic loss of water across the gills.

The skin acts as a passive osmoregulatory defense in aquatic animals, providing a critical physical defense against osmotic pressures, in addition to protection from injury and infection. Unlike mammals, the outer layer of cells in the skin of fish is living and actively secreting protective substances that make up the outer cuticular layer which includes the mucous layer (secreted by mucous cells). The skin may also play an important role in sensing changes in chloride levels and triggering hormones that participate in osmoregulation.

In the gills (and other osmoregulatory organs), movement of sodium, chloride, and potassium occurs by ionocytes known as mitochondria-rich cells, formerly named chloride cells. These cells can be seen histologically in the gill epithelium, at the base of the secondary filaments. The details of ion transport remain an area of active research, and the details of how some function remain uncertain. Ionocytes in freshwater fish gills actively uptake Na^+ and Cl^- on the apical membrane driven by Na^+/K^+ -ATPase on the basolateral membrane. Such apical NaCl transporter mechanisms may include a Na^+-Cl^- cotransporter and a Na^+/H^+ exchanger, among others. While marine fish have similar cells, they may have each type in different proportions where the function is secretory rather than uptake. These types of cells are also present in other osmoregulatory organs. Though the cells present in the gills typically face larger fluctuations in osmolality, stress due to rapid environmental changes can impact the transporter activity of these cells in all the osmoregulatory organs. The cellular mechanisms that function to move ions in these cells continue to be studied, and it is thought that amphibian skin functions similarly to the gill of freshwater fish for osmoregulation. While this general scheme between freshwater and seawater fish may be similar, much variation exists between species due to various adaptations to their environment. Since only a few species have been extensively studied thus far, there remains much to learn about the broad diversity likely to exist in aquatic animals.

The primary adaptation of teleosts to life in freshwater is the ability to filter large volumes of water and excrete it from the body as dilute urine to compensate for being hyperosmotic to their environment. As such, the glomerulus maintains a high filtration rate. Resorption of sodium occurs in the tubules as well as the bladder, since the bladder in fish has a mesodermal rather than endodermal origin.

It is thought that fish first evolved in seawater, then adapted to life in freshwater. This may explain the complicated and varied mechanisms for osmoregulation in freshwater fish. The mitochondria-rich cells of saltwater fish gills use potassium channel-coupled Na/K^+ -ATPase transporters on the basal membrane and cystic fibrosis transport regulator Cl^- channels on the apical membrane surface that function together in NaCl excretion.

When marine fish ingest seawater, salt begins to diffuse out across the lining of the esophagus and stomach. Most of the water and salt uptake occurs in the small intestines through Na^+Cl^- cotransport and water follows osmotically. When present, the glomerulus in the kidney is reduced in comparison with freshwater species, the flow rate is slow, and urine resorption may even occur to excrete urine that is isotonic to the environment. The excess salts absorbed in the intestines are excreted renally (via urine) or extra-renally by the gills.

Ionocytes can rapidly adapt to changes in osmolality by shifting the transporter types on the cell membranes. More chronic changes will lead to larger, long-term changes such as shifts in epithelial cell types and even renal changes such as glomerular atrophy. As anadromous fish prepare to trade a freshwater life for a marine existence, they undergo a period of "smoltification" which includes major physiological changes in the gill epithelium. When working with anadromous species, it is recommended to explore these adaptations further and become familiar with how they may impact the health of cultured fish. Diseases may occur concurrent with stress during this and other life stage changes, as well as stress related to extra environmental osmoregulatory demands in general.

Kidneys Teleost kidneys are a combination of renal, hematopoietic, reticuloendothelial, and endocrine tissues (Figure 2.6). Fish retain their mesonephros (second kidney), unlike mammals, which have the metanephros (third kidney). In many species, the pronephros (head kidney) is

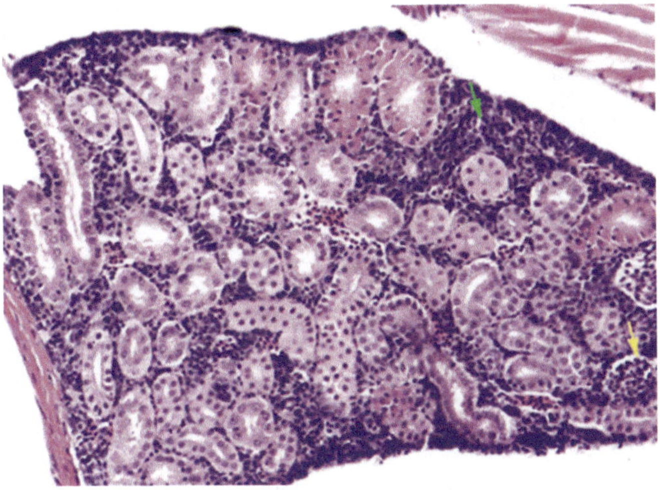

Figure 2.6 Channel catfish fry, mesonephros. Green arrow indicates the hematopoietic tissue, and yellow arrow a glomerulus. Many tubules are present throughout. Wes Baumgartner hematoxylin and eosin stain.

retained, but usually only contains hematopoietic tissue and not nephrons. The organ is retroperitoneal, and is tightly adherent to the vertebrae. Fish glomeruli and tubules are generally similar to mammals, however fish are able to regenerate tubules throughout life. Some fish have no glomeruli. Renal tubules vary considerably by species, but generally have proximal, intermediate, and distal segments, ending in the collecting ducts. Ureters drain collecting ducts and can empty into a bladder, or continue to urinary ducts near the anus.

Hematopoietic, Lymphoid and Immune Systems Fish lack lymph nodes and bone marrow. The spleen, thymus, kidneys, and mucosa-associated lymphoid tissues (MALT; gut, skin, nasal, gill) are the organs of hematopoiesis and lymphomyeloid function in fish. Hematopoiesis is predominantly in the spleen and kidneys, while the thymus is the primary lymphoid organ, with spleen and MALT as secondary lymphoid tissues. A detailed description of the immune system is available in Chapter 5.

The spleen is located in the central aspect of the viscera; it is generally deep red and ovoid. Enlarged spleens are generally significant, especially in cases of bacterial infection. The main element of the spleen are the ellipsoids (Figure 2.7), which are thick-walled blood filtration vessels that branch from the arterioles. Each ellipsoid is ensheathed by layers of macrophages. Macrophages that become filled with phagocytic debris will congregate into melanomacrophage centers. In time, an abundance of such centers may grossly discolor the spleen (and kidneys) gray. The thymus is located in the dorsal aspect of the branchial cavity.

Endocrine System Endocrine physiology is in many ways similar to that in mammals, but the distribution of endocrine tissues is quite different in fish. Fish do have discrete pituitaries, but the thyroid, adrenal cortex, adrenal medulla, endocrine pancreas, and thyroid C cells are located within or around other organs, and are not easily appreciated.

The interrenal and chromaffin tissues (adrenal cortex and medulla) are in a perivascular location within the pronephros. The thyroid is spread within the tissues surrounding the aorta

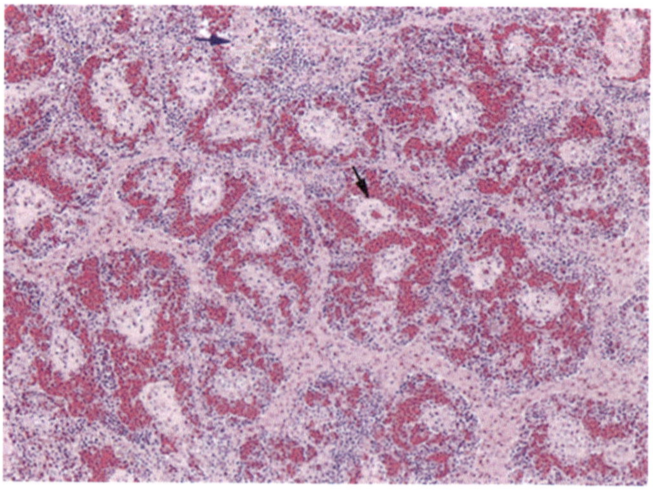

Figure 2.7 Channel catfish spleen, contracted state. Black arrow indicates an ellipsoid, and blue arrow a melanomacrophage center. Red pulp sinuses are subdivided by smooth muscle bands. Wes Baumgartner hematoxylin and eosin stain.

in the lower jaw. The endocrine islets are distributed in the mesentery, with the exocrine pancreas. In some species, discrete nodules of endocrine tissue are evident. Calcitonin secreting cells are present in the ultimobranchial gland, which is situated in the transverse septum between the heart and liver. In addition, the corpuscles of Stannius, which regulate blood calcium in concert with the ultimobranchial gland, are found along the lateral aspects of the mesonephros.

Reproductive System Reproductive patterns in fish are highly variable, and while most species have male and female sexes, hermaphroditism, bisexuality, parthenogenesis (development from unfertilized ovum) and other variations are well known. Fertilization may be external or internal, with delivery of fertilized eggs or live young.

Male fish have paired testes in the caudal abdomen; they are often elongate and vary markedly in size depending on the season. Blind seminiferous tubules are filled with sperm that empty into a duct at the posterior pole, which ends at the genital pore. Testosterone is produced by the interstitial cells of the testis.

Female fish have paired ovaries in the caudal abdomen, which, like testes, also vary markedly in size (up to 70% body weight) depending on the season. The ovary is a sac into which developing ova mature along fine lamellae. The central aspect of the ovary is a cavity, into which the ova are carried to the oviduct and then to the genital pore. Fish lack a uterus and vagina; the ovary supplements the function of both organs and, in addition, can store spermatozoa. In some species, ova are secreted into the abdomen, with eventual exit via the genital pore. Degenerate/unexpelled ova are a frequent occurrence; they are digested by macrophages and, in time, inflammation can lead to fibrosis.

Nervous System and Special Senses The central nervous system of fish is composed of a brain and spinal cord, which are comparable to those seen in mammals. The telencephalon is much smaller, however, and the mesencephalon (*optic tectum*) larger (Figure 2.8). Fish have 10 cranial nerves.

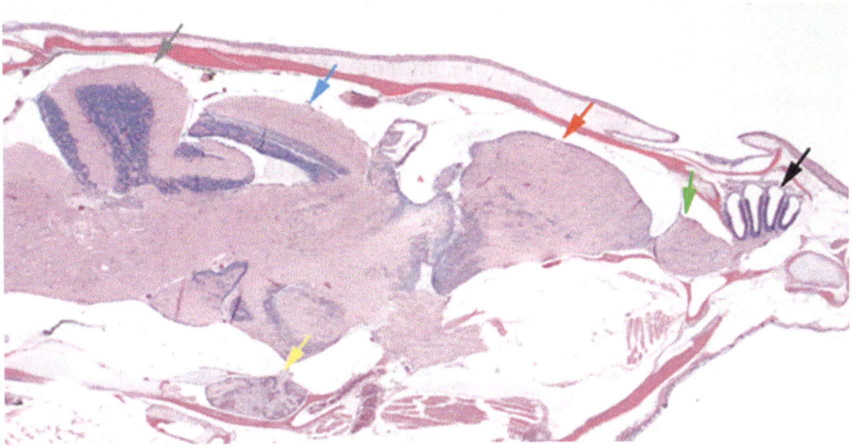

Figure 2.8 Zebrafish sagittal section of the head. Black arrow indicates the nasal pit/lamellar organ, green arrow indicates the olfactory lobe, red arrow the telencephalon, blue arrow mesencephalon (optic tectum), gray arrow the cerebellum, and yellow arrow the pituitary. Wes Baumgartner hematoxylin and eosin stain.

Fish lack eyelids and the sclera is supported by cartilage or mineralized cartilage/bone. Iris movement is minimal and the lens is inelastic; to accommodate this issue, fish have a muscle (*retractor lentis*) that moves the lens (Roberts and Ellis, 2012).

Fish have nasal pits with lamellar organs that function in olfaction as well as immune surveillance. Fish have inner ears, complete with otoliths and semicircular canals; they are embedded in the skull in association with the vertebrae. In addition to the auditory and vestibular systems that are present in mammals, fish also have mechanosensory and electrosensory systems in the skin. Many free neuromasts are scattered throughout the skin, following species-specific patterns. Neuromasts are similar to those seen in the inner ear of mammals, and also occur within canals just beneath the skin (the lateral line system).

The lateral line system is a series of fine canals in the skin, with periodically occurring neuromasts and surface openings. It is mechanosensory and the canal patterns are quite elaborate; they predominate in the head and cranial trunk.

Electrogenesis and electrical reception elements are less common, but are seen in eels, catfish, and knifefish.

2.3.2 Amphibians

2.3.2.1 Classification of Amphibians

The term amphibian is derived from the Greek word *amphibios*, meaning "double life", referring to the generalized life traits of aquatic larvae metamorphosing into terrestrial adults. Some species of amphibians are permanent land dwellers, others are 100% aquatic, while some species use both terrestrial and aquatic habitats. There are species of amphibians which remain entirely arboreal or even fossorial. These amphibians, however, still require high humidity levels and/or water for reproduction – even if it is water retained in a bromeliad leaf reservoir. All amphibians are ectothermic, carnivorous vertebrates with soft, scaleless, permeable skin covered with a protective mucus.

The class Amphibia contains three orders: Anura (frogs and toads), Caudata (salamanders and newts), and Gymnophiona (caecilians). The order Anura contains 54 families, which may be arboreal, fossorial, terrestrial, semi-aquatic, or aquatic by nature. There are only five anuran families containing species that are 100% aquatic. The order Caudata contains ten families, of which nine contain aquatic species. Caudata larva are completely aquatic and possess external gills that are lost as they metamorphose into adults. Some species of caudates are neotenic and do not lose their external gills as adults. The order Gymnophiona contains 10 extant families, most of which are fossorial. Only one family, *Typhlonectidae*, contains aquatic and semiaquatic species and are found in the tropical and temperate forests of northern South America, have tracheal lungs, and are viviparous.

A taxonomy chart is available in the website materials accompanying this text.

2.3.3 Reptiles

2.3.3.1 Classification of Reptiles

Reptiles are heterothermic vertebrates which have keratinized scales and skin. During the Mesozoic era, reptiles dominated the world where the giant dinosaurs prevailed. Most reptiles became extinct in the late Cretaceous period, leaving only four orders of modern reptiles: Chelonia, Squamata, Rhynchocephalia, and Crocodilia. Aquatic reptilian species are not found within the order Rhynchocephalia.

2.3.3.1.1 Chelonia

Order Chelonia (testudines) includes turtles, tortoises, and terrapins, with 10 families of aquatic species. In general, turtles and tortoises are the most commonly referred subdivisions, so it is important to know that (in American vernacular) tortoises are all exclusively land-dwelling while turtles all have some degree of aquatic lifestyle. Phylogenetically, the testudines are the second oldest group of reptiles (only surpassed by the Rhynchocephalia) and is divided into two suborders: Pleurodira and Cryptodira. These divisions are primarily based on the structure of their neck vertebrae. Whereas all extant species of testudines have eight cervical vertebrae, Cryptodira have wide and flat cervical vertebrae and double articulations on cervical vertebrae 6/7 and 7/8, allowing for ginglymoidy, the ability to fold their head and neck in a dorsoventrally aligned sigmoid shape in front of their body. Pleurodira, in contrast, have long and narrow cervical vertebrae and withdraw their head and neck laterally within the margin of the shell. An additional major difference between these suborders is that all Pleurodira species have 13 plastronal scutes, while all Cryptodira only have 12.

There are 14 families in the order Chelonia, with 10 aquatic Cryptodira families: *Chelydridae* (snapping turtles), *Dermatemydidae* (river turtles), *Kinosternidae* (mud turtles), *Cheloniidae* (sea turtles), *Dermochelyidae* (leatherback turtles), *Platysternidae* (big-headed turtles), *Emydidae* (pond turtles), *Geoemydidae* (Asian river turtles), *Carettochelydidae* (pignose turtles), and *Trionychidae* (softshell turtles). All three families of Pleurodira have aquatic components: *Chelidae* (Austro-American sideneck turtles), *Pelomedusidae* (African sideneck turtles), and *Podocnemididae* (Madagascan and South American sideneck turtles). All families except *Testudinidae* have partially or completely aquatic lifestyles.

2.3.3.1.2 Squamata

Order Squamata is the largest and most diverse reptilian group and includes three suborders: Amphisbaenia (worm lizards), Sauria (lizards), and Ophidia (snakes). Most Squamate families contain aquatic species. The saurian family, *Iguanidae*, contains marine iguanas. The ophidian families *Elapidae*, contains sea snakes, *Homalopsidae*, the tentacled snake, *Boidae*, contains anacondas, and *Acrochordidae*, includes the elephant trunk snake. Many other families of squamates include genera that are at least partially aquatic, such as amphisbaenids, lizards, and snakes.

2.3.3.1.3 Crocodilia

Order Crocodilia includes three families: *Alligatoridae* (alligators and caimans), *Crocodylidae* (crocodiles), and *Gavialidae* (gharials). All Crocodilia are aquatic species.

A taxonomy chart is available in the website materials accompanying this text.

2.3.4 Aquatic Avian Species (Class Aves)

A taxonomy chart is available in the website materials accompanying this text.

2.3.5 Aquatic Mammals (Class Mammalia)

Aquatic mammal species do not belong to a single taxonomic unit. The group generally covers the mammal species which spend most or all of their life time in marine or freshwater habitats. This group comprises four orders: Cetacea, Sirenia, Pinnipedia, and Carnivora.

A taxonomy chart is available in the website materials accompanying this text.

Species identification is important for research, protection and conservation purposes. After identification of the species, check the conservation status from the International Union for Conservation of Nature website and, if necessary, give information to local authorities.

For the purposes of this text, the focus is on those aquatic mammals which physiologically must spend the majority of their time in the water. Descriptions found below point out some of the differences between these species and the typical terrestrial forms.

2.3.5.1 Cetacea

Order Cetacea (whales, dolphins, and porpoises): cetaceans are found in coastal and offshore waters. They are fully adapted to the aquatic environment and have developed a fusiform body shape (Kinze *et al.*, 2001). They have a streamlined spindle-shaped torso, flattened paddle-like fore flippers, a telescoped skull, a nasal opening on top of the head, a well-developed blubber layer under the skin, and reproductive organs inside the body (Jefferson *et al.*, 1993). There are no external ears and fur (except in some species, during early development stages), hind limbs are vestigial and only found in the body or lacking completely. The front limbs developed into flippers and most of them have a dorsal fin (Kinze *et al.*, 2001). The dorsal fin and tail flukes lack bones (Jefferson *et al.*, 1993).

Depending on the species, the adult size varies between 1.5–33 meters. (Kinze *et al.*, 2001). Those with a body length over 10 meters are classed as large, - 4–10 meters are classed as medium, less than 4 meters are small cetaceans (Kinze *et al.*, 2001). Cetaceans can be further subdivided into two groups: the toothed whales (suborder Odontoceti), with teeth and a single blowhole, and the baleen whales (suborder Mysticeti), with baleen plates in the mouth and a double blowhole. Mysticetes are large whales, with an asymmetrical skull and a sternum consisting of a single bone. All small-sized species, some of the medium and a few large-sized species are found under Odontoceti (Kinze *et al.*, 2001). Colorations and patterns, tail fluke markings, as well as wound scars are useful for identification purposes.

2.3.5.2 Order Sirenia

Sirenians are herbivorous marine mammals Sirenians have a robust body, thickened skin, short hair, two nostrils on top or at the front of a thick muzzle, no ear pinnae, no hind limbs, mammary nipples located near the axillae, forelimbs modified into flippers, horizontally flattened tail and dense bones (Jefferson *et al.*, 1993).

2.3.5.3 Order Carnivora – Pinnipedia Group

The group Pinnipedia includes the families *Otariidae*, *Phocidae*, and *Odobenidae*. The *Otariidae* family comprises 14 species of sea lions and fur seals, called “eared” or “walking seals”. The *Phocidae* family comprises 19 species of true seals, sometimes called “earless”, “true”, or “crawling seals”. The walrus is the only existing member of the *Odobenidae* family (Jefferson *et al.*, 1993). All have fur and also use blubber for thermoregulation, have fore and hind flippers, long whiskers, nasal openings at the tip of the snout, and reduced or lost ear flaps (Jefferson *et al.*, 1993). The color of the fur is important because it is used for identification of individuals and age stage evaluation.

A general consideration on the digestive system in aquatic animals is available in the website materials accompanying this text.

References

Caceci, T., Neck, K.F., Lewis, D. H. and Sis, R.F. (1988). Ultrastructure of the hepatopancreas of the Pacific white shrimp. *J. Marine Biology* 68: 323–337.

De Gryse, G.M.A., Thuong, V.K., Descamps, B. *et al.* (2020). The shrimp nephrocomplex serves as a major portal of pathogen entry and is involved in the molting process. *PNAS* 117: 28374–28383.

Demski, L.S., Gerald, J.W. and Popper, A.N. (1973). Central and peripheral mechanisms of teleost sound production. *American Zoologist* 13: 1141–1167.

Fricke, R., Eschmeyer, W., and van der Laan, R. (2021). *Eschmeyer's Catalog of Fishes: Genera, Species, References.* http://researcharchive.calacademy.org/research/ichthyology/catalog/fishcatmain.asp (accessed 14 September 2021).

Holthius, L.B. (1980). Shrimps and Prawns of the World: An annotated catalogue of species of interest to fisheries. FAO Fisheries Synopsis No. 125, Volume 1. FAO Species Catalogue. Rome: Food and Agriculture Organization of the United Nations.

Jefferson, T.A., Leatherwood, S. and Webber, M.A. (1993). *Marine Mammals of the World.* FAO Species Identification Guide. Rome: Food and Agriculture Organization of the United Nations.

Kinze, C.C., Carpenter, K.E. and Niem, V.H. (eds). (2001). *FAO Species Identification Guide for Fishery Purposes. The Living Marine Resources of the Western Central Pacific. Volume 6. Bony Fishes Part 4 (Labridae To Latimeriidae), Estuarine Crocodiles, Sea Turtles, Sea Snakes and Marine Mammals.* Rome: Food and Agriculture Organization of the United Nations.

Le, H.T.M.D., Shao, X., Krogdahl, A. *et al.* (2019). Intestinal function of the stomachless fish, ballan wrasse (Labrus bergylta). *Front Marine Sci* 6: 140.

Myers, P. (2001). Crustacea. *Animal Diversity Web.* University of Michigan, Museum of Zoology. https://animaldiversity.org/accounts/Crustacea (accessed 20 April 2021).

National Center for Biotechnology Information. (2020). NCBI Taxonomy Browser. Crassostrea gigas. https://www.ncbi.nlm.nih.gov/Taxonomy/Browser/wwwtax.cgi (accessed 20 April 2021).

Roberts, R.J. and Ellis, A.E. (2012). The Anatomy and Physiology of Teleosts. In: *Fish Pathology*, 4e (ed. R.J. Ellis), 17–61. Oxford: Blackwell Publishing.

Rojo-Arreola, L., García-Carreño, F., Romero, R. and Díaz Dominguez, L. (2020). Proteolytic profile of larval developmental stages of *Penaeus vannamei*: an activity and mRNA expression approach. *PLoS One* 2020;15(9): e0239413.

Shimada, A., Kawanishi, T., Kaneko, T. *et al.* (2013). Trunk exoskeleton in teleosts is mesodermal in origin. *Nature Communications* 4: 1639.

Sis, R.F., Lewis, D.H. and Means, J.E. (1992). Shrimp: an anatomical study. IAAAM 1992: Proceedings of the International Association for Aquatic Animal Medicine. https://www.vin.com/apputil/content/defaultadv1.aspx?id=3981482&pid=11110& (accessed 20 April 2021).

Tacon, A.G.J. (1987). Nutrient sources – composition of feedstuffs and fertilizers. In: *The Nutrition and Feeding of Farmed Fish and Shrimp: A training manual. 2: Nutrient Sources and Composition*, ch. 3. Rome: Food and Agriculture Organization.

Tsing, A., Arcier, J-M. and Brehelin, M. (1989). Hemocytes of Penaeid and Palaemonid shrimp: morphology, cytochemistry, and hemogram. *Journal of Invertebrate Patholog.* 53: 64–67.

Ulloa, E.P., Peña, A.A., Lizama, C.D. *et al.* (2013). Growth response and expression of muscle growth-related candidate genes in adult zebrafish fed plant and fishmeal protein-based diets. *Zebrafish* 10: 99–109.

WoRMS. 2020. The World Register of Marine Species (WoRMS). www.marinespecies.org, (accessed 30 December 2020).

3

Husbandry and Industries

Trista Becker, Olanike K. Adeyemo, Erdem Danyer, and Nicholas Saint-Erne

Learning Objectives
To better understand health issues that may arise from husbandry and nutrition, the student should become familiar with the standard of care in large and small scale production systems.

3.1 Introduction to chapter

Large-scale production systems to rear fish have been around for over a century. Theories behind each system have changed over the years, but in general there is a global increase in production of fish for both the pet trade and food industry. As systems become more complex, there can be an increase in husbandry-related disease problems. Understanding these systems is important to identify monitoring checkpoints for early detection of health issues that can impact the wellbeing of aquatic organisms and also lead to large economic losses for a producer. Husbandry and nutrition are very important components of preventive medicine. Breeding performance can increase with better management of husbandry and nutrition topics.

3.2 Husbandry and Industry

3.2.1 Culture Environment

Managed ecosystems form the basis for aquaculture production, which has been widely offered as a means to compensate and ultimately supplement traditional fisheries. Unlike fisheries, inputs, production processes and quality of output of managed ecosystems can be at least partially controlled, and ownership, care and environmental responsibility might be more easily established. By removing natural constraints to survival and productivity, and improving husbandry and management, production need to be limited only by availability of simple inputs such as land, water, fish, brood stock quality, food source, and appropriate climate for species.

Aquatic animal husbandry needs will vary with the industry and its goals. The private home aquarium with few fish will be managed much differently than a 20-acre catfish pond. Regardless

Fundamentals of Aquatic Veterinary Medicine, First Edition. Edited by Laura Urdes, Chris Walster, and Julius Tepper.

Companion website: www.wiley.com/go/urdes/aquatic-veterinary-medicine

of whether the client is interested in individual or population health, aquatic animals need adequate food and clean water. Of course, fish and other gill-breathing organisms will need water with adequate oxygen, while aquatic mammals will need a habitat that provides enough clean air for oxygen intake. Obtaining a thorough history that includes effective communication of the clients' goals is important to developing a health management plan that will be effective as well as practical.

3.2.2 Types of Aquaculture Systems

As shown in Chapter 1, aquaculture is the farming of aquatic organisms. Farming also implies individual or corporate ownership of the stock being cultivated. Aquatic ecosystems provide the basis for aquatic production. The worldwide practice of aquaculture runs the gamut from low-technology extensive methods to highly intensive systems.

Fish can be cultured in systems that use water in different ways. Common types are complete flow through, large pond, recirculation and net pen. Each type of system comes with advantages and challenges, making one type more appropriate for certain species of aquatic animals based on their biology.

3.2.2.1 Extensive Culture System

Extensive aquaculture is characterized by low to no inputs (food, fertilizer, etc.) and low stocking densities. Extensive aquaculture is practiced in lakes, reservoirs and lagoons.

3.2.2.1.1 Ponds

A common production system in use are ponds that can be unlined (earthen) or lined with concrete or vinyl. Earthen ponds are extremely popular among fish growers due, in part, to ease of construction, low maintenance, relatively small area requirements and the ability to grow a wide variety of species. Additionally, because earthen ponds mimic nature, they may produce fish of an overall healthier appearance than other techniques. A natural supply of food is often available in earthen ponds, which may lead to better fish health. Pond culture can vary from all life stages naturally occurring in a single pond to elaborate systems with discrete ponds for holding brood stock, spawning, rearing, growing and catch-out or harvest. However, earthen ponds can harbor disease organisms following a viral or bacterial outbreak as they cannot be disinfected. An effective disease management plan can include a fallowing period as part of the pond rotation schedule to allow for desiccation of infectious organisms.

3.2.2.1.2 Tanks

These essentially act as ponds but are generally constructed of concrete or fiberglass. Wood can also be used but must first be treated to prevent rotting. Concrete tanks have the advantage of being less expensive, easily constructed and formed into various shapes. Concrete tanks must be maintained and can breakdown over time with repeated disinfection and pressure washing.

Plastic, fiberglass or glass tanks are ordinary tanks which are either designed and constructed for rearing fish or used for storing water. This is becoming prominent in many countries. They can be moved from one place to another. They can be used outdoors or inside buildings where the environmental conditions are easier to maintain year around and algae growth can be reduced.

Wooden troughs are constructed with planks. They vary in size and depth. After construction, the tank is lined with nylon to prevent leakage. It can be moved from one place to other.

3.2.2.2 Semi-Intensive Culture System

Semi-intensive aquaculture is distinguished by increased stocking rates and the requirement for some level of input, such as food, fertilizer, chemicals, aeration.

3.2.2.2.1 *Cage Culture*

This strategy uses existing water resources (i.e., lakes or ponds) but encloses the fish in a cage or basket, which allows water to pass freely between the fish cage and the pond or lake. One of the main advantages is the ease of harvesting. Food is often obtained from the natural water, but additional feeding is usually necessary because of the density of the fish in the cage.

3.2.2.2.2 *Fish Pens*

Pens are enclosures installed in open waters that are not too deep for raising fish. The fish has access to the water bottom unlike in cages. Pen culture is not common in certain areas (it is uncommon in Nigeria for instance).

3.2.2.2.3 *Rafts, Trays or Long Lines*

These are mostly used for oyster culture. They provide an easily accessible site for oysters or other mollusks to attach to while growing and to feed on the natural organisms in the water.

3.2.2.2.4 *Makeshift Containers*

Some improvised containers such as bathroom tubs, big plastic containers, abandoned plank canoe, earthen pots etc. are used to culture fish where the farmer cannot afford the conventional rearing facilities.

3.2.2.3 Intensive Culture System

With intensive aquaculture, animals are grown in systems such as concrete tanks and raceways, where the support parameters are carefully controlled and dependence on the natural environment is minimal. Such systems require a high degree of management and usually involve substantial investment and operating costs, resulting in high yields per unit area. These systems usually require electricity to operate water pumps and filtration systems, water heaters or chillers, and aeration equipment.

3.2.2.3.1 *Recirculating Systems*

Recirculating systems filter and reuse all or a portion of their water. Although this technique is associated with high start-up and maintenance costs, its use is growing in popularity. It has several advantages in areas where a constant water supply may be questionable or a discharge is not appropriate. Additionally, other advantages of this type of system are the ability to incorporate the growth of a second product through hydroponics (aquaponics) and the use of settled material as fertilizer. As the technology evolves and water withdrawal and discharge requirements become more stringent, this technique is bound to see an increase in use. Biofilters remove dissolved metabolites and convert ammonia, which is lethal to fish, to nitrate. A secondary settling chamber may be employed to remove suspended materials that may pass through the biofilter.

3.2.2.3.2 *Ponds and Tanks*

Round ponds, especially when used in conjunction with a water reuse system that can recirculate water back into the supply, may be more ideal for areas with limited water availability (Figures 3.1–3.3). The benefit of water savings must outweigh the other challenges often faced with the designs such as high maintenance and water quality monitoring requirements. Round ponds with a reuse system are more popular in newer production facilities as water availability declines and waste discharge allowances become increasingly strict.

3.2.2.3.3 *Raceways*

Flow-through raceways (Figure 3.4) used in large-scale production have a simple design that provides good oxygen flow as water comes in one end and leaves the other at roughly the same speed, taking with it some waste products. Fresh water is added continuously, but these types of systems require large volumes of water with high flows. Raceways are a challenge when water supplies are limited.

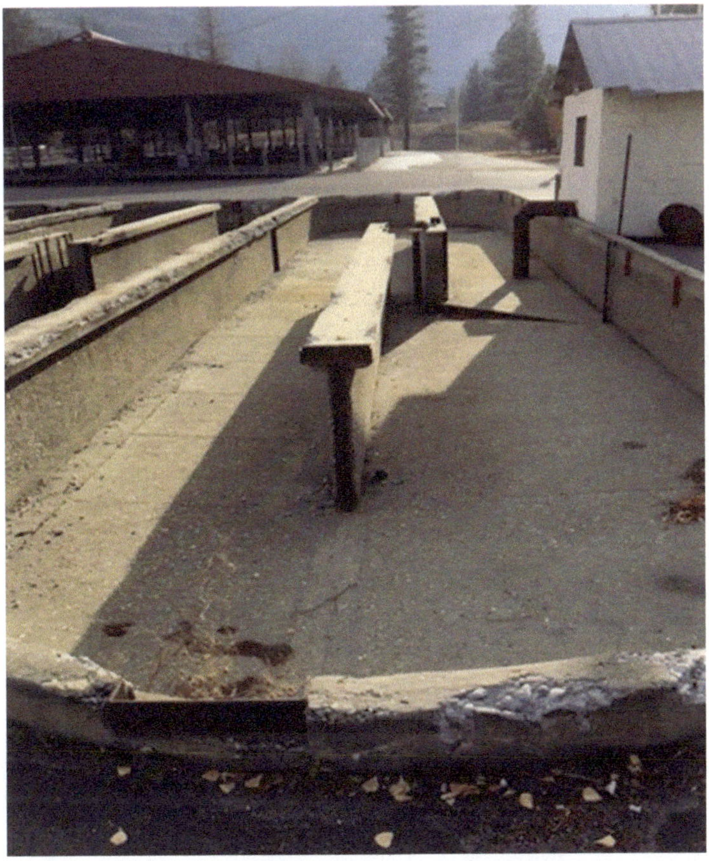

Figure 3.1 Example of a round pond. This is a Foster-Lucas-style round pond, an early style center drain round pond. This was an early prototype to the round ponds in use today. Plumbing for this pond has been removed, but would have consisted of an external pipe entering the top center of the pond and distributing water in opposite directions creating a circular flow. *Source:* photo by T. Becker.

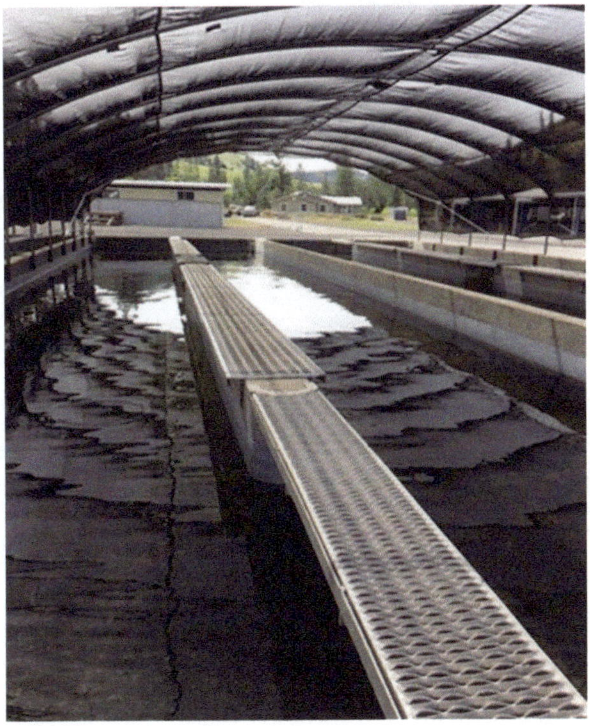

Figure 3.2 Another early style of round pond still in use at some salmonid hatcheries. These Burrows-style ponds have a center drain but the plumbing feeds water in at each end of the pond rather than at the center, creating a circular flow. Note the coverings providing shade to young fish. Source" photo by T. Becker.

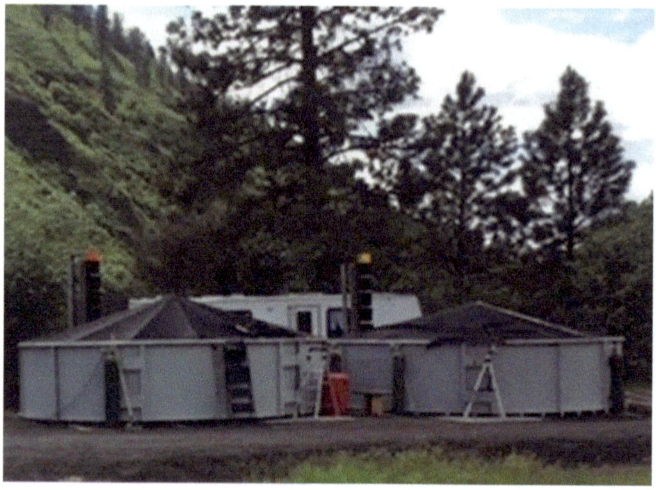

Figure 3.3 Fiberglass round tanks are more popular in new designs and can be partially buried or fully above ground. These tanks usually require protective coverings from predators and inclement weather, and are ideally constructed inside fully enclosed buildings for improved environmental control. *Source:* photo by T. Becker.

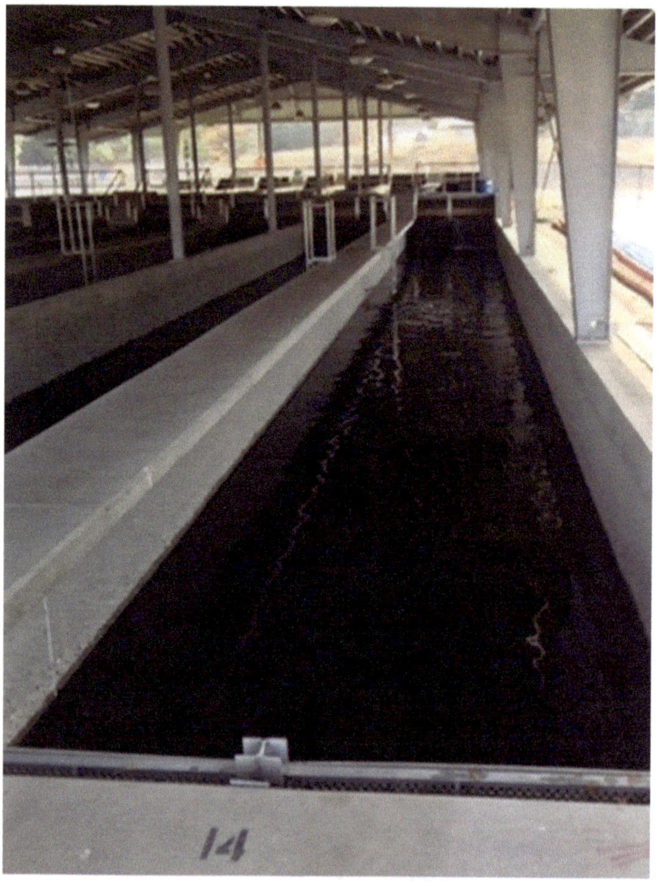

Figure 3.4 Example of a standard flow-through raceway with rectangular shape. This particular bank is designed with the ability for serial reuse of water from a raised bank of raceways above. *Source:* photo by T. Becker.

3.2.3 Management of Culture Environment

Proper management of culture environment offers optimum environmental conditions for the growth and better health of the cultivated fishes. It also strengthens the defense mechanism of the fish body to fight against invading disease producing organisms. Eradication of predatory and competitor fishes, disinfection, selection of quality and healthy seed for stocking, maintaining proper species ratio and stocking density, water quality regulation, proper feeding and proper handling are the various steps of this management measure (see Chapter 1).

3.2.3.1 Selection of Stocking Materials and Population Regulation

It is advisable to stock the pond only with healthy and genetically vigorous fry and fingerlings so that they may have better immunological status, better growth rate and resistance toward some diseases. Before stocking, a representative sample size of the fish should be examined to check their health status. Overcrowding may lead to biological degradation resulting in waste build-up, decreased availability of food and oxygen, deterioration of water quality and so on, and hence it is advisable to stock 5000–6000 fingerlings in each hectare of water spread area. Exact quantity will vary depending on water quality, temperature, food availability, and species of fish.

3.2.3.2 Proper Feeding

Proper management of the natural (undrainable) pond ecosystem ensures sustained production of natural fish food organisms. However, the amount is often not enough to support the high stocking density of fish in complex fish culture and hence an adequate amount of quality feed needs to be supplemented. Supplementary feeding at 2–3% of body weight on a daily basis might be necessary for proper health and faster growth of fish. Any reduction in quantity and the quality deterioration of feed may cause various deficiency and nutritional diseases, at the same time it can increase the susceptibility to infections.

3.2.3.3 Reduction of Handling Stress

The rougher the handling is when netting or otherwise capturing and handling aquatic animals, the greater the stress and risk of disease outbreak. Proper care should be taken not to break the protective mucous coating of the skin. Extreme (high or low) temperature causes additional stress and hence hauling, netting or transporting should be avoided during extreme weather conditions. Other stressors when fish are handled could include biopsy for disease diagnosis, applying medication, and vaccination. Through careful planning, the frequency and length of handling events can be reduced or even avoided altogether.

There are potential environmental problems associated with aquaculture. Most of the fish that are raised are genetically altered or hybridized for quick growth. If they escape into the wild, they compete against and can crowd out smaller or less voracious native fish. In addition, the large amounts of water that are used in aquaculture become laden with fish feces and unconsumed food that, if not removed through treatment or used as agricultural fertilizer, can add injurious amounts of nitrogen and phosphorus to a river or stream when the water is returned to it. Development of improved recirculating tank technologies, however, may lead to a reduction in such pollution threats, as well as allowing the spread of aquaculture to areas where large volumes of water are not available in the environment.

Concerns have been raised about disease transfer from farmed to wild stocks. Fish farm antibiotic and pesticide use has also raised concerns about impacts to natural ecosystems and human health. The risk of human exposure to antimicrobial drug residues in marketed farmed fish appears to be slightly higher than for terrestrial species. The probability of human exposure to tissue residues of antimicrobial drug residues in wild species captured near fish farms is low. Exposure will be largely restricted to areas in close proximity to farms and within narrow time frames. However, drugs used by aquaculture operations could move beyond the immediate vicinity of treated farms if fish escape before the drug withdrawal period expires or if mobile species such as wild fish or crustaceans ingest sufficient drug to develop harmful tissue residues.

3.2.4 Natural History and Aquaculture

Attributes of a species that can impact the type of husbandry system are feeding behavior, intra- and interspecific competition, life-history traits at different life stages (such as reproduction/breeding and early development), physiological demands of the temperature range, oxygen consumption and waste excretion, and region specific disease risks. Some species may be housed together, for example, herbivores that use different food sources, while others, such as predatory species, may need to be housed separately or only with like species.

Knowledge about the life history of a species is important to understand the requirements of feeding and nutrition at different life stages to assure energy needs are met for maintenance and growth. Feeding strategies and other aspects of husbandry that maintain water quality (e.g. cleaning and pathogen removal) are limited by the type of culture system. Brooming or vacuuming of raceways in a flow-through system must be done frequently for removal of feces. Monitoring feed consumption is important during feeding and prior to waste removal. Excess feed left after feeding can be due to poor palatability, inadequate feed distribution, or alternatively an early sign of disease. Feed consumption will often decline in animals experiencing illness. Also, excess feed in a pond/raceway will cause poor water quality, which will lead to poor gill health, and can eventually lead to disease outbreaks.

3.2.5 Environmental and Social Acclimation

Water temperature changes should occur slowly to allow animals time to acclimate with the least amount of stress as possible and should not be allowed to exceed the range of tolerance for that species. A good rule of thumb for salmonids is no more than 2.5 degrees C temperature change per hour, which may fluctuate for some species at the extreme ends of tolerance. Salmonids can generally better handle a change to cooler water than from cold to warmer. Sudden, large changes in dissolved oxygen, salinity, pH, alkalinity and hardness should also be avoided.

For anadromous species, such as chinook salmon and steelhead trout, fish must "imprint" to a water body in order to return from the ocean for spawning at maturity. One common approach with state and federal hatcheries is to utilize groundwater, or "pathogen free" water, for the early rearing stages (egg, fry, parr) to avoid diseases at the young immune susceptible stages. To allow for imprinting to the stream of origin for a particular stock, these fish will be moved to a site for rearing and "acclimation" on surface water when they are older and the environmental conditions at the site are more favorable (often in the fall and winter). Depending on the geographic location, many other factors may need to be considered and a thorough discussion with the program managers is always recommended to determine potential health impacts of these movements.

3.2.6 Animal Transport

Groups of fish can be transported in various types of containers, from a small plastic bag to a large tank or even a tanker truck. Ornamental fish are often shipped long distances overseas in small plastic bags with added oxygen. The size of the fish and the transport time will determine the size of the container and the amount of water needed, with care taken to allow enough space for additional oxygen. For large tanks, ideally monitoring equipment should be installed that is easily viewed inside the vehicle and include at a minimum water temperature and dissolved oxygen measurements (and possibly pH). Long road trips may require water exchanges, ice, or refrigeration to prevent temperature elevation or oxygen depletion if supplemental oxygen is not available. Ideally, supplemental oxygenation of the water or container should be considered standard. Generally, fish will be calmer in the dark so tanks and transport containers are usually designed to keep out sunlight. As oxygen depletes in the tank or container over time without water exchanges, and the length of time in a confined space may lead to increased stress, the route of travel should be planned to reduce the transit time as much as possible. Extreme weather conditions may interfere with safe transport and should be avoided. If a large truck is to be used, a commercial drivers' license may be required and the amount of time the driver can spend behind the wheel may need to be factored into the trip, especially in the event of large moves with multiple trips. As transport is most often highly stressful for both the animal and the handlers, ideally it should be planned to minimize the time and number of handling events/moves as much as possible. Sedatives and other water conditioners are commercially available and may be added to reduce the stress of handling and transport, but fish should be regularly monitored in such cases.

If animals to be moved are highly active and the risk of injury is high during transport (especially for larger animals), then sedation may be a good option. Very few options are available for food fish species, as the withdrawal time required preempts the use for euthanasia in animals to be consumed. Contact your national drug approval organization or a local aquatic chemical supplier to find out what options may be available in your country. National veterinary medical associations may have lists of mechanical methods considered humane in food animals.

Transport of marine mammals has been made for a variety of reasons: mercantile purposes between aquariums, moving of the pool, or transporting stranded animals from the shore to rehabilitation centers (Antrim and McBain, 2001). Overland transport of species like pinnipeds and otariids can be relatively easy as these species are more adapted to land compared with cetaceans. However, overland transport is a significant stress factor in cetaceans because they rely on the support of the natural buoyancy gained in their aquatic habitat (Suzuki *et al.*, 2008). Internal organs, especially lungs and muscles of cetaceans can be compressed and damaged by pressure while out of the water. It also becomes difficult for cetaceans to regulate body temperature out of the aquatic environment where some complications such as dehydration, hyperthermia, dryness of skin, trauma, myopathy, myoglobinuria, and stress can be observed (Noda *et al.*, 2007; Herráez *et al.*, 2007, 2012; Suzuki *et al.*, 2008).

The two main methods for the transportation of marine mammals are dry or wet. In the wet method, the cetacean is placed in a water-filled tank on a stretcher and secured with appropriate holes for fins. This requires stretchers made from a material (strong enough and non-abrasive) that permits the animal to be constantly kept comfortable and wet within water tanks designed according to animal's length and height (Figure 3.5).

By using the wet method, the risk of complications like hyperthermia, the difficulty of breathing and crushing the internal organs is minimized by the help of the buoyancy. Constantly keeping the animal in water prevents skin drying. The animal is kept wet and pectoral fins are kept in natural position; therefore, the animal is more comfortable during transport, (Geraci and Lounsbury, 2005). The wet method is expensive, requires special equipment, and is not suitable for emergency operations. The dry method of transportation is most often used for emergency rescue operations with relatively short distances. Individuals are laid on a wet towel or inflatable mattress. Cold water is sprayed on cetacean species, but it is not obligatory for pinniped and otariid species.

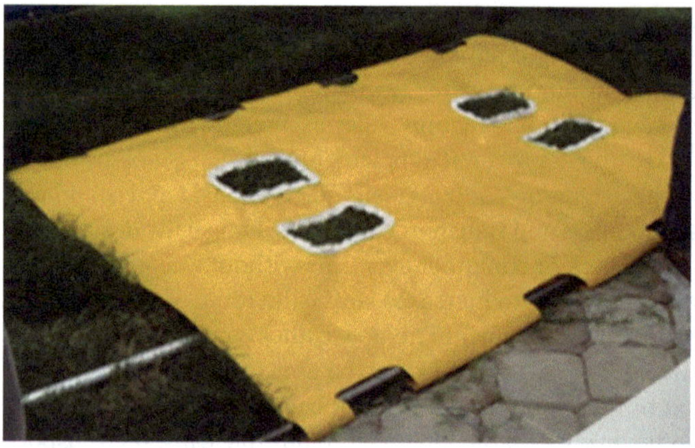

Figure 3.5 Canvas stretcher used in the transportation of cetaceans. *Source:* photo by E. Danyer.

3.2.7 Ornamental Fish Culture

Import data (2018) show the European Union as the largest importer at US$84.2m (UK, Germany, Netherlands, France and Italy comprise 85% of the market), followed by the United States US$65.3m, China US$29.1m, Japan US$15.6m and Singapore US$12.9m. Markets in India and the middle East are growing. Asia continues to remain the major supplier for fish. Note that the values quoted also include trade in zebrafish and public aquaria specimens.

Freshwater species constitute 80% of the ornamental trade and marines constitute 20%. Trending are smaller aquaria and nanotanks, with plants and aquascaping, housing small species including freshwater shrimp. Marines are growing as there has been technological advances in equipment and lighting to allow for these more sensitive species to be kept.

Most freshwater tropical fish sold in the United States are produced by aquaculture on fish farms. About 40% of those are from US fish farms, primarily in Florida, and about 60% are imported, mostly from Asian countries such as Singapore, Thailand, Sri Lanka, Taiwan, China (including Hong Kong) and Japan. A small percentage of freshwater aquarium fish (5–10%) are still collected from the wild in South America, Africa, and Southeast Asia.

Marine aquarium fish are still mostly collected from coral reefs; however, over 233 species have been captive bred. Over 100 species of marine fish are commercially available for sale as captive-bred specimens. The most abundant species are in the families angelfish, blennies, damselfish, cardinalfish, clownfish, dottybacks, gobies, and seahorses. To sustain marine aquarium fish keeping economically and environmentally, it is important that more species of fish and invertebrates are produced by aquaculture, as they are in the freshwater fish industry.

Freshwater tropical fish traditionally have been bred with extensive culture systems in open ponds outdoors (Figure 3.6). This production method is cost effective if it is used in areas with warm weather, inexpensive land, abundant water, and low-cost labor. Florida has been the primary site in the United States for tropical aquarium fish aquaculture and Arkansas for goldfish culture. Ponds dug in the sandy soil in Florida naturally fill with water; however, increased cost of land and lowered underground water tables have caused some small ornamental fish farms to sell out to commercial developers. The larger farms have efficiently increased capacity to make up for the growing demand and fewer suppliers. Modern techniques, such as indoor intensive culturing and covered lined ponds have increased the production of fish in less space (Figure 3.7). This efficiency comes with an increased cost in materials, though it is ultimately offset by greater production capacity. Large amounts of capital are needed for this endeavor, making it practical for only farms with high production (Saint-Erne, 2013).

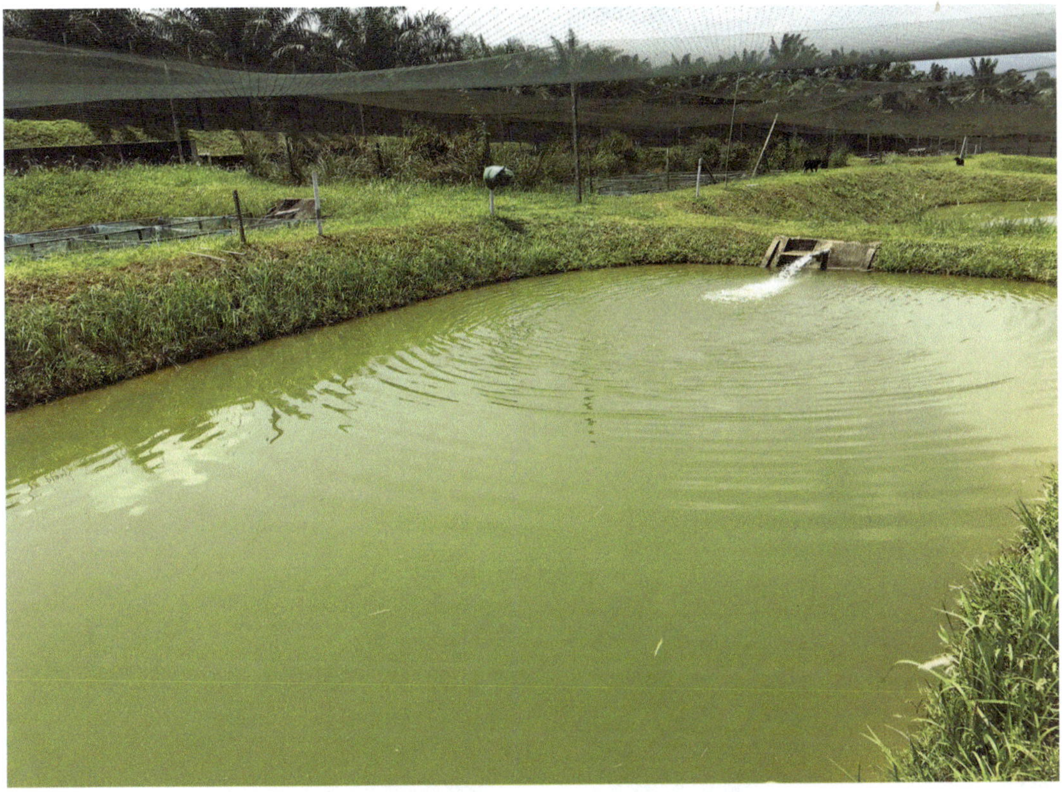

Figure 3.6 Traditional dirt-bottomed fishpond in Malaysia. *Source:* photo by N. Saint-Erne.

Traditional extensive culture system ponds have no filtration, but often use aerators to keep the water oxygenated. Some fresh water is added each day and the excess water overflows into the standpipe. This method has allowed for fish production with limited investment where land and water are available and labor costs are low.

Indoor aquaculture involves considerable expense in building costs, vats or containers for fish production, and filtration systems for water quality control (Figure 3.8). Most of these systems use recirculating water rather than flow-through water. This allows for the maintenance of proper water quality by mechanical and biological filtration. The number of fish produced in an indoor tank with water filtration and recirculation can compare to the production from a large outdoor pond (Figure 3.9).

After the fish are produced at the tropical fish farm, they are shipped in plastic bags or boxes to an export center where they are checked for health, given a water change, and then repacked in plastic bags with one-third water and two-thirds oxygen added (Figure 3.10). The bags are packed in insulated boxes and shipped to a distributor, often in a different part of the world (Figure 3.11). At the distributer, the fish are unpacked into aquariums, again checked for health, treated with medications as necessary, and fed if not going to be shipped again right away (Figure 3.12). They may stay in that location for as little as a day, or for many weeks. When a retail pet store orders the fish, they are again packed and then shipped to the store for display in the retail aquarium (Figure 3.13). Customers finally select fish form the retail store to take home to their aquarium – sometimes many months after the fish were first sent out from the farm (Figure 3.14).

The typical journey for aquarium fish from producer to customer can pass through as few as three steps (producer – retailer – customer) or as many as seven steps for the fish:

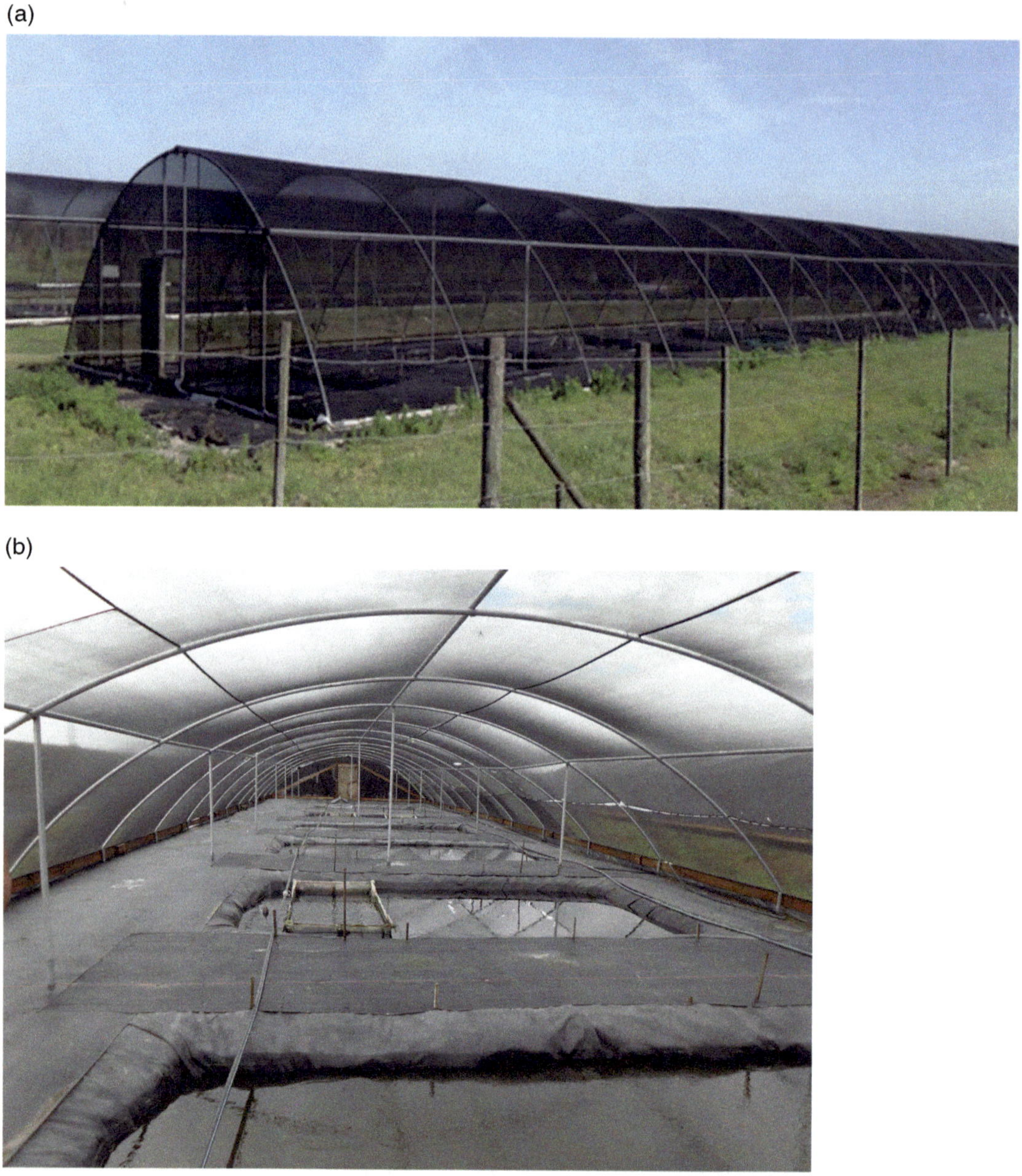

Figure 3.7 (a,b) Covered pond in Florida completely lined to eliminate weeds, water loss, and to reduce predation. *Source:* photo by N. Saint-Erne.

1) Fish producer or collector
2) 95% are from fish farms: 60% farmed in Asia; 35% the United States
3) 5% wild collected, mostly in South America, Africa and Asia
4) Exporter – importer – wholesaler
5) Distribution center
6) Pet store
7) Customer's aquarium

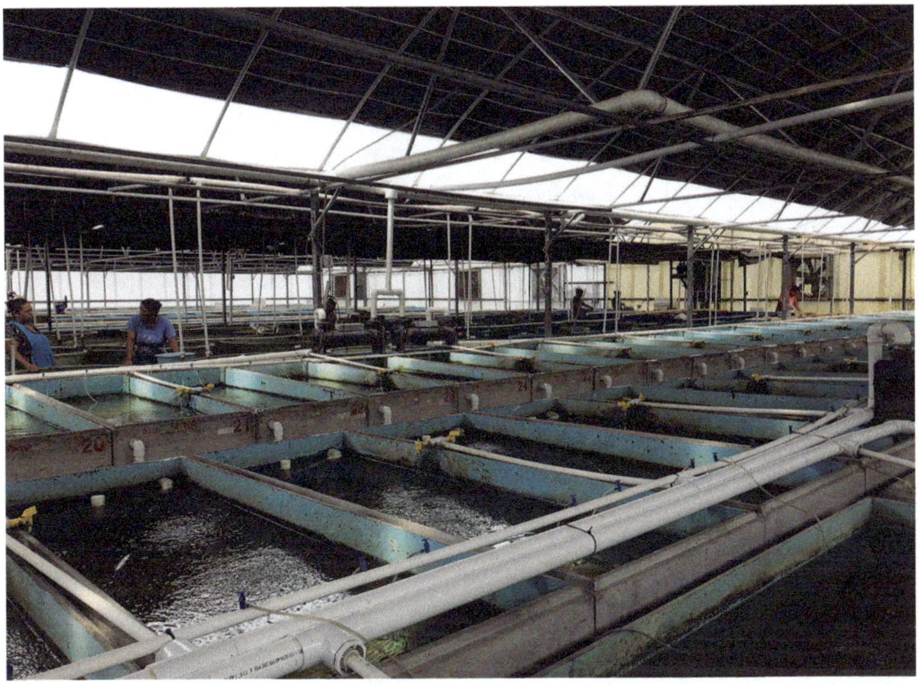

Figure 3.8 Indoor production facility for tropical fish in Florida. *Source:* photo by N. Saint-Erne.

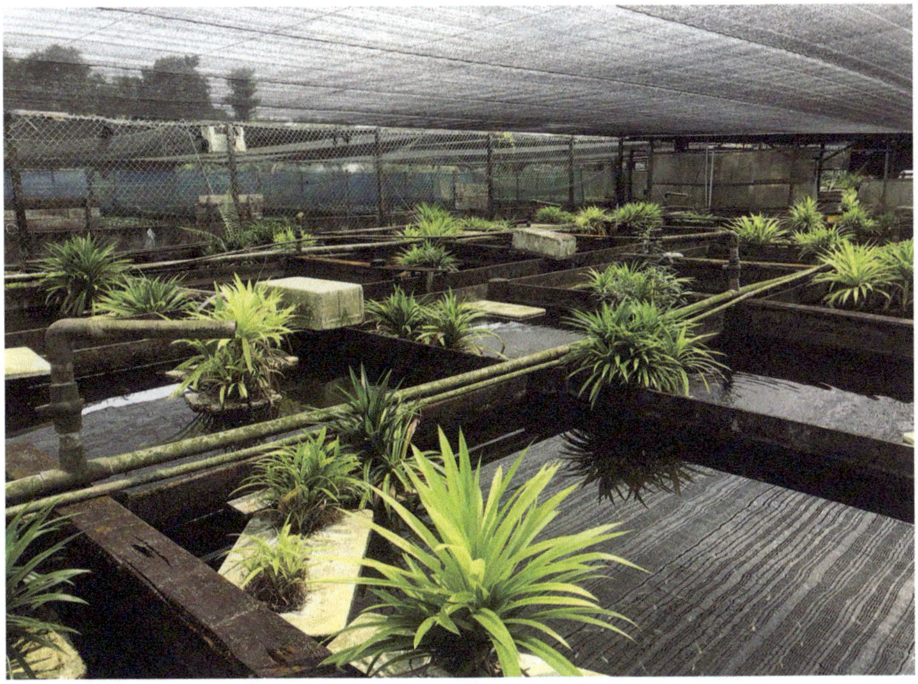

Figure 3.9 Angelfish farm in Singapore. *Source:* photo by N. Saint-Erne.

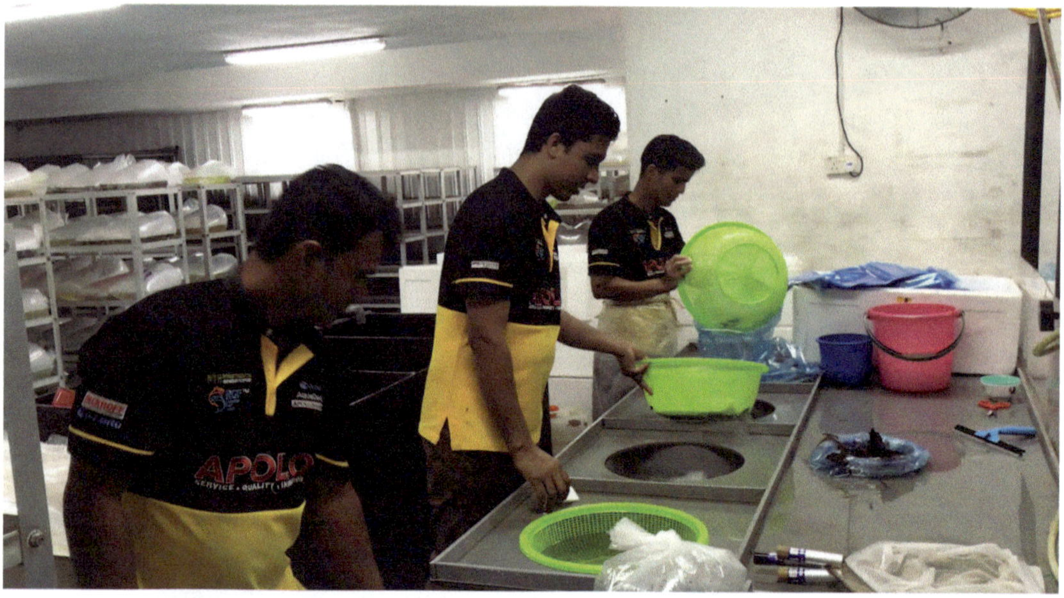

Figure 3.10 Export facility personnel inspecting fish coming in from farm ponds in Singapore. *Source:* photo by N. Saint-Erne.

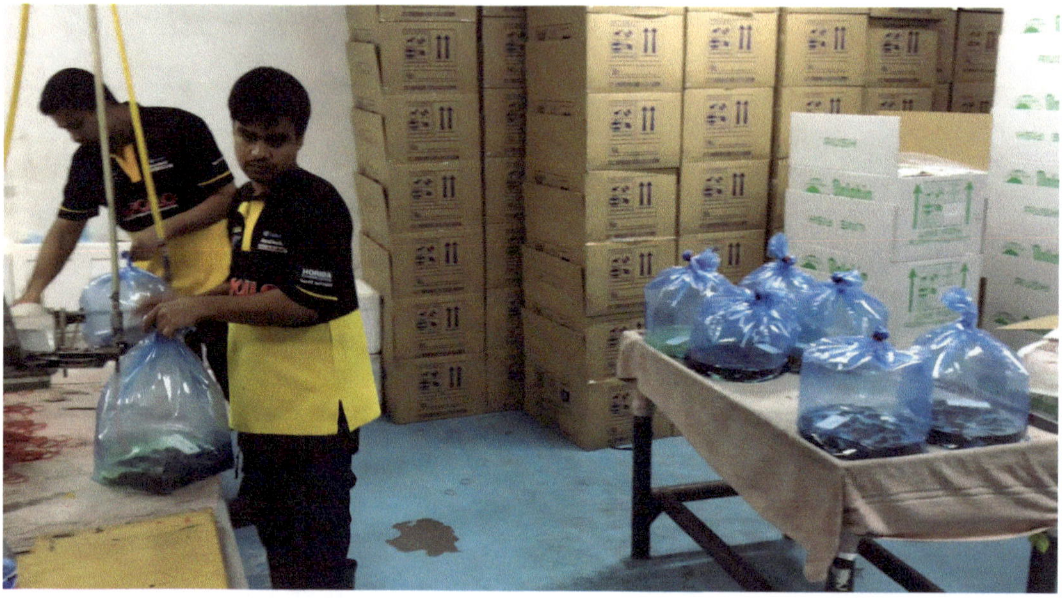

Figure 3.11 Exporter repacking fish in Singapore to air ship to the United States. *Source:* photo by N. Saint-Erne.

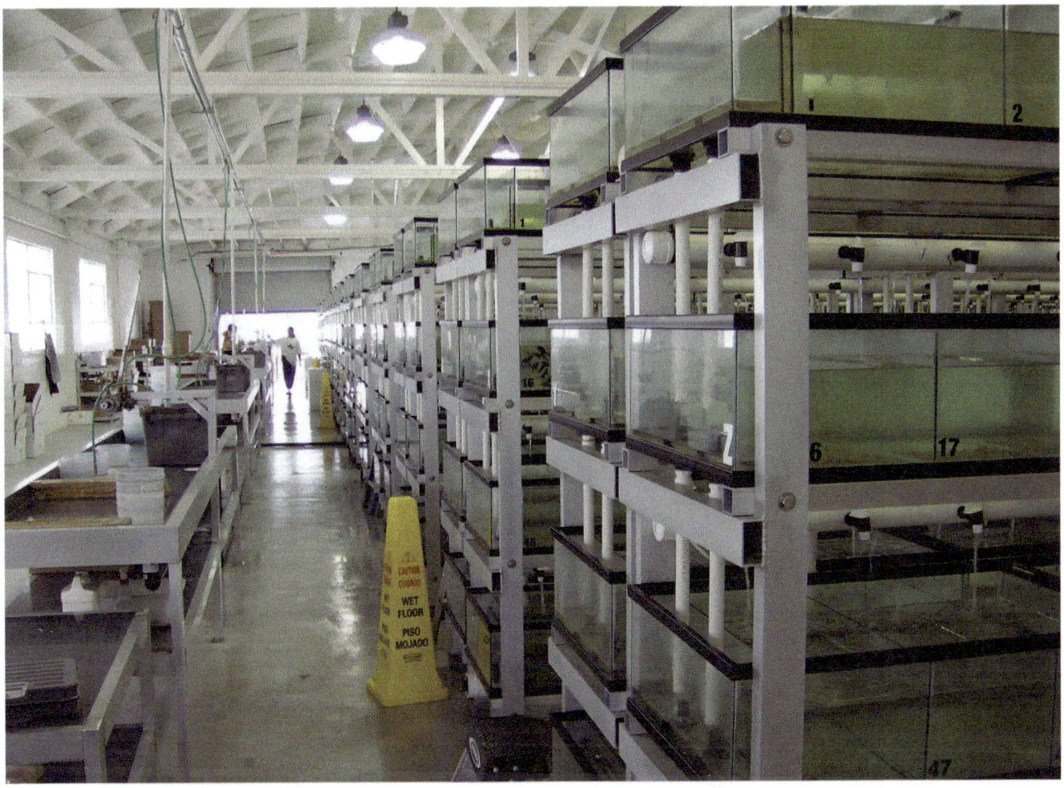

Figure 3.12 Wholesale facility in California. *Source:* photo by N. Saint-Erne.

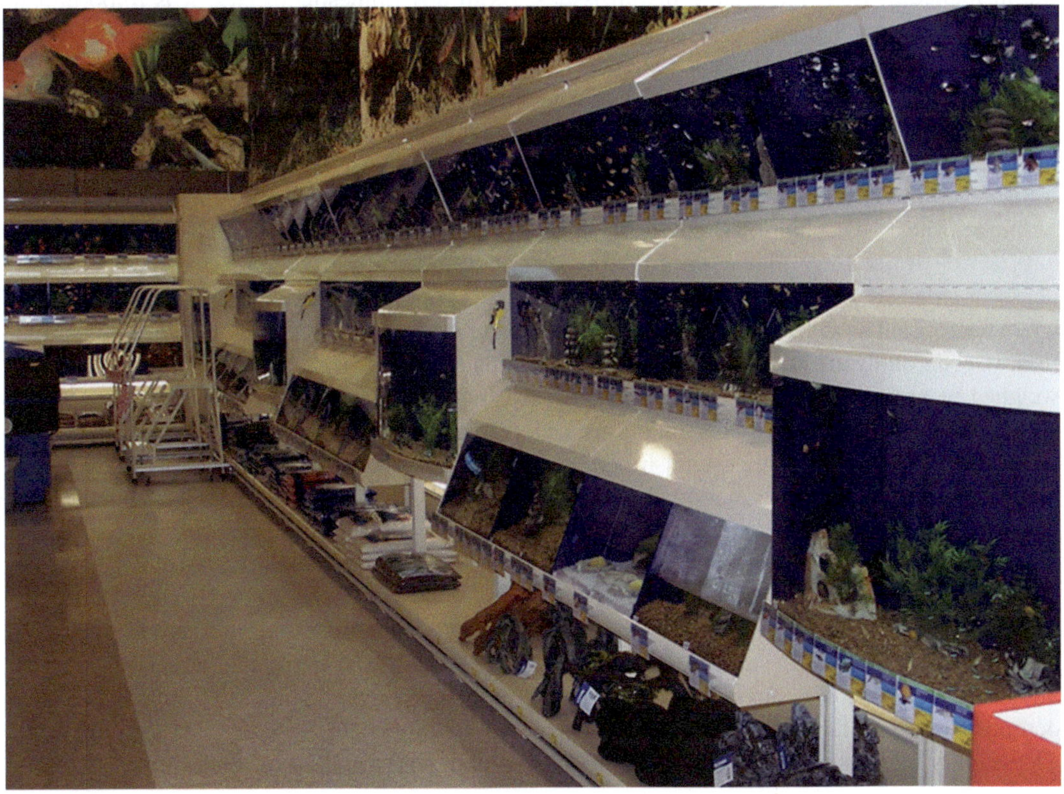

Figure 3.13 Retail pet store display. *Source:* photo by N. Saint-Erne.

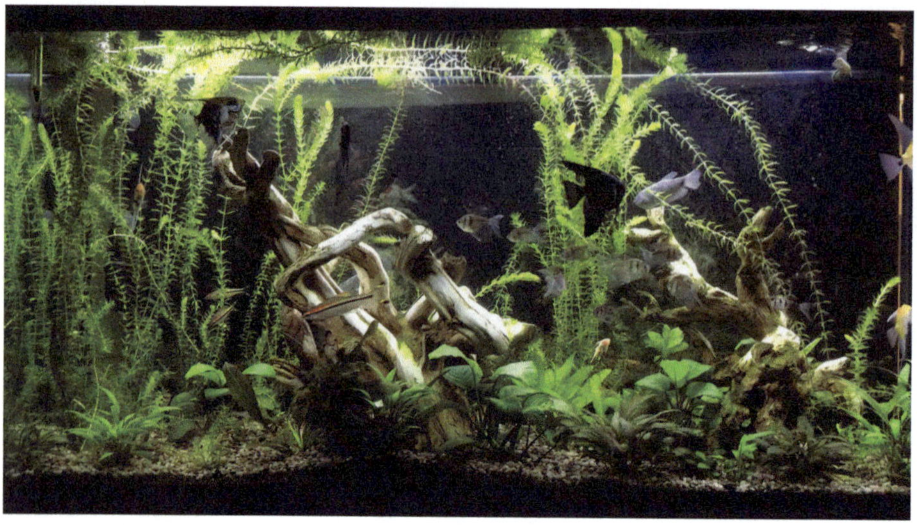

Figure 3.14 Fishes' final home: customer's aquarium. *Source:* photo by N. Saint-Erne.

3.3 Nutrition

3.3.1 Feeds and Feeding

The development of complete pelleted feeds for common captive fish species has greatly reduced the incidence of nutrition-related health issues. As in any domestic species, it is important to assure that nutrients are being provided in the correct proportion for those specific taxa and life stage. Young growing salmonids, for example, have higher protein requirements at the first-fed fry stage. Also not to be overlooked are mechanical restrictions such as mouth size and feeding behaviors. A diet with pieces too small may be just as difficult to consume as pellets too large for a fish's mouth. Feed of the wrong size or an excess amount can lead to waste and poor water quality.

Fish accumulate most fat stores around their viscera and to some extent under the skin and within muscle. Body condition can be assessed from above and the sides, although even an observer with a well trained eye may have difficulty externally determining condition beyond average, obese, or emaciated. The Goede index has been used in salmonid species to assign fat scores to fish when necropsied, which can be used in an overall examination of the health of a cultured population, (Goede and Barton, 1990). For small, young fish in large-scale production, fish are often weighed in groups and the weight reported in fish per pound or kilogram. Larger fish may be weighed individually in pounds or kilograms. Determination of the body condition score of marine mammals is necessary for the establishment and follow-up of the nutrition program. Body condition score also provides information about physiological and health changes in individuals. Since the weighing of cetaceans is not practical compared to otariids and pinnipeds, the body condition score makes it easier for the examination of general health conditions and it is used as one of the most important criteria about whether individuals are ready to be released back to the wild.

Marine mammals are widespread in the oceans and can consume different nutrient sources in different regions. Through stomach content studies of marine mammals, an idea can be obtained about the feeds and specific species needs. Various feed sources like anchovy, horse mackerel, octopus, and squid have been found in stomach content studies. However, due to economic and accessibility reasons, usually frozen fish (mackerel, cod, etc.) are used in rehabilitation centers.

It should be noted that naturally marine mammals live in unlimited space and they become stressed in the relatively small pool environment. Stress can result in decreased immunity and increased susceptibility to pathogens and secondary infections. Daily ration planning should be done separately for each individual. Buckets can be separated for each individual to monitor the individual's consumption of fish, since they may or may not like the variety of fish being fed, and each food fish has a different nutritional value. Feeding is recommended to be done 5–10 times a day to simulate natural behavior (Gage and Whaley, 2009). In the beginning, it is normal for marine mammals to not want to consume dead fish. For this reason, tube feeding can be easier in the first days. The daily consumption of fish from an adult cetacean may vary individually. Daily ration should be increased slowly until the average amount of fish consumed is found. It is a good indication of health and acceptance if the record shows a consistent increase in fish consumption. When creating a diet for marine mammals, it is useful to create a program with different food fishes if possible, considering the individual's body condition score, age, activity, and nutrient values of the fish used.

3.3.2 Feed Storage

Appropriate storage of feed is crucial to maintain freshness. Important conditions to consider when evaluating feed storage are temperature, humidity, and avoiding oxygen and sunlight exposure (see further considerations on mycotoxicosis in Chapters 4 and 8). Warm temperatures, especially in high humidity, may encourage bacterial and mold growth and lead to oxidation of nutrients. Some feeds are stable at room temperature while others require refrigeration or freezing. Feed that does not require refrigeration or freezing should generally be kept in a cool dry area. Heat and humidity cause premature nutrient breakdown. Pelleted dry feeds for fish such as salmonids are packaged to be kept cool and dry. Freezing these types of feeds will cause nutrient breakdown and is not typically recommended.

Even when retained in airtight packaging, commercial feeds have a shelf life that should not be exceeded. Check with the feed manufacturer for recommendations on storage and shelf life (expiration date). The storage period of feed is considered reasonable for three months (Saint-Erne, 2010). Opened bags or boxes of feed should be fed out as quickly as possible and examined regularly for unusual textures, pellet sizes and/or shapes, smells, or other atypical characteristics that may indicate an error in the manufacturing process. Also, pests such as flies and rodents should be kept out of the feed storage area and floors kept free of spills or anything else that may attract rodents or other pests. Feed containers should be regularly checked for tears and chew marks from rodents.

In marine mammal nutrition, strict hygienic conditions of the fish to be used in feeding should be practiced. In general, fish that humans would not consume should not be offered to marine mammals in rehabilitation. Preparing daily food in an easy to clean and sanitized industrial kitchen, free from cross-contamination, will improve feed safety. Fish should be stored in the freezer and thawing of frozen products should be done at room temperature or with water. Thawing in tap water can lead to a decrease in beneficial nutrients such as minerals and vitamins passing into the water by diffusion and this will reduce the nutritional value of the fish. Since feeding is carried out in the open air, it is not appropriate to refeed leftover fish in the next feeding session due to the possibility that the fish may deteriorate from external influences and microbial contamination may occur. Apart from this, the food buckets should be disinfected after every feeding session.

3.3.3 Nutrient Analysis

Regular sampling of pelleted feeds is recommended for quality assurance of the feed as well as the storage conditions. Sampling of newly opened bags or containers should be done on a quarterly basis. Ideally, each type of feed (and size) used should be analyzed regularly for consistency of size, shape, texture, and odor, as well as nutrient composition. Such elements as proteins, lipids, ash, and moisture are given on pelleted feed products on the label in the guaranteed analysis as a percent of total ration. Also, labels should provide a production or expiration date and be adequately sealed to prevent air oxidation of lipids. Containers that have been punctured or otherwise broken open should be refused or returned as the vitamins will oxidize quickly and breakdown. Lipids exposed to air or moisture will become rancid over time. Rancidity can be tested through various means by commercial labs to assure that fats have not deteriorated through oxidation or hydrolysis.

3.3.4 Nutrient Requirements

Consider the life stage of the animals when calculating the amount of nutrients that will be required. The energy requirements of many fish species are lower than mammals due to such factors as higher protein to muscle conversion efficiency, passive ammonia loss through the gills and ectothermy (lower metabolic demands than endotherms since there is no need to maintain a high internal temperature). Basic fish nutritional requirements are shown in Table 3.1. Primarily, it is recommended to use fish protein sources. However, many new commercial foods have been developed with plant-based proteins as well as insects as the protein source. If a plant-based protein source needs to be used, soybean is a nutritious source. Carbohydrates should be starch-based. The indigestible carbohydrates (fiber) should be no more than half of the total carbohydrate level. The ration should contain up to 1% sodium chloride, 0.3% phosphorus, and 1% vitamins (A, C, D, E, K and B vitamins).

3.3.5 Nutritional Deficiencies and Toxicities

Fish can develop disease symptoms from either too much or too little of a nutrient. Some micronutrients, such as selenium and other minerals, can cause disease in both cases. Signs of nutritional disease will often be general in nature and can be due to nutrient excess, deficiency, or imbalance. In populations of fish where growth and performance are measured, deficiencies will often be a result of multiple nutrients and present as poor growth and/or feed conversions (a measure of how

Table 3.1 Fish nutrition requirements (adapted from Corcoran and Roberts-Sweeney, 2014)

	Herbivore and omnivore (%)	Carnivore (%)
Protein	35–45	40–55
Fat	15–25	15–25
Carbohydrate	25–40	<20
Fiber	<5	<5

much growth is gained for the amount of feed fed during a given period) and even an increase in susceptibility to disease. Deficiencies can be complex and very difficult to pinpoint. Identifying the offending feed and changing it out is often the most reasonable option, but it can be a challenge. If the feed is obtained from a reputable source, problems due to storage (high humidity and/or temperature) are often the cause of degradation in feed quality leading to disease issues.

Inadequacy in fish feeds can lead to insufficient growth, slow growth and reduced egg quality (Snieszko, 1975). Nutritional deficiencies sometimes cause secondary diseases and may mask the main cause of malnutrition (Hardy, 2012). Nutritional diseases encountered in the aquarium sector are usually based on inadequacies. This may be due to lack of feed or a missed feeding event, inability to reach the food due to crowded conditions or poor feed dispersal, poor palatability and feeding methods that are incompatible with the animals' behavior, as in the case of non-domesticated wild fish and mammals being held in captivity for the first time.

Proteins are essential for survival, growth, reproduction, cell repair, amino acid synthesis, and energy metabolism (Hardy, 2012). It is especially important in larvae rearing. Deficiency of proteins can lead to a lack of micronutrients such as specific amino acids. Larva production significantly decreases with a lack of sufficient nutrients and deficiency in amino acids. The protein and amino acid requirements of fish in different age groups will also vary, but the essential amino acids of most monogastric animals are the same. Ten essential amino acids need to be added to the fish diet: arginine, histidine, isoleucine, leucine, lysine, methionine, phenylalanine, threonine, tryptophan, and valine (Saint-Erne, 2010; Hardy, 2012; Halver, 1976; Ketola, 1983; Walton *et al.*, 1982; Mazid *et al.*, 1978). Since their deficiency will affect the synthesis of proteins, it should be ensured that they are present at a sufficient level when creating diets. The main symptom of amino acid deficiency is reduced growth rate (Hardy, 2012), such as reported with lysine and methionine (Halver, 1976). Other lesions that may be seen are fin erosion with lysine deficiency (Hardy, 2012; Walton *et al.*, 1984), as well as scoliosis and lordosis with tryptophan and histidine deficiency in Atlantic salmon (Roberts, 2002).

Protein requirements are higher for salmonids in saline conditions, but protein excess may also lead to toxic effects in fish. For example, high amounts of valine and isoleucine levels three times greater than leucine may impede growth (Halver, 1976). Therefore, the amount of amino acids in the feed should be balanced properly.

Adequate amounts of energy should be given to convert amino acids into proteins (Halver, 1976). The requirements of energy in feed depends on many factors in fish. Water temperature, salinity, fish size, and feeding type all change the amount of digestible energy obtained from feed. For example, metabolism and feed consumption increases with increasing water temperatures (Bureau *et al.*, 2002). The energy requirements of fish are lower than mammals because they can remove ammonia from the body without converting it to uric acid or urea, and it is sufficient to feed 3–5% of the fishes' body weight per day as their ration (Lovell, 1991; Corcoran and Roberts-Sweeney, 2014). An excessive feeding regimen can lead to obesity and water pollution, which can in turn lead to health and disease issues.

Meeting the energy needs of marine mammals has an important role in maintaining daily activities and aiding in recovery during rehabilitation. Energy needs should be determined by considering the size of the body, daily activity, water temperature, and pregnancy (Worthy, 2001). The fat and protein content of the feeder fish should meet the energy needs in the fish for which the diet will be prepared. Since it is not known when an individual, released back into the wild, will start hunting its own feed, it is necessary to release it back with sufficient energy stores. Body condition score is a good indicator of whether the amount of energy in the diet is sufficient.

Fats are valuable as an energy source for young fish in rapid growth states. They also contribute to the development of fish color and are incorporated into cell structure and hormone production. In particular, the lack of essential oils may result in slow growth, decreased absorption of vitamins A, D, E and K, fin erosion, and neuromuscular effects (Saint-Erne, 2010). It is desirable that 15–25% of the diet consists of fats (Lall and Tibbetts, 2009) and 1% consists of omega-3 and omega-6 fatty acids (Roberts, 2002; Saint-Erne, 2010).

In contrast to mammals, 18 : 2 and 18 : 3 omega-3 fatty acids are needed in fish nutrition and 20 : 5 and 22 : 6 omega-3 fatty acids in marine aquariums, (Corcoran and Roberts-Sweeney, 2014). Predatory fish have very little need for carbohydrates. Herbivorous species may be able to use carbohydrates more effectively for energy. Since the digestion rate of carbohydrates is around 34%, it is not a nutrient source that fish can metabolize well and it is recommended that the ratio in the diet is between 25% and 40% (Saint-Erne, 2010). Carbohydrates are not high among the natural nutrient sources of fish and excess intake can lead to degeneration of liver cells from hepatic lipidosis (Saint-Erne, 2010). In general, among animals, fish require less carbohydrates and more protein. Adjusting the blood glucose level in fish is not very important and, unlike mammals, studies are indicating that fish can be insulin resistant and 10% starch level in the ration has been determined as the optimum value (Hemre *et al.*, 2001; Oliva-Teles, 2012). The presence of 25–40% carbohydrates for omnivores and herbivores and 20% for carnivores is recommended (Lall and Tibbetts, 2009). Water-soluble vitamins are very important for fish and there are situations in which aquarium conditions need to be supplemented with vitamins. Fat-soluble vitamins are frequently supplemented because they can be stored in the liver and other organs. Common signs of vitamin deficiency include decreased appetite and slow growth. A common problem of koi fish is vitamin C deficiency, which interrupts bone development and leads to scoliosis and anatomical disorders of the spinal canal. Floating vitamin tablets, orange slices added to the pond, or periodically using a pelleted feed that is soaked in orange juice are simple methods that can be used in koi fish (Saint-Erne, 2010). Similar effects appear in salmon (Roberts, 2002).

Vitamin E deficiency is characterized by muscle loss in the posterior part of the body in koi fish. A feed rate of 50 mg vitamin E and 100 g of food has been reported to be therapeutic (Saint-Erne, 2010). Since corneal opacity can be due to vitamin deficiency, mixed vitamin supplements are recommended in such cases (Maclean, 2010). Temperature affects the stability of vitamins. At low temperatures, the need for vitamin E increases and deficiency manifests itself with cardiomyopathies (Roberts, 2002). Coenzymes of water-soluble vitamins work as they do in other animals, but because the body temperature of fish varies according to water temperature, the work of enzymes does not remain constant as in mammals.

Preserved forms of vitamin A (vitamin A acetate, palmitate, propionate) reduce the risk of insufficiency because they are not oxidized, and in general vitamin A (retinol) deficiency is not a problem in fish diets (Roberts, 2002). Vitamin D (cholecalciferol) is very important for calcium metabolism and when deficiencies in calcium metabolism are seen, the total body ash, calcium, and potassium values are decreased. Vitamin D deficiency can occur in water containing less calcium. Vitamin K deficiency causes an increase in clotting time and a decrease in hematocrit value (Roberts, 2002). In marine mammals, although vitamin D is usually adequate due to subcutaneous adipose tissue deposits, vitamins A, C, and E may require addition in the diet. Especially in vitamin C deficiency, anorexia, weight loss, necrotic stomatitis, and gingivitis may be observed. Vitamin C deficiency can be prevented by supplementing the food with 200–250 mg/day. To treat vitamin C deficiencies, 1000 mg/day ascorbic acid can be administered (Worthy, 2001).

Deficiency of water-soluble B and C group vitamins normally is not observed in marine mammals (Roberts, 2002). Necrotic stomatitis (Figure 3.15), gingivitis, necrosis of the gums, and anorexia due to ascorbic acid deficiency may be seen in marine mammals, characterized by weight

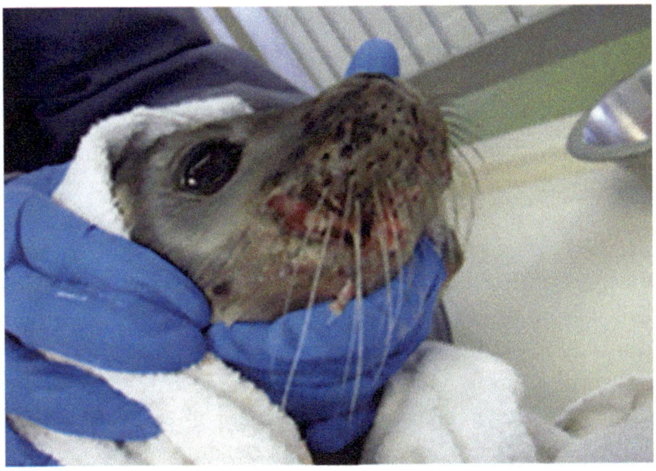

Figure 3.15 Necrotic stomatitis in a seal related to malnutrition (Vitamin C deficiency). *Source:* photo by E. Danyer.

loss. For marine mammals, the addition of 1000 mg/day ascorbic acid to the diet is recommended for treatment and prevention (Worthy, 2001). Thiamine deficiency occurs due to the effects of thiaminase in fish feeding. Thiamine deficiency is not observed in wild animals because of the variety of fish consumed (Worthy, 2001). For this reason, different food fish species should be used when planning daily diets for marine mammals. Thiamin deficiency translates to neurologic symptoms, such as tremors and headshaking (Worthy, 2001). In the case of mammals housed in rehabilitation and captivity facilities, a variety of fish food and thiaminase-based additives should be provided.

Pantothenic acid deficiency can be seen in young fish and may result in extreme hypertrophy and synechia of gill tissue. Niacin deficiency can manifest as dorsal and pectoral fin erosion. Choline requirements are higher in fish and deficiency may slow development (Roberts, 2002).

Mineral element needs of fish are generally the same as in other vertebrates. Although many mineral requirements can be met by absorption from untreated groundwater, the use of deionized and distilled water in aquariums may cause mineral imbalances (Lovell ,1991; Lall and Tibbetts, 2009; Oliva-Teles, 2012). Calcium, chloride, cobalt, iodine, iron, magnesium, phosphorus, potassium, sodium, and zinc can be absorbed through the gills, but other minerals need to be in the ration (Saint-Erne, 2010). Hyponatremia is characterized by an absence of plasma sodium, chloride, and potassium exchange, and is associated with anorexia, followed by muscle tremors and incoordination in marine mammals. While sodium chloride is consumed naturally by fish in the wild, losses can occur during freezing, thawing, and soaking processes when they are used as food fish in captivity. As prevention, 3 g NaCl/kg food fish/day can be given in the fish (Worthy, 2001).

Fish can absorb copper from water, so copper insufficiency is uncommon (Roberts, 2002). Copper is an essential trace metal necessary for growth and metabolism of all living organisms, including fish, as copper forms part of many enzymes and glycoproteins and is necessary for hemoglobin synthesis (Nordberg *et al.*, 2007). Sources such as urban runoff, pesticides and mining can lead to toxic levels of copper that interfere with olfaction in salmonid species (Baldwin *et al.*, 2011). Copper is also used as an algaecide and to control parasites in aquatic systems. The most bioavailable and therefore most toxic form of copper is the cupric ion (Cu_2^+). Copper at a dosage rate of 0.15–0.20 mg/l Cu_2^+ is effective for control of fish parasites, many species of algae, and unwanted invertebrates in marine aquariums. By contrast, in freshwater systems, measured alkalinity is normally used to calculate dosage rate. The toxicity of copper to fish increases as the total alkalinity decreases. A good rule of thumb for fresh water copper use is to divide the total alkalinity (in parts per million) by 100 to get the concentration of copper sulfate to use in parts per million (milligram/liter; Watson and Yanong, 1989).

Excess levels of copper in the water can lead to toxicity and fish death. Fish and crustaceans are more sensitive to the toxic effects of copper than are mammals. Even for more tolerant species, chronic copper use can damage the gills, kidney and spleen, and it will depress the immune system. Copper can also damage the beneficial bacteria in the biofilter. Activated carbon and water changes can be used to remove copper from the aquarium water.

Although phosphorus is required for growth, deficiency is rare because it is typically present in sufficient amounts in the feed (Roberts, 2002). Reduced levels may lead to reductions in growth rates. It is important that a soluble form of phosphorus is used in fish feed (Lovell, 1991). Excess phosphorus in the water can lead to abundant algae and cyanobacteria growth. Commercial chemicals can be used to precipitate phosphorus from solution to assist its removal from the aquarium water.

Dwarfism, growth restriction and cataracts are seen with manganese deficiency (Roberts, 2002). Zinc deficiency is characterized by poor growth, skin and fin disorders, and bilateral cataracts (Roberts, 2002). The amount of mineral and trace elements of the aquarium or pond water should be measured every one to two weeks to ensure that the fish can get enough minerals (Corcoran and Roberts-Sweeney, 2014). The balance of trace elements in the ration is important for their interactions with each other. It should be noted that absorbability, toxicities, drug–nutrient interactions, environmental conditions, and metabolism play an important role in mineral deficiency cases (Chanda *et al.*, 2015).

3.3.6 Water

Freshwater fish generally do not drink water and remove excess water from the body through the kidneys by producing copious urine. Saltwater fish do drink water to replace body fluids lost by osmosis into the more concentrated sea water in which they live. They have specialized cells in their gills that excrete the excess salts consumed with sea water ingestion. Marine mammals meet their water needs primarily from the water contained in their food, from the water released through catabolism and by direct drinking. The most important of these is the 60–80% water per fish that is obtained from their prey (Rosen and Worthy, 2018). Since commercial feeds containing more than 9–10% moisture will degrade more quickly, it is recommended to store such types of moist feed refrigerated or frozen (Saint-Erne, 2010).

3.3.7 Therapeutic Diets

3.3.7.1 Principles and Techniques of Therapeutic Diet Administration During Treatment and Recovery

Many medications that can be given orally can be included in a therapeutic diet. For instance, heat stable medications can be included directly into the extrusion process for pelletized diets, those that are not can be top-coated afterwards (check if legal in your jurisdiction). Aquatic gel foods have been developed for many species which can easily be used to mix and deliver medications. Adding a few drops of, for example, aniseed and other compounds to the water can stimulate appetite.

Stranding and maintenance in captivity are sources of stress in marine mammals, especially for cetaceans. This may cause hypoglycemia, vomiting and loss of appetite. During hypoglycemia, administration of 20 ml of 40% glucose solution to seals has proved beneficial (Barnett *et al.*, 2013). Vomiting causes loss of nutrients requiring immediate treatment. Considering the stress they will have during rehabilitation, additional hydration should be provided by injecting 50–100 ml of potable fresh water into the food fish during forced feeding in individuals who are not eating.

3.3.7.2 Prebiotics, Probiotics, and Other Feed Additives

The colors of aquarium fish are important for breeders. Carotenoid pigments are the most commonly used food additives to enhance skin color of ornamental fish. Beta-carotene and xanthophylls highlight yellow-orange and capsicum produce red-orange pigmentation (Saint-Erne, 2010). In addition, over 700 carotenoid definitions have been made and these are grouped as melanin, pterin, purine, and carotenoid (Yeşilayer, 2008). Besides coloration, carotenoids also have effects such as enhancing immunity, supporting reproduction, and replacing provitamin A (Yeşilayer, 2008). Crustaceans, vegetable products, algae, yeasts, and synthetic products can also be used as pigment sources. Ration components capable of photosynthesis (plants and algae) produce red, orange and yellow colors. The type of feed and the amount of fat it contains can affect the bioavailability of carotenes and xanthophylls (Yonekura and Nagao, 2007).

Prebiotics and probiotics have become an indispensable part of animal nutrition. Prebiotics are defined as cultures that help the digestive system develop non-digestible, beneficial bacterial colonies when they are used (Gibson and Roberfroid, 1995). The use of probiotics is also increasing in the fish industry. Probiotic usage reduces antibiotic use, improves feed efficiency and reduces stress. *Lactococcus lactis*, *L. plantarum* and *L. fermentum* can reach the intestines without being affected by the acidic environment and bile acids in the stomach (Corcoran and Roberts-Sweeney, 2014). Live feed sources can also be used to increase dietary diversity. Precautions should be taken to minimize the risks of microbial, bacterial and parasitic contamination of food sources.

Supplementary materials available online

- Bibliographic references.
- Further reading.
- Further resources.
- Acknowledgements.

References

Antrim, J. and McBain, J.F. (2001). Marine mammal transport. In: *CRC Handbook of Marine Mammal Medicine*, 2e (ed. L.A. Dierauf and F.M.D. Gulland), 881–891. New York, NY: CRC Press.

Baldwin D.H., Tatara C.P. and Scholz N.L. (2011). Copper-induced olfactory toxicity in salmon and steelhead: extrapolation across species and rearing environments. *Aquatic Toxicology* 101: 295–297.

Barnett, J., Knight, A. and Stevens, M. (2013). *British Divers Marine Life Rescue Marine Mammal Medic Hand Book*, 7e. Horsham, UK: The Printed Word.

Bureau, D.P., Kaushik, S.J. and Cho, C.Y. (2002). Bioenergetics. In: *Fish Nutrition*, 3e (ed. J.E. Halver, J. E. and Hardy, R. W. (eds), 1–59. New York, NY: Academic Press.

Chanda S., Paul B.N., Gosh K. and Giri S.S. (2015). Dietary essentiality of trace minerals in aquaculture: a review. *Agricultural Reviews* 36:100–112.

Corcoran, M. and Roberts-Sweeney, H. (2014). Aquatic animal nutrition for the exotic animal practitioner. *Veterinary Clinics of North America Exotic Animal Practice.* 17: 333–346.

Gage, L. and Whaley, J.E. (2009). *Marine Mammal Response, Rehabilitation, and Release: Standards for release.* Silver Spring, MD: NOAA National Marine Fisheries Service Marine Mammal Health and Stranding Response Program.

Geraci, J R. and Lounsbury, V.J. (2005). *Marine Mammals Ashore: A field guide for strandings, 2e.* Baltimore, MD: National Aquarium in Baltimore.

Gibson, G.R., and Roberfroid, M.B. (1995). Dietary modulation of the human colonic microbiota: introducing the concept of prebiotics. *Journal of Nutrition* 125: 1401–1412.

Goede, R.W. and Barton, B.A. (1990). Organismic indices and an autopsy-based assessment as indicators of health and condition in fish. In: *Biological Indicators of Stress in Fish* (ed. S.M. Adams), 93–108. Bethesda, MD: American Fisheries Society.

Halver, J.E. (1976). Formulating practical diets for fish. *Journal of the Fisheries Research Board of Canada* 33: 1032–1039.

Hardy, R.W. (2012). The nutritional pathology of teleosts. In: *Fish Pathology*.4e (ed. R.J. Roberts), 402–424. Chichester: Wiley-Blackwell.

Hemre, G.I., Mommsen, T. and Krogdahl, Å. (2002). Carbohydrates in fish nutrition: effects on growth, glucose metabolism and hepatic enzymes. *Aquaculture Nutrition* 8: 175–194.

Herráez, P., Sierr, E., Arbelo M. *et al.* (2007). Rhabdomyolysis and myoglobinuric nephrosis (capture myopathy) in a striped dolphin. *Journal of Wildlife Diseases* 43: 770–774.

Ketola, H.G. (1983). Requirement for dietary lysine and arginine by fry of rainbow trout. *Journal of Animal Science* 56: 101–107.

Lall, S.P. and Tibbetts, S.M. (2009). Nutrition, feeding, and behavior of fish. *Veterinary Clinics of North America Exotic Animal Practice.* 12: 361–372.

Lovell, R.T. (1991). Nutrition of aquaculture species. *Journal of Animal Science* 69: 4193–4200.

Maclean, B. (2010). Ornamental fish. In: *Manual of Exotic Pets* 5e (ed. A. Meredith and C. Johnson-Delaney), 267–279. London: BSAVA.

Mazid, M.A., Tanaka, Y., Katayama, T. *et al.* (1978). Metabolism of amino acids in aquatic animals-iii indispensable amino acids for *Tilapia zillii*. *Bulletin of the Japanese Society of Scientific Fisheries* 44: 739–742.

Noda, K., Akhiyoshi, H., Aoki M. *et al.* (2007). Relationship between transportation stress and polymorphonuclear cell functions of bottlenose dolphins (*Tursiops truncatus*). *Journal of Veterinary Medical Science* 69: 379–383.

Nordberg, G.F., Fowler, B.A., Nordberg, M *et al.* (2007). *Handbook in the Toxicology of Metals*. 3e. New York, NY: Elsevier.

Oliva-Teles, A. (2012). Nutrition and health of aquaculture fish. *Journal of Fish Diseases* 35: 83–108.

Roberts, R.J. (2002). Nutritional pathology. In: *Fish Nutrition*, 3e (ed. J.E. Halver and R.W. Hardy), 453–504. Academic Press.

Rosen, D.A.S. and Worthy, G.A.J. (2018). Nutrition and energetics. In: *CRC Handbook of Marine Mammal Medicine* (ed. L.A. Dierauf and F.M.D. Gulland), 695–736. New York, NY: CRC Press.

Saint-Erne, N. (2013). Freshwater and marine ornamental fish industry. American Veterinary Medical Association Convention, Lecture Event ID# 14338, Chicago, IL.

Saint-Erne, N. (2010). *Advanced Koi Care for Veterinarians and Professional Koi Keepers*. Glendale, AZ: Erne Enterprises.

Snieszko, S.F. (1975). History and present status of fish diseases.*Journal of Wildlife Diseases* 11: 446–459.

Suzuki, M., Hirako, K., Saito, S. *et al.* (2008). Usage of high-performance mattresses for transport of indo-pacific bottlenose dolphin. *Zoo Biology* 27: 331–340.

Walton, M.J., Cowey, C.B. and Adron, J.W. (1984). Effects of biotin deficiency in rainbow trout, *Aquaculture* 37: 21–38.

Walton, M.J., Cowey, C.B. and Adron, J.W. (1982). Methionine metabolism in rainbow trout fed diets of differing methionine and cystine content. *Journal of Nutrition* 112: 1525–1535.

Watson, C. and Yanong, R.P.E. (1989). *Use of Copper in Freshwater Aquaculture and Farm Ponds.* FA-13, UF/IFAS Extension Service. Gainesville, FL: University of Florida.

Worthy, G.A.J. (2001). *Nutrition and energetics. CRC Handbook of Marine Mammal Medicine*, 2e (ed. L. Dierauf and F.M.D. Gulland), 791–827. New York, NY: CRC Press.

Yeşilayer, N. (2008). The use of natural carotenoid sources in fish feed. *Journal of Fisheries Sciences* 2: 241–251.

Yonekura, L. and Nagao, A. (2007). Intestinal absorption of dietary carotenoids. *Molecular Nutrition and Food Research* 51: 107–115.

4

Pathology of Aquatic Animal Diseases

Wes Baumgartner, Acacia Alcivar-Warren, Farah Gonul Aydin, Kelly Bateman, Morag Clinton, Pádraig Duignan, Mansour El-Matbouli, María J. Forzán, Leo Foyle, Soliman Hatem, Gregory Lewbart, Richmond Loh, and Nicole Marie Nemeth

LEARNING OBJECTIVES
Understanding of environmental conditions and pathogens that cause diseases in teleost fish, the pathological changes and clinical signs that these pathogens cause, needed to determine the cause of the disease and the course of action or treatment, as well as to assess the risk of contagion.

4.1 Introduction

A good understanding of aquatic animal diseases provides a sound basis for clinical reasoning and postmortem diagnoses. This chapter provides a concise review of the pathological changes that occur in teleost fish.

4.2 Infectious Diseases

4.2.1 Mycobacteriosis

- Overview/etiology: *Mycobacterium marinum*, *M. fortuitum* and several other species are the cause of common, chronic, severe granulomatous, systemic disease in fish, amphibians, and other aquatic animals. These agents may be zoonotic, causing dermatitis in humans. Additional information can also be found in Chapters 5 and 8.
- Host range and transmission: Any species of fish (as well as amphibians, reptiles, birds, and mammals), marine or freshwater, can be considered susceptible. Transmission is horizontal; diseased fish may shed bacteria into the water chronically. Distribution is worldwide.
- Signs/diagnosis: Infection leads to progressive granulomatous disease, where fish remain asymptomatic until late in the course. Animals lose condition (Figure 4.1), develop ulcers (Figure 4.2), exhibit exophthalmia, develop ascites, and may have altered pigmentation due to spinal cord involvement. Internally, granulomas efface organs, particularly spleen and kidney, however

Fundamentals of Aquatic Veterinary Medicine, First Edition. Edited by Laura Urdes, Chris Walster, and Julius Tepper.

Companion website: www.wiley.com/go/urdes/aquatic-veterinary-medicine

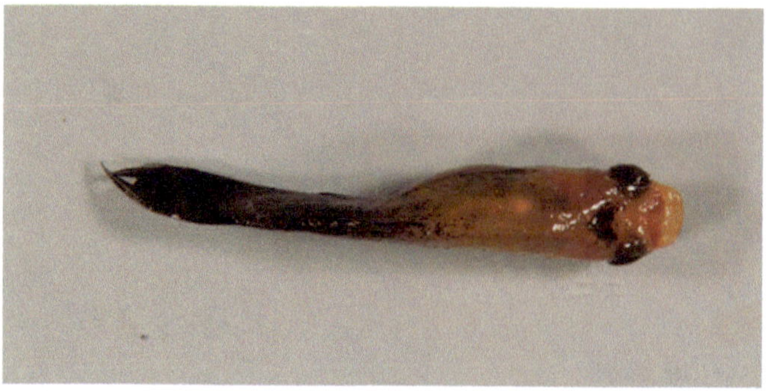

Figure 4.1 Mycobacteriosis, caudal peduncle atrophy in a molly (*Poecilia sphenops*).
Source: W. Baumgartner.

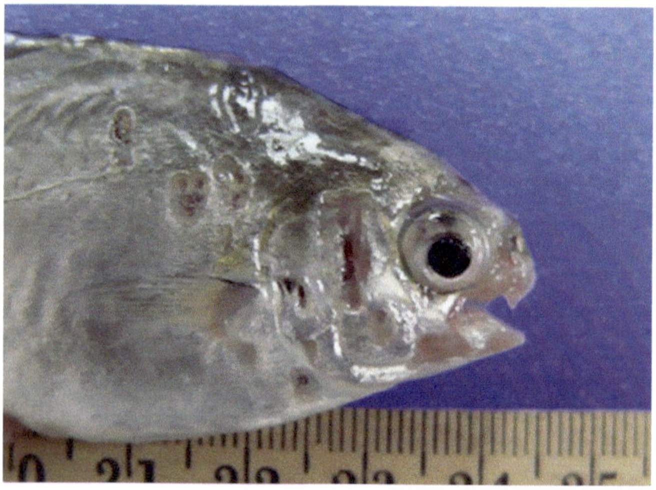

Figure 4.2 Mycobacteriosis, ulcerative dermatitis in a Florida pompano (*Trachinotus carolinus*).
Source: LADDL and W. Baumgartner.

many organs tend to be affected (Figure 4.3). In some species (amphibians in particular), mucopurulent discharge may develop as a sign. Any fish with chronic disease should be suspected of having mycobacteriosis.

Bacteria can be cultured on blood agar, although specialized media (Lowenstein-Jensen, Middlebrook) are preferred. Growth may take as little as two weeks, but some species may take months for colonies to develop. Histology or cytology smears of granulomas show acid-fast rod bacteria (not a specific test, as *Nocardia* spp. may also be acid fast). Acid-fast staining often shows many organisms, although in some cases few or no bacteria are seen; if any acid-fast organisms are evident, the diagnosis can be made. If no acid-fast organisms are seen, then mycobacteriosis cannot be excluded completely. Keep in mind that many aquarium fish and other species may harbor mycobacterial granulomas as background lesions; other causes of morbidity should be sought if the infection is mild.

- Differentials: Any granulomatous condition. *Nocardia* can mimic the infection, requiring culture to discriminate.

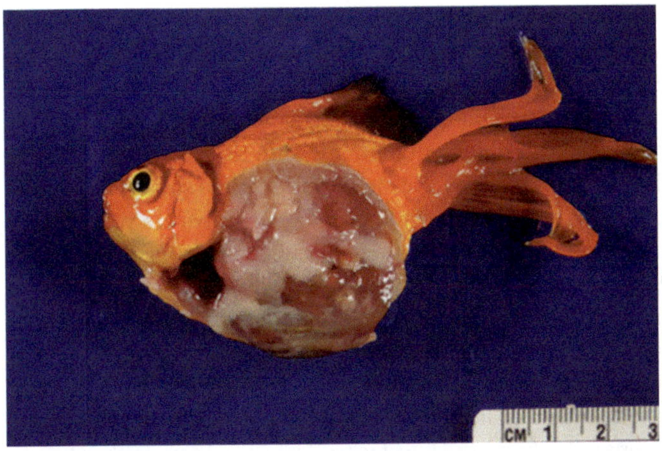

Figure 4.3 Mycobacteriosis, granulomatous peritonitis in a goldfish. *Source:* W. Baumgartner.

- Management: None. Depopulate to eradicate. The bacterium is difficult if not impossible to eliminate from some systems. Reduction in fish density, removal of fomites, frequent water changes, and reduced stress may slow disease progression in valuable animals.

4.2.2 Columnaris Disease (*Flavobacterium columnare*)

- Overview/etiology: A common acute to chronic skin and gill infection of freshwater fish that is often associated with mortalities. The bacterium attaches rhamnose binding receptors on fish skin and gills to establish an infection and produce biofilms, leading to marked necrosis. Outbreaks are typically in warmer months, generally 25–32°C. Younger fish are more susceptible. Mixed infections with other bacteria or parasites are common (Figure 4.4). *F. columnare* is a Gram-negative, slender, non-flagellated rod; wet mounts show a gentle gliding motility and the formation of irregular clumps (haystacks).

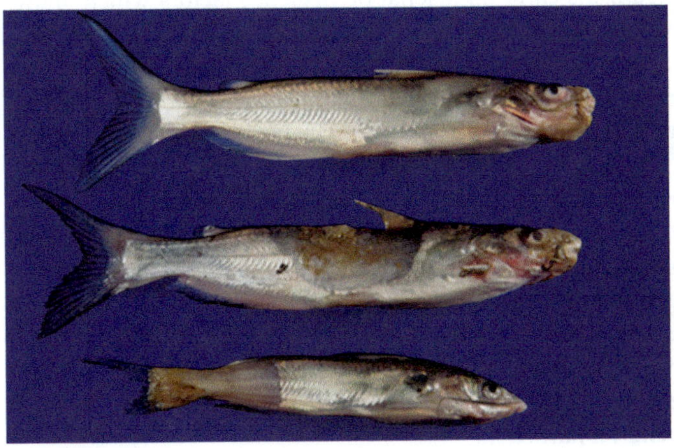

Figure 4.4 Columnaris disease, with secondary *Saprolegnia* and emaciation in a channel catfish. *Source:* W. Baumgartner.

- Host range and transmission: Any freshwater fish is susceptible. Transmission is horizontal and disease is often associated with stressful events. Fish that survive outbreaks can shed bacteria for up to 140 days at 5000 cells/ml/hour. The bacteria can survive at 25°C for 16 days, given a high organic load in the water and pH above 7; with low organic content and reduced pH, survival decreases.
- Signs/diagnosis: The disease is characterized by depigmentation and skin necrosis of the mouth, fins, and gills. The skin becomes milky (edema, necrosis) and sloughs, leading to superficial ulcers. The bacterium secretes a flexirubin pigment, which is pale yellow; infection imparts a yellow, dirty tinge to the tissues. Infections may start around the fin base and will spread centrifugally and caudally, following the flow of water and mucus off the body (saddleback lesions). Gill lesions are often multifocal, well demarcated; they comprise several adjacent filaments, white/tan, and ragged due to necrosis. Presumptive diagnosis can be made from wet mounts of yellow mucus, which show many gliding long rod bacteria that form "haystacks" within minutes. Darkfield microscopy provides superior resolution of the bacteria, and examination along the margins of mucus, at the interface with the wet-mount saline, generally shows the haystacks. Bacteria adhere to the slide or coverslip glass readily, and adjustment of the focus will usually show numerous organisms. For culture, bacteria require specialized media (selective cytophaga agar with neomycin 5 µg/ml and polymyxin B 200 iu/ml), forming yellow/orange colonies at 4–36°C.
- Differentials: None.
- Management: Reduce environmental stressors. Sensitivity-based antimicrobial therapy is effective. Potassium permanganate.
- For Epitheliocystis go online:

4.2.3 Motile Aeromonad Septicemia

- Overview/etiology: A common worldwide Gram-negative infectious septicemia known by many names (hemorrhagic septicemia, infectious dropsy, red pest, red sore). *Aeromonas hydrophila* is most often associated with disease, outbreaks, but *A. sobria* and *A. caviae* are often associated with lower level mortalities. Generally, epizootics occur where significant additional stressors or infections (parasites, high ammonia, low oxygen, temperature stress, handling, etc.) occur. Recently, a strain of *A. hydrophila* with acquired virulence factors has caused severe mortalities in the US catfish industry. Outbreaks are more frequent in warmer months. There are many strains of motile aeromonad septicemia, and these organisms carry an arsenal of virulence factors which allows them to take advantage of immunocompromised animals. See also Chapter 8 (Bacterial zoonoses).
- Host range and transmission: Any species of freshwater, brackish water, or marine warmwater fish. Transmission is horizontal. Aeromonads survive as facultative anaerobes in the water, mud, and detritus ubiquitously; organisms can be cultured from healthy fish. Aeromonads can infect mammals.
- Signs/diagnosis: Hyperemia, hemorrhage, edema, and necrosis are characteristics of infection. Exophthalmia, ascites, hemorrhage, and ulceration (sometimes deep) of the fins, muscle, and skin are typical (Figure 4.5). Internal organs are hemorrhagic. In peracute cases, signs may not be evident. With chronicity, skin ulcers progress to exposure of muscle and bone. Secondary oomycete/fungal infections may develop. Motile aeromonad septicemia can also develop as a secondary infection. Aeromonads can be grown on standard media and identified by biochemical testing; they have a temperature range of 18–39°C and grow well at 25–30°C.
- Differentials: Any Gram-negative bacterial pathogen.
- Management: Vaccines may be available, depending on the fish species. Antimicrobial sensitivity testing and administration of antibiotics and/or antiseptics are effective. Bath treatments with 1–3% NaCl or 2–4 mg potassium permanganate/liter can treat early skin infections.

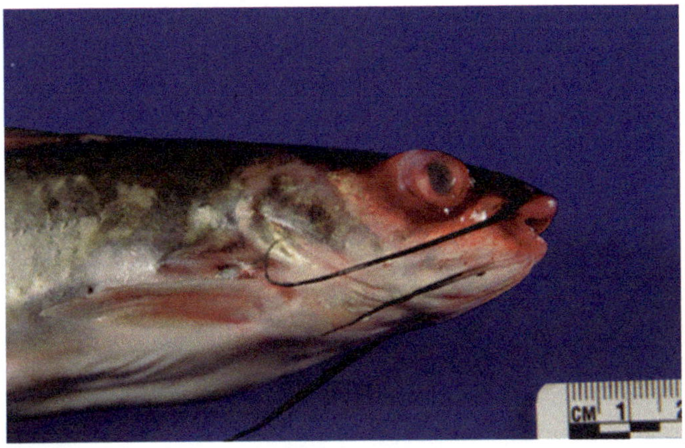

Figure 4.5 *Aeromonas hydrophila* septicemia in a channel catfish. *Source:* W. Baumgartner.

4.2.4 Furunculosis

- Overview/etiology: *A. salmonicida* is an important worldwide pathogen of salmonids. It causes septicemia and characteristic skin ulcers and furuncles (furunculosis). Currently, it is absent in salmonid culture in Australia, New Zealand, and Chile. *A. salmonicida subsp. salmonicida* is a Gram-negative, non-motile, facultative anaerobe rod bacterium which is classically rather homogeneous, but atypical strains (found in salmonids and non-salmonids) are known that do not fit into the current subspecies classification.
- Host range and transmission: Salmonids (Atlantic, Pacific), cyprinids (goldfish, carp, minnows), catfish, trout, char, turbot, cod, agnathans, perch, bream, pike, sole, halibut, among others. Bacteria are transmitted horizontally, in some cases from oozing skin lesions and possibly sea lice. The bacterium can persist in organic sediments.
- Signs/diagnosis: While skin ulcers and liquefactive necrosis of muscle (furuncles is a misnomer) are classically described, skin and fin lesions are not regular features of outbreaks. Acute and chronic disease occurs, often prompted by stressors of various sorts. Acute disease causes rapid death, sometimes without prior signs. Chronically infected fish exhibit signs typical of bacterial sepsis; lethargy, poor appetite, dark skin, pale gills, petechiae around the fins, exophthalmia. Liquefactive necrosis of the muscle causes bulging, soft skin lesions that ooze watery, flocculent, red/tan fluid filled with bacteria. Other signs include ascites, splenomegaly, and hemorrhage in the viscera. Ruptured furuncles form large ulcers. Kidney culture on tryptic soy agar or brain–heart infusion agar at 22°C.
- Differentials: Other aeromonads and *Vibrio* species.
- Management: Vaccination is available. Multidrug-resistant isolates are well known, making therapy a challenge. Probiotic use has inconsistent results.
- For Francisellosis go online:

4.2.5 Bacterial Kidney Disease

- Overview/etiology: Bacterial kidney disease is a chronic, granulomatous disease affecting freshwater and marine salmonids naturally (*Oncorhynchus*, *Salmo*, *Salvelinus* and *Thymallus* spp.) and a wider range of species experimentally. Given the chronicity of the disease, diagnosis is usually made in fish older than one year, and it represents a significant financial burden in these larger stock. Bacterial kidney disease has previously been called salmonid kidney disease and corynebacterial kidney disease.

- Host range and transmission: The infection can be found throughout many salmonid producing countries in the Northern hemisphere (Europe, North America, Japan). It is not present in Australia and New Zealand but is found in Chile.
- Signs/diagnosis: Mortalities are chronic in nature, and increase over a long period of time. Bilateral exophthalmia and ascites as a consequence of renal damage and compromised osmoregulation are accompanied by hyperpigmentation, lethargy, anemia and branchial pallor. Cystic cavities, vesicular lesions and hemorrhage appear in the musculature and skin. Local infections are seen in some fish, with lesions noted in the eyes and brain. Internal examination reveals large, granulomatous, greyish masses in the kidney which may extend to the liver. Histopathology reveals renal and hepatic granuloma with large numbers of bacteria. Kidney impression smears or sections will reveal Gram-positive bacteria. Culture is slow, taking 6–19 weeks at 15°C in a medium containing cysteine and serum. Direct and indirect fluorescent antibody tests, enzyme-linked immunosorbent assays (ELISA) and PCR are available.
- Differentials: Proliferative kidney disease (*Tetracapsula bryosalmonae*), nephrocalcinosis, Gram-positive bacteria, fungal infections causing granuloma, mycobacteriosis.
- Management: There is no vaccination, and fish are too far affected to treat effectively. Surveillance and attention to biosecurity are useful for limiting spread.

4.2.6 Vibrionaceae Diseases

- Overview/etiology: Bacteria in this group (*Listonella anguillarum*, *Vibrio alginolyticus*, *V. ordalii*, *V. parahemolyticus*) are a major cause of disease in warmwater marine caged fish species (especially yellowtail, red sea bream, flounder, and horse mackerel), and should be included as a differential for any marine species. Elasmobranchs are also highly susceptible. Outbreaks occur as a result of stress, and vibriosis may be a secondary infection in many cases. *Vibrio* infection has been associated with sleepy-grouper disease.
- Host range and transmission: Transmission is horizontal; the organisms are present ubiquitously in marine environments. Bacteria may enter fish through the skin or gills, and can be shed from the intestine or from any ulcerative lesions. There are no known limits to the range of species affected.
- Signs/diagnosis: Lesions may differ according to the *Vibrio* species, the fish infected, and environment. The disease can present anywhere from peracute to chronic morbidity and mortality. In peracute disease, there is sudden death, often with very high mortality, without signs. Hemorrhagic septicemia is typical. Externally, skin ecchymosis around the mouth and fins develop in early stages, and ulcers develop subsequently. Hemorrhage is extensive in the viscera; the liver, kidney, and spleen become swollen and friable or liquefied. The gastroenteric form is less common, with no prior skin lesions. Bacteria are present throughout diseased tissues, and can be cultured from the skin or internal lesions (*Vibrio*-selective agar). Presumptive diagnosis can be made based on the following features of the bacteria: Gram-negative, short curved rods, polar flagella/motile, cytochrome oxidase-positive, glucose fermenter without gas production. As these bacteria are ubiquitous, they may be cultured from the gut of normal fish (commensals).
- Differentials: *Mycobacterium*, *Lactococcus*, *Photobacterium*, *Nocardia*, *Listonella*, *Tenacibaculum*.
- Management: Good husbandry; reduce stress. Vaccination has been proposed. Sulfa drugs have been used successfully.

4.2.7 Edwardsiellosis

- Overview/etiology: *Edwardsiella* (*E. ictaluri*, *E. tarda*, *E. anguillarum*, *E. piscicida*) are Gram-negative bacteria, and are causative agents of septicemic disease.
- Host range and transmission: Ictalurid catfish (*E. ictaluri*, *E. piscicida*, *E. tarda*), eels (*E. anguillarum*), cultured marine fish (*E. tarda*), and others such as zebra fish, tilapia (*E. ictaluri*).
- Signs/diagnosis: Skin ulcers and hemorrhage (*E. ictaluri*, *E. piscicida*, *E. anguillarum*), hepatitis, enteritis. Early lesions start as hyperemia and petechiation of the skin (Figures 4.6, 4.7), soon developing abdominal hyperemia, ascites, and granulomatous inflammation in the viscera (Figure 4.8). Bacterial dissemination in the blood leads to lodgment in the dermis, forming "buckshot" ulcers (*E. ictaluri*). Survivors may develop encephalitis, which can lead to ulcers (hole-in-the-head lesions), particularly evident in catfish (*E. ictaluri*, *E. piscicida*; Figure 4.9). Such lesions are characteristic, but are not specific for edwardsiellosis. *E. tarda* is associated with

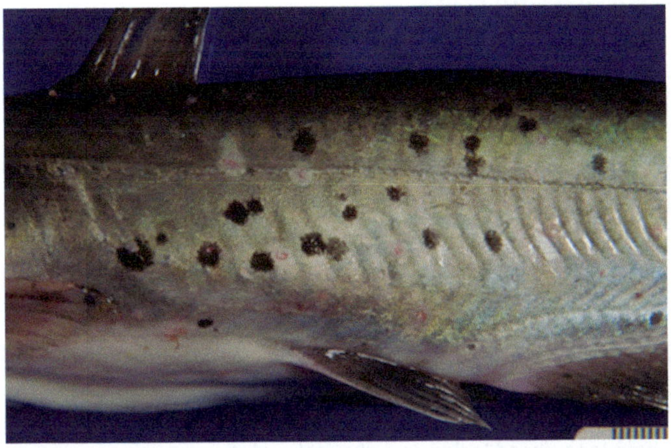

Figure 4.6 *Edwardsiella ictaluri* infection, skin ulcers in a channel catfish. *Source:* W. Baumgartner.

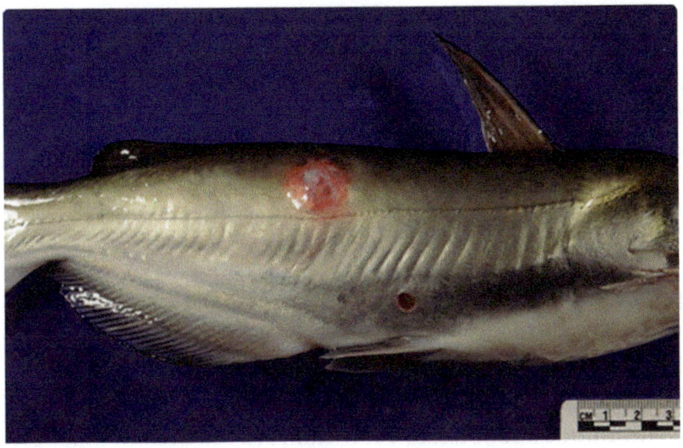

Figure 4.7 *Edwarsiella piscicida* infection, skin ulcer and furuncle, in a channel catfish. *Source:* W. Baumgartner.

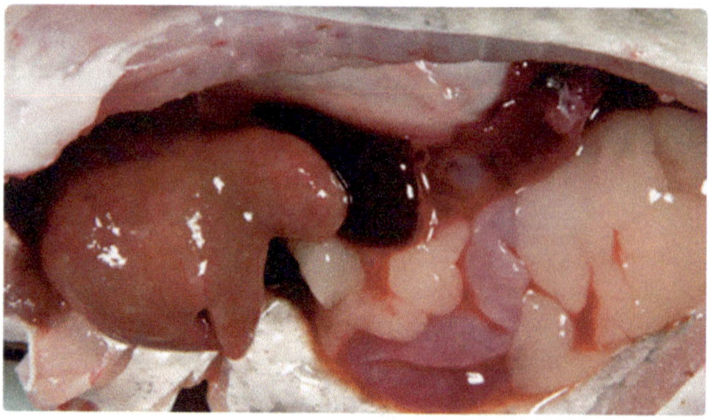

Figure 4.8 *Edwarsiella ictaluri* infection, hepatic necrosis, splenomegaly, bloody ascites, in a channel catfish. *Source:* W. Baumgartner.

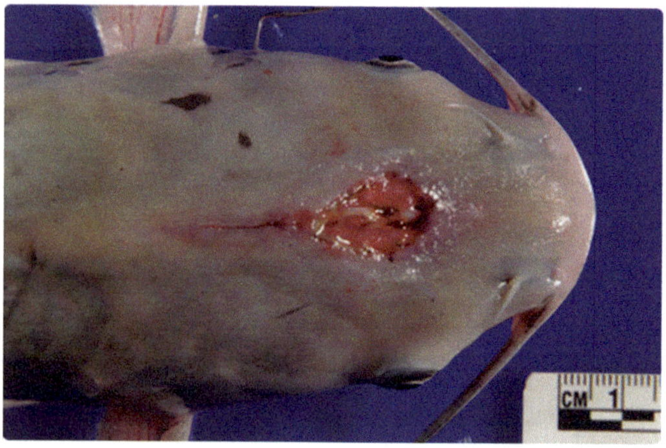

Figure 4.9 *Edwardsiella ictaluri* infection, hole in the head lesion, in a channel catfish. *Source:* W. Baumgartner.

large necrotizing skin and muscle lesions. Bacterial culture of liver, spleen, or kidney on blood agar produces small, white non-hemolytic colonies in one to two days.

- Differentials: Any cause of bacterial sepsis.
- Management: Antibiotic medicated feed is effective; florfenicol, tetracyclines, oxolinic acid/trimethoprim. Vaccines have been developed in catfish and eel.

4.2.8 Streptococcosis

- Overview/etiology: *Streptococcus* species, including *S. iniae* and *S. agalactiae*, are diseases of major importance in marine and freshwater species. Outbreaks can be severe, and often occur during high temperatures and stress.
- Host range and transmission: Many species can be affected, including tilapia, European sea bass, red drum, grouper, chinook salmon, barramundi, rabbitfish, yellowtail, red sea bream, Japanese flounder, Japanese sea perch, rockfish, and horse mackerel. Horizontal transmission by contact and contaminated feed. Distribution is worldwide.

- Signs/diagnosis: Bacteria are ingested and can rapidly proliferate in the gut, with systemic spread. Ophthalmitis and endomeningitis are characteristic in tilapia. In other species, ocular disease, erratic swimming, hemorrhage, and necrosis in the viscera and muscle are reported. Granulomas may develop in abdominal organs. Diagnosis is by blood agar (or other standard media) culture from internal organs or periorbital tissues. Streptococci are Gram-positive, non-motile bacteria less than 2 microns wide, and can form chains in liquid media. Many species are facultative anaerobes.
- Differentials: Sepsis (especially aeromonads), mycobacteriosis, viral infection, toxicosis.
- Management: Reduce stress. Antimicrobials, including erythromycin, have been effective.

4.2.9 Nocardiosis

- Overview/etiology: An uncommon, chronic granulomatous disease that appears similar to mycobacteriosis.
- Host range and transmission: *Nocardia kampachi* is a severe pathogen of yellowtail, amberjack, and striped jack in East Asia. Transmission is likely horizontal, via direct contact.
- Signs/diagnosis: Disease may be seasonal. Early signs include loss of condition, skin ulcers/nodules, anorexia. Culture of diseased organs (brain–heart infusion, tryptone soy agar, nutrient agar) reveals filamentous, branched, or beaded bacteria that are acid fast.
- Differentials: Mycobacteriosis.
- Management: None.

4.2.10 Pseudomoniasis (*P. fluorescens*)

- Overview/etiology: Pseudomonads are ubiquitous and opportunistic pathogens that cause septicemia. Organisms are present in gut flora normally. The disease is in many ways similar to aeromoniasis.
- Host range and transmission: Tilapia, carp. Horizontal transmission.
- Signs/diagnosis: Exophthalmia, ascites, edema, hemorrhage, ulcers. Internal organs are effaced by inflammation and necrosis. Pseudomonas can be cultured on standard media and identified with routine testing. They are Gram-negative, have one to three polar flagella and grow best at 20–25°C.
- Differentials: Any bacterial cause of septicemia.
- Management: None.
- For Infection with Lymphocystis go online:
- For Infection with Megalocytivirus go online:

4.2.11 Viral Hemorrhagic Septicemia

- Overview/etiology: Viral hemorrhagic septicemia (VHS) is one of the most threating systemic notifiable diseases of various salmonid and a few non-salmonid fish species worldwide (McAllister, 1990). The causative agent is a bullet-shaped, negative-sense, enveloped single-stranded RNA virus, assigned formerly as viral hemorrhagic septicemia virus and recently as piscine novirhabdovirus, that belonging to genus *Novirhabdovirus*, within the family Rhabdoviridae (Tordo *et al.*, 2005; Adams *et al.*, 2017). The piscine novirhabdovirus genome encodes six proteins: a nucleoprotein, N, a phosphoprotein, P, a matrix protein, M, a

Table 4.1 Geographical distribution of piscine novirhabdovirus genotypes.

Genotype	Distribution
Ia	Continental Europe
Ib	Northern Europe (Marine)
Ic	Continental Europe
Id	Scandinavia, Baltic Sea (fresh water)
Ie	Black Sea area
II	Baltic Sea (marine)
III	North Sea, Scotland, Ireland and Norway (marine)
VIa	North American Pacific Coast
VIb	Great Lakes region in North America
IVc	Atlantic coastal regions of North America

glycoprotein, G, a non-virion protein, NV and a polymerase, L (Walker *et al.* 2000). Comparisons of the N-gene, G-gene and NV-gene sequences of many piscine novirhabdovirus isolates revealed four major genotypes (I–IV), related to geographical location (Table 4.1) than host species (Snow *et al.*, 1999, 2004; Einer-Jensen *et al.*, 2004, 2005; Olesen and Skall 2013).

- Host range and transmission: VHS can occur at any age, but younger fish appear to be most susceptible. Rainbow trout (*Oncorhynchus mykiss*) are among the most affected species, with losses also occurring in farmed Japanese flounder (*Paralichthys olivaceus*) and turbot (*Scophthalmus maximus*; Smail, 1999; Ross *et al.*, 1994; Isshiki *et al.*, 2001). Piscine novirhabdovirus established a wide range of more than 80 species, fish species for which there is scientific evidence of susceptibility are listed in Table 4.2. Piscine novirhabdovirus is transmitted by direct contact with infected fish or with water containing virus particles, which shed in urine, reproductive fluids and feces, or by oral ingestion of infected materials (Neukirch, 1985; Kurath and Winton, 2011; Schönherz *et al.*, 2013). Predators and asymptomatic carriers act as mechanical vectors, transferring piscine novirhabdovirus into new areas (Peters and Neukirch, 1986; Goodwin and Merry, 2011).
- Signs/diagnosis: By penetration and multiplication of the piscine novirhabdovirus in endothelial cells of blood capillaries, leukocytes, hematopoietic tissues, and nephron cells, the virus induces the clinical signs that may appear on infected fish (Evensen *et al.*, 1994). Impairment of the osmotic balance in the presence of edema and hemorrhages can lead to death of the infected fish. VHS diseased fish exhibited clinical signs in the early stages of infection that may be non-specific and include rapid onset of mortality, lethargy, anemia, exophthalmia, darkening of the skin, hemorrhages at the base of fins, gills, internal organs and eyes, distended abdomen. Abnormal neurological signs such as severely abnormal swimming behavior (spiral or flashing swimming) can be evident. Postmortem finding of the VHS include petechial hemorrhage in the muscle tissue (Figure 4.10), especially in the dorsal muscle, splenomegaly, pale and mottled liver, dark red kidney, pale hind gut, which is mostly devoid of food, and the body cavity may be filled with ascetic fluid (Smail and Snow, 2011).

Table 4.2 Fish species susceptible to piscine novirhabdovirus according to the World Organisation for Animal Health (2019).

Common name	Scientific name
Rainbow trout	*Oncorhynchus mykiss*
Coho salmon	*Oncorhynchus kisutch*
Chinook salmon	*Oncorhynchus tshawytscha*
Brown trout	*Salmo trutta*
Atlantic salmon	*Salmo salar*
Grayling	*Thymallus thymallus*
Whitefish	*Coregonus* spp.
Atlantic herring	*Clupea harengus*
Pacific herring	*Clupea pallasii*
European sprat	*Sprattus sprattus*
South American pilchard	*Sardinops sagax*
Muskellunge	*Esox masquinongy*
Northern pike	*Esox lucius*
Atlantic cod	*Gadus morhua*
Poor cod	*Trisopterus minutus*
Norway pout	*Trisopterus esmarki*
Whiting	*Merlangius merlangus*
Blue whiting	*Micromesistius poutassou*
Norway pout	*Trisopterus esmarkii*
Alaska Pollock	*Theragra chalcogramma*
Fourbeard rockling	*Enchelyopus cimbrius*
Burbot	*Lota lota*
(North) Pacific hake	*Merluccius productus*
Dab	*Limanda limanda*
Flounder	*Platichthys flesus*
European plaice	*Pleuronectes platessa*
Greenland halibut	*Reinhardtius hippoglossoides*
Atlantic halibut	*Hippoglossus hippoglossus*
Turbot	*Scophthalmus maximus*
Japanese flounder	*Paralichthys olivaceus*
Lesser argentine	*Argentina sphyraena*
Surf smelt	*Hypomesus pretiosus*
Sand eel	*Ammodytes* spp.
Sand goby	*Pomatoschistus minutus*
Round goby	*Neogobius melanostomus*
Shiner perch	*Cymatogaster aggregata*
Freshwater drum	*Aplodinotus grunniens*
Chub/Pacific mackerel	*Scomber japonicus*
Yellow perch	*Perca flavescens*
European seabass	*Dicentrarchus labrax*
Three-spined stickleback	*Gasterosteus aculeatus*
Fathead minnow	*Pimephales promelas*

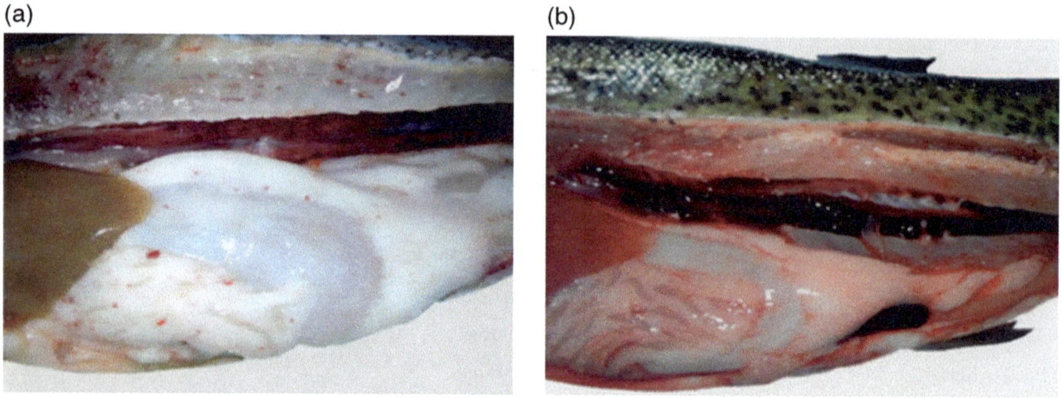

Figure 4.10 Rainbow trout infected with hemorrhagic septicemia virus. Internal gross lesions included widespread petechiae of the pyloric region (a) and in the musculature (a, b), severe congestion of the kidney (a, b), and pale enlarged liver (a). *Source:* Adapted from Ahmadivand *et al.* (2016) with permission.

- Differentials: VHS should be differentiated from other diseases which demonstrate a similar clinical picture in fish, such as infectious hematopoietic necrosis, furunculosis, and enteric red mouth disease. Bacteriological investigation can identify *A. salmonicida* as the causative agent of furunculosis diseases and *Yersinia ruckeri* as the causative agent of the enteric red mouth disease, and can differentiate them from piscine novirhabdovirus. In addition, virological isolation and confirmation using ELISA, immunofluorescence or reverse transcription PCR (RT-PCR) can differentiate the piscine novirhabdovirus from the salmonid novirhabdovirus (formerly known as infectious hematopoietic necrosis virus), the causative agent of the infectious hematopoietic necrosis virus.
- Management: Currently, there are no effective antiviral agents and no commercial vaccines exist to control VHS. Piscine novirhabdovirus can persist for long periods in the bottom of farm ponds if the ponds are not dried and disinfected. Strict biosecurity measures should be applied for fish, eggs, water sources, equipment, vehicles, vectors, and people working on the farm to avoid infection. Piscine novirhabdovirus is highly thermolabile and is inactivated by drying, pH 2.5 or 12.2, ultraviolet C (200–280 nm), or in the presence of disinfectants, including iodophor disinfectants, formalin, sodium hypochlorite, and sodium hydroxide.

4.2.12 Infectious Hematopoietic Necrosis

- Overview/etiology: Infectious hematopoietic necrosis (IHN) is one of the most serious notifiable diseases for salmonid fish, as it causes more than 80% losses depending on the species and size of the fish, the virus strain and environmental conditions (Wolf, 1988; Bootland and Leong, 1999). IHN was originally endemic in the Pacific Northwest of North America (Walker and Winton, 2010). The causative agent was described as IHN virus (IHNV) and then assigned as salmonid novirhabdovirus (Adams *et al.*, 2017). IHNV was firstly recognized in sockeye salmon (*Oncorhynchus nerka*) in 1950s and then emerged in 1970s to become an important pathogen of farmed rainbow trout (*O. mykiss*) in the United States (Yasutake and Mead, 1969). Subsequently, the virus was spread by the movement of contaminated eggs to several countries of Western Europe and East Asia, where it emerged to cause severe losses in farmed rainbow trout (Walker and Winton, 2010). As a member of the genus *Novirhabdovirus* in the family Rhabdoviridae, salmonid novirhabdovirus is a bullet-shaped virion containing a non-segmented, single-stranded, negative-sense RNA genome of approximately 11 000 nucleotides which encodes six proteins in the following order: a nucleoprotein (N), a phosphoprotein (P), a matrix protein (M), a glycoprotein (G), a non-virion protein (NV), and a polymerase (L) Kurath and Leong, 1985; Kurath *et al.*, 1985). Phylogenetic analysis of the G genes sequences has revealed five major genogroups denoted with U, M, L, E and J, correlating with the geographic ranges among worldwide isolates of IHN (Kurath *et al.*, 2010; Penaranda *et al.*, 2011; He *et al.*, 2013). Genogroups U, M and L are designated according to their geographic occurrence in North America (Kurath *et al.*, 2003). Genogroup J is mainly constituted by virus isolates from Japan and South Korea, whereas genogroup E is restricted to Europe (Haenen *et al.*, 2016). Water temperature is the most important factor affecting the progress of IHN. Experimental trials have demonstrated that salmonid novirhabdovirus can produce mortality from 3°C to 18°C, although clinical disease typically occurs at 8–15°C under natural conditions (Bootland and Leong, 1999).

- Host range and transmission: Most salmonid species are susceptible to salmonid novirhabdovirus. Fry and small fingerlings are the most highly susceptible fish stages. Fish become increasingly resistant with age until spawning, when they become highly susceptible and may shed large amount of virus in sexual products (World Organisation for Animal Health, 2019). The most susceptible and occasionally infected fish species with salmonid novirhabdovirus are listed in Table 4.3. Salmonid novirhabdovirus transmitted either horizontally by contact between fish and virus particles shed by the infected juveniles in the faeces, urine and external mucus, or through invertebrate vectors, vertical transmission, egg-associated transmission, have been also recorded (Bootland and Leong, 1999).
- Signs/diagnosis: Clinical signs of IHN appear in young salmonid, while infection in adults is subclinical and more frequently results in development of a chronic infection of carrier state (Wolf, 1988). During outbreaks, fish demonstrated behavioral changes such as lethargy interspersed with spiral swimming and flashing. Clinical signs (Figure 4.11) also include darkening of the skin, pale gills, ascites, distended abdomen, exophthalmia, petechial hemorrhages, and trailing fecal cast is observed in some species (Bootland and Leong, 1999). Gross pathological signs include yolk sac hemorrhages in fry, hemorrhages in the abdomen, around the eye pupil, and in the fatty tissue and muscle surrounding the organs and stomach wall, bleeding at the base of the fins. The stomach is empty and filled with a gelatinous substance and there are spinal deformities in surviving fish.
- Differentials: IHN should be differentiated from similar diseases that demonstrate a similar clinical picture, such as enteric red mouth disease, epizootic hematopoietic necrosis, furunculosis, infectious pancreatic necrosis, infectious salmon anemia, VHS, whirling disease. Tissue impression stained with Gram-stain can demonstrate the Gram-negative *Aeromonas salmonicida*, the causative agent of furunculosis or *Yersinia ruckeri*, the causative agent of the enteric red mouth disease, and can distinguish them from IHN. Virus isolation and confirmation with ELISA and/or RT-PCR can differentiate between salmonid novirhabdovirus and infectious pancreatic necrosis, infectious salmon anemia and VHS. DNA extraction from internal organs and cartilages can be used to differentiate between salmonid novirhabdovirus, epizootic hematopoietic necrosis virus, and *Myxobolus cerebralis*, the causative agent of whirling disease, respectively, by PCR using specific primers for each pathogen.

Table 4.3 Principle hosts and occasionally infected fish species with salmonid novirhabdovirus.

Common name	Scientific name
Rainbow trout	*Oncorhynchus mykiss*
Coho salmon	*Oncorhynchus kisutch*
Chinook salmon	*Oncorhynchus tshawytscha*
Sockeye salmon	*Oncorhynchus nerka*
Chum salmon	*Oncorhynchus keta*
Japanese amago	*Oncorhynchus rhodurus*
Masu salmon	*Oncorhynchus masou*
Atlantic salmon	*Salmo salar*
Occasionally infected species:	
Brown trout	*Salmo trutta*
Cutthroat trout	*Oncorhynchus clarki*
Arctic charr	*Salvelinus alpinus*
Lake trout	*Salvelinus namaycush*
Brook trout	*Salvelinus fontinalis*
White-spotted charr	*Salvelinus leucomaenis*
Ayu	*Plecoglossus altivelis*
European eel	*Anguilla anguilla*
Pacific herring	*Clupea pallasi*
Atlantic cod	*Gadus morhua*
Northern pike	*Esox lucius*
Sturgeon	*Acipenser transmontanus*
Shiner perch	*Cymatogaster aggregata*
Tube-snout	*Aulorhynchus flavidus*

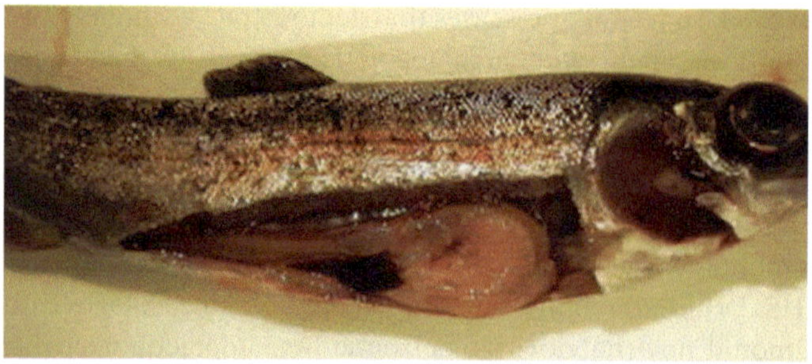

Figure 4.11 Gross pathology of infectious hematopoietic necrosis in rainbow trout. Typical gross appearance, including darkening of the skin, pale gills, exophthalmia, petechial hemorrhages, empty gut and ascitic fluid. *Source:* Adapted from Dixon *et al.* (2016) with permission (CC BY 4.0).

- To control IHN, general husbandry practice should include the use of spring water that is free of the virus, using of ultraviolet light or ozone to disinfect surface water source, disinfection of eggs to block vertical transmission, the use of common disinfectants and drying to inactivate salmonid novirhabdovirus (Winton, 1991; Bovo *et al.*, 2005; Wolf, 1988). Some autogenous, killed, and DNA vaccines have been licensed for commercial use in Atlantic salmon net-pen aquaculture on the west coast of North America but in Europe and the United States, its commercialization is restricted due to safety concerns.
- For Salmonid Novirhabdovirus disease go online:

4.2.13 Infectious Pancreatic Necrosis

- Overview/etiology: Infectious pancreatic necrosis is a contagious systemic viral disease of freshwater and marine fish, mollusks, and crustaceans (Hill, 1982; Wolf, 1988; Olesen *et al.*, 1988; Mortensen *et al.*, 1990; Saint-Jean *et al.*, 2003). The causative agent is a double-stranded bi-segmented RNA virus belonging to the family Birnaviridae. Virulent isolates that produce disease in salmonid fish are called infectious pancreatic necrosis virus (IPNV), while avirulent isolates for salmonid fish that are usually isolated from other teleosts or from aquatic invertebrates are named aquatic birnaviruses (Hill and Way, 1995; Reno, 1999). Serologically, IPNV is divided into two-distinct serogroups (A and B) which do not cross-react with each other in serum neutralization tests (Underwood *et al.*, 1977; Olesen *et al.*, 1988; Ahne *et al.*, 1989). IPNV serogroup A contains nine different serogroups, most associated with fish diseases, such as the most virulent serotype Sp and the lowest virulent serotype Ab, in addition to the serotypes WB, He, Te, Can.1, Can. 2, Can. 3, and JA, while serogroup B contains only a single serotype (B1) with small number of isolates (Jørgensen and Kehlet, 1971; Hill and Way, 1995).
- Host range and transmission: IPNV affects mainly various species of salmonid including the rainbow trout (*Oncorhynchus mykiss*), brown trout (*Salmo trutta*), Atlantic salmon (*S. salar*), and brook trout (*Salvelinus fontinalis*; Wolf and Quimby, 1962, 1971). The susceptibility to IPNV decreases with the age; fry and fingerlings are highly susceptible, while the infection in the older fish be inapparent (Smail and Munro, 1989). The virus was also detected in marine fish such as Atlantic cod (*Gadus morhua*), turbot (*Scophthalmus maximus*), yellowtail (*Seriola quinqueradiata*), and halibut (*Hippoglossus hippoglossus*; Nakajima *et al.*, 1993; Castric *et al.*, 1987; Mortensen *et al.*, 1990; Novoa *et al.*, 1993; Rodger and Frerichs, 1997). The avirulent isolate aquatic birnavirus was isolated from different fish species such as white suckers (*Catostomus commersonii*), Japanese eels (*Anguilla japonica*), Senegalese sole (*Solea senegalensis*), sea bream (*Pagrus aurata*), rockfish (*Sebastes schlegelii*), ayu (*Plecoglossus altivelis*), spikes dogfish (*Squalus megalops*), ling (*Genypterus blacodes*) and tilapia (*Oreochromis niloticus*).

  The disease is transmitted horizontally by direct contact between healthy and infected fish, ingestion of contaminated feces, urine, by fomites, or via contact of fish gills or eggs with contaminated water (Frantsi and Savan, 1971; Desautels and MacKelvie, 1975; Ahne *et al.*, 1989). IPNV accumulate in the marine bivalve mollusks, which act as reservoirs for the virus (Dobos *et al.*, 1979; Lo *et al.*, 1998; Mortensen *et al.*, 1990, 1998). Surviving fish of an infectious pancreatic necrosis outbreak become lifelong carriers and continuously shed and transmit IPNV to other healthy fish (Bootland *et al.*, 1991; Dorson, 1982; Wolf, 1988). Transmission can also occur via predatory birds and mammals, which can transport and excrete viable IPNV (Peters and Neukirch, 1986; McAllister and Owens, 1992). Vertical transmission has been reported for rainbow trout and brook trout but not for Atlantic salmon (Ahne *et al.*, 1989; Ahne and Negele, 1985; Dorson and Torchy, 1981).

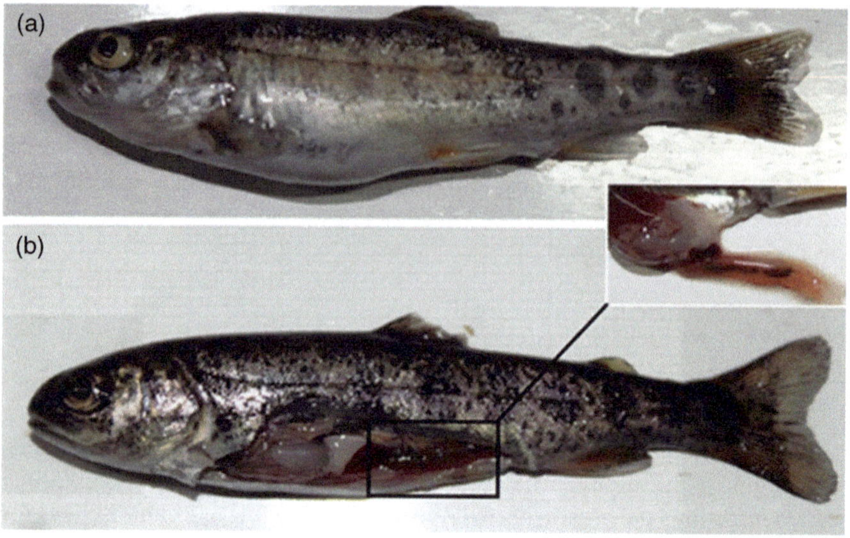

Figure 4.12 Gross lesions in infected rainbow trout with infectious pancreatic necrosis virus. (a) Abdominal distension. (b) Yellow mucoid fluid in the gastrointestinal tract. *Source:* Adapted from Zhu *et al.* (2017).

- Signs/diagnosis: Sudden and progressive increase in daily mortality is the first sign of an outbreak of infectious pancreatic necrosis in salmonid fry (Hill, 1982; Reno, 1999). Clinical signs of include behavioral changes ranging from lethargy to short bursts of corkscrew swimming interspersed with ataxia (Wood *et al.*, 1955). The affected fish exhibit a variety of clinical signs such as exophthalmia, darkening of skin, pronounced abdomen ascites (Figure 4.12a), pale gills, petechiae in the ventral area and at the base of the fins, and the presence of cast-like pseudofeces (Wolf, 1988). Internally, postmortems finding include pale and enlarged liver, kidney, spleen and heart, the presence of ascetic fluid in the body cavity, the presence of milky cohesive mucus in the lumen of the stomach and intestine (Figure 4.12b), and petechial hemorrhages throughout the visceral mass (Wolf, 1988).
- Differentials: Infectious pancreatic necrosis should be differentiated from other fish diseases that cause similar behavioral changes and clinical signs such as IHN, infectious salmon anemia, VHS, and salmonid alphavirus. Virus isolation and characterization by RT-PCR or immunofluorescence assays can differentiate IPNV from other similar diseases.
- Management: Rapid and sensitive diagnosis is essential to control the spread of the virus by restriction the movement of infected fish eggs, fingerlings, adults, and asymptomatic carriers. After an outbreak, all equipment and holding facilities should be disinfected to inactivate IPNV using ozone, iodine chlorine, or formalin (Economon, 1973; Hamor, 1996; Liltved *et al.*, 1995; Øye and Rimstad, 2001). Fertilized eggs must be originated from disease-free brood stock and a protected water supply such as a spring or borehole pond should be used. Vaccines designed for Atlantic salmon smolts after sea transfer are available but with unreliable results (Christie, 1997).
- See also Chapter 5 and the further information available in the website materials accompanying this text).

4.2.14 Salmonid Alphavirus

- Overview/etiology: Salmonid alphavirus is the causative agent of the two serious notifiable diseases pancreas disease and sleeping disease of farmed Atlantic salmon (*Salmo salar*) and rainbow trout (*Oncorhynchus mykiss*) in Europe (Boucher and Baudin-Laurencin, 1996; McLoughlin and Graham, 2007). Salmonid alphavirus is a spherical, enveloped, single-stranded positive-sense RNA virus with a 12 kb genome that belonging to genus *Alphavirus*, family Togaviridae (Strauss and Strauss, 1994; Weston *et al.*, 1999; Powers *et al.*, 2001). The salmonid alphavirus genome codes for eight proteins: four nonstructural proteins (nsP1–4) by the 5′ end and four structural capsid glycoproteins (E1, E2, E3 and 6K) by the 3′ end (Strauss and Strauss, 1994, Powers *et al.*, 2001). Based on the nucleic acid sequences of the proteins E2 and nsP3, six salmonid alphavirus subtypes have been identified (subtypes 1–6; Fringuelli *et al.*, 2008). The geographic distribution and species affected by each subtype are presented in Table S4.1 (online only). Subtype 2 is divided into two variants: the freshwater variant (SAV-2 FW), which typically causes sleeping disease (Graham *et al.*, 2007; Lewisch *et al.*, 2018; Deperasińska *et al.* 2018) and the marine variant, (SAV-2 MW), which typically causes pancreas disease (Jansen *et al.*, 2017). The other subtypes (SAV-1, 3, 4, 5 and 6) cause pancreas disease in seawater Atlantic salmon and rainbow trout (Deperasińska *et al.*, 2018; World Organisation for Animal Health, 2019).
- Host range and transmission: All life stages of Atlantic salmon and rainbow trout are susceptible to infection with salmonid alphavirus (Kerbart Boscher *et al.*, 2006; McVicar, 1990). Other fish species such as the Arctic charr (*Salvelinus alpinus*) and common dab (*Limanda limanda*) are susceptible to salmonid alphavirus (Bruno *et al.*, 2014; Lewisch *et al.*, 2018). However, salmonid alphavirus RNA was detected in tissues of some fish species with no signs of active infection, including brown trout (*Salmo trutta*), European flounder (*Platichthys flesus*), Argentine hake (*Merluccius hubbsi*), Norway pout (*Trisopterus esmarkii*), herring (*Clupea harengus*), haddock (*Melanogrammus aeglefinus*), sculpin species (*Myoxocephalus octodecemspinosus*), cod (*Gadus morhua*), saithe (*Pollachius virens*), and whiting (*Merlangius merlangus*; World Organisation for Animal Health, 2019).

  The mechanism of transmission appears to be horizontally via water currents (Graham *et al.*, 2007, 2012; Jansen *et al.*, 2010; Kristoffersen *et al.*, 2009; Viljugrein *et al.*, 2009) and movement of infected fish across longer distances (Kristoffersen *et al.*, 2009; Rodger and Mitchell, 2007). The possibility of vertical transmission is negligible (McLoughlin and Graham, 2007; Bratland and Nylund, 2009; Kongtorp *et al.*, 2010).
- Signs/diagnosis: Clinical signs are not pathognomonic. Outbreaks of salmonid alphavirus infection lead to increased mortality and reduced growth; they affect feed conversion and eventually lead to low product quality. Clinically diseased fish may be observed swimming slowly at the water surface, lying on their side on the bottom of the tank (sleeping), increased number of fecal casts, and in the later stages of disease, long slender fish (runts) with low condition are typically observed (Figure 4.13; McLoughlin *et al.*, 2002; McLoughlin and Graham, 2007). Postmortem changes, which are also not pathognomonic, include pale hearts or heart ruptures, small ascites, petechial hemorrhages, reddening of the pancreatic region between the pyloric caeca, and yellow mucoid gut contents (McLoughlin and Graham, 2007).
- Differentials: Careful diagnosis is necessary to determine the involvement of salmonid alphavirus and to rule out other pathogenic agents. Salmonid alphavirus diseases should be differentiated from infectious pancreatic necrosis, cardiomyopathy syndrome, and heart and skeletal muscle inflammation. Virus isolation in cell culture and then characterization by RT-PCR or

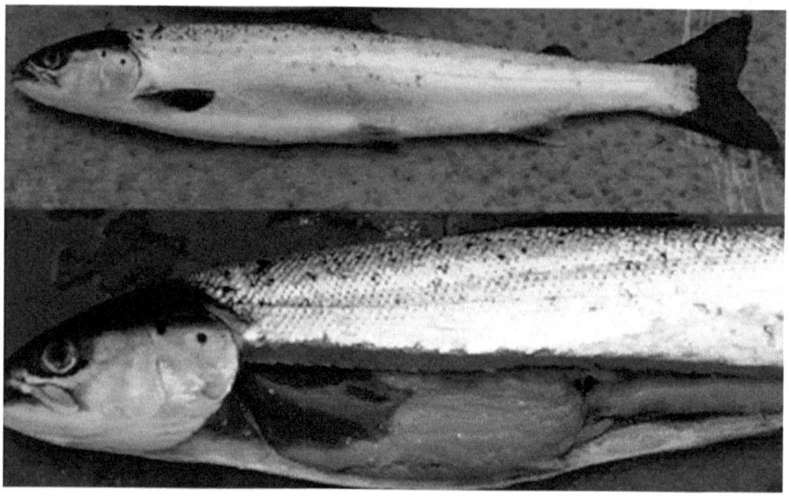

Figure 4.13 Salmonid alphavirus subtype 1-infected Atlantic salmon. A typical pancreas disease runt fish with minimal body and caecal fat. *Source:* photograph courtesy of Tom Turnbull. Adapted from McLoughlin and Graham (2007) with permission.

immunofluorescence assay can differentiate salmonid alphavirus from IPNV and piscine myocarditis virus, the causative agents of salmonid alphavirus and cardiomyopathy syndrome, respectively. The histopathological lesions in the heart and red skeletal muscles in the absence of histopathological changes in the pancreas distinguish heart and skeletal muscle inflammation from salmonid alphavirus.

- Management: Biosecurity protocols play an important role in preventing disease outbreaks and the spread of pathogens both on and between farms. A high level of site biosecurity should be maintained, with emphasis on personnel visitors and equipment. Salmonid alphavirus was rapidly inactivated after five-minute exposure to pH 4 or 12, or after one hour of exposure to 60°C (Graham *et al.*, 2007). Common disinfectants such as Virex®, Virkon-S®, or chloramine-T are effective in the inactivation of salmonid alphavirus. Management strategy also includes monitoring of pancreas disease and sleeping disease using sensitive diagnostic tools for early detection and application of control measures. DNA-based and virus-inactivated vaccines against salmonid alphavirus are commercially available, which can be used as a preventive measure.
- See also Chapter 5 and the further information available in the website materials accompanying this text).

4.2.15 Infectious Salmon Anemia

- Overview: Infectious salmon anemia is a serious notifiable disease of sea-farmed Atlantic salmon (*Salmo salar*) characterized by severe anemia, variable hemorrhages, and necrosis in several organs (Thorud and Djupvik, 1988). The causative agent was isolated and identified as infectious salmon anemia virus (ISAV), which belongs to the genus *Isavirus*, family Orthomyxoviridae (Dannevig *et al.*, 1995). ISAV is an enveloped virus, with a genome consisting of eight single-stranded, negative-sense RNA segments (Mjaaland *et al.*, 1997). There are two major lineages of ISAV: the European genotype (genotype I) and the North American genotype (genotype II; Blake *et al.*, 1999; Kibenge *et al.*, 2001). The European genotype is more widespread and shows greater genetic variation and virulence variation than the North American genotype (Kibenge *et al.*, 2006, 2007, 2009; Nylund *et al.*, 2007; Christiansen *et al.*, 2011). Within these genotypes there are various clades. A highly polymorphic region (HPR) of the viral hemagglutinin esterase on viral segment 6 can be used to classify ISAV into numbered groups (Kibenge *et al.*, 2009). The presence of a nonpathogenic HPR0 ISAV genome has been reported in both apparently healthy wild and farmed Atlantic salmon, but has not been detected in diseased fish, with clinical disease and pathological signs consistent with infectious salmon anemia (Cunningham *et al.*, 2002; McBeath *et al.*, 2009; Nylund *et al.*, 2007; Christiansen *et al.*, 2011; Lyngstad *et al.*, 2012).

- Host range and transmission: Based on the World Organisation for Animal Health (2019) criteria, Atlantic salmon, brown trout (*S. trutta*) and rainbow trout (*Oncorhynchus mykiss*) are susceptible hosts for ISAV. Several cases have been reported in freshwater stages of Atlantic salmon, but most outbreaks are reported in seawater cages (Nylund *et al.*, 2003; Rimstad *et al.*, 2011). Subclinical infections have been reported from amago trout (*Oncorhynchus masou*) and Atlantic herring (*Clupea harengus*), also the virus was isolated from coho salmon (*Oncorhynchus kisutch*).

  In marine environment, infectious salmon anemia can be transmitted by cohabitation with infected live fish or infected biological materials which establish reservoirs of infection (Vagsholm *et al.*, 1994; Shannon, 1998; Murray *et al.*, 2002). Horizontal transmission is likely to be occur in both marine and fresh water environments by direct contact, fish to fish, or indirectly in water, or on fomites as the virion shed with gut content, mucus, blood, and urine (Totland *et al.*, 1996; Rolland and Nylund, 1998). Vertical transmission of the ISAV has not been demonstrated (Melville and Griffiths, 1999). Sea lice (*Caligus elongatus* and *Lepeophtheirus salmonis*) could increase the susceptibility of fish to infectious salmon anemia by increasing stress, and may also act as mechanical vectors during epidemics (Nyland *et al.*, 1994). As ISAV can infect fresh water brown trout, sea trout, and rainbow trout without producing disease, these fish species act as carriers and serve as a reservoir for ISAV (Nylund *et al.*, 1995a, 1997; Nylund and Jakobsen, 1995; Rolland and Nylund, 1999).
- Signs/diagnosis: Infectious salmon anemia is characterized by high mortality with exophthalmia, pale gills due to anemia, ascites, darkened skin, and jaundice on the ventral portion of the body (Thorud, 1991). Postmortem lesions include an enlarged and congested spleen; enlarged, congested liver, in some cases covered with thin layer of fibrin; dark, swollen kidney; congested gastrointestinal tract without free blood in the lumen; yellow or blood-tinged fluid may be found in the peritoneal cavity and pericardial cavity, and petechiae in various organs, visceral fat and the skeletal muscles (Figure 4.14; Hovland *et al.*, 1994; Thorud and Djupvik, 1988; Evensen *et al.*, 1991).
- Diferentials: Infectious salmon anemia should be differentiated from other fish diseases that causes septicemia and anemia, such as winter ulcer, vibriosis, furunculosis and VHS. Bacterial isolation and identification can differentiate from the Gram-negative bacteria, such as *Vibrio* spp., the causative agent of vibriosis, *Aeromonas salmonicida*, the causative agent of furunculosis and *Moritella viscosa*, the causative agent of winter ulcer disease. Isolation of the ISAV in specific cell culture and identification by RT-PCR or immunofluorescence can differentiate ISAV from VHS.
- Management: Vaccination against infectious salmon anemia has been carried out in North America since 1999 and in the Faroe Islands since 2005. In Norway, vaccination was carried out for the first time in 2009 in a region with a high rate of outbreaks. Chile started vaccinating

(a)

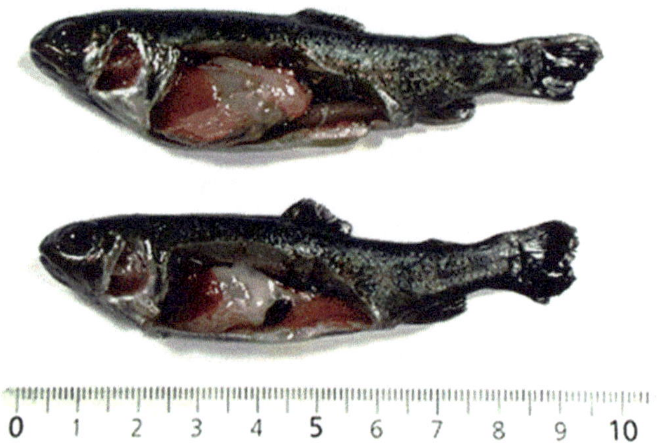

(b)

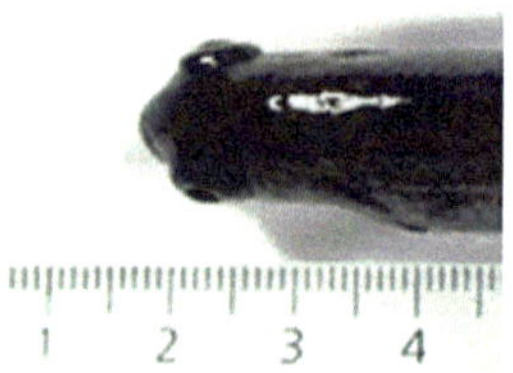

Figure 4.14 (a) Lesions of infectious salmon anemia in experimentally infected rainbow trout (clone A22, mean weight 6.2 g) by the waterborne route (bottom): note the pale gills, dark liver, moderate splenomegaly and scarce petechiae. The upper fish is a mock-infected control. (b) Exophthalmos in diseased fish. *Source:* Adapted from Biacchesi *et al.* (2007) with permission.

against infectious salmon anemia in 2010. The strategy to control infection involves screening brood fish and conducting proper egg disinfection, destruction of infected populations, disinfection and fallowing of contaminated sites, control of ships/wellboats and personnel movement among sites, trials for selection of infectious salmon anemia-resistant Atlantic salmon strain (Eide, 1992; Hill, 1994; Nylund *et al.*, 1995b; Dahle *et al.*, 1996; Jarp and Karlsen, 1997; Mullins, 1998; Murray, 2001). Variety of disinfectants can inactivate ISAV including ultraviolet C irradiation, ozone, extremely acid (pH 4) or basic (pH 12), Virkon® S, sodium hypochlorite, chlorine dioxide, formaldehyde, formic acid, iodophor, and chloramine-T when used according to the manufacturer's instructions (Smail *et al.*, 2001; Rimstad *et al.*, 2011).

- See also Chapter 5 and the further information available in the website materials accompanying this text).

4.2.16 Viral Erythrocytic Necrosis Virus

- Overview: Viral erythrocytic necrosis is also known as piscine erythrocytic necrosis, classified as an iridovirus (Emmenegger *et al.*, 2014). The disease was observed in the late 1960s and was first reported in Atlantic cod (*Gadus morhua*; Laird and Bullock, 1969). The disease can cause severe blood abnormalities, and is characterized by destruction of red blood cells and the presence of cytoplasmic inclusion bodies within affected erythrocytes, leading to anemia. The virus particles have icosahedral symmetry, 150–360 nm, depending on the fish species. Viral erythrocytic necrosis has been observed in several marine and anadromous species in the North Atlantic and North Pacific oceans. The infection can cause mortality in both farmed and wild fish populations. It is not considered as an economically important infection for aquaculture. The severity of disease can range from a benign infection to a highly fatal disease associated with osmoregulatory difficulties, loss of stamina, and greater susceptibility to secondary infections or environmental stressors.

- Host range and transmission: The host range and geographic distribution is widely diverse. Although primarily reported from salmonoids and herring, the host range extends to more than 20 species. Marine and anadromous species like Atlantic cod, coho, chum, pink, and Chinook salmon, and steelhead trout have been reported as naturally susceptible to the disease. Disease outbreaks periodically occur in populations of Pacific herring, particularly juveniles. Geographically, the virus has been found in the North Atlantic and North Pacific oceans, around Taiwan and the UK. In the Mediterranean area, the infection also has been detected in wild and reared European sea bass (*Dicentrarchus labrax*). In addition, molecular analysis showed that the virus is closely aligned to erythrocytic iridoviruses that infect terrestrial reptiles. Horizontal transmission may be the main route of spread, and fish surviving the infection are considered to become carriers to young fish. Although vertical transmission has not been reported, some studies have shown that the fry of infected bloodstock can also be affected. Vector-borne transmission should also be considered.
- Signs/diagnosis: Juvenile fish are more susceptible to disease and the inclusion bodies can be observed in peripheral erythrocytes within the two to seven days. External signs are not precise. The clinical signs in affected fish are related to anemia and the ensuing disruption of physiology and homeostasis. Pale gills are evident on examination and the hematocrit (packed red blood cell volume) can be dramatically reduced to 10% over several weeks, as a result of severe blood dyscrasias. Pale heart, liver, and gastrointestinal tract have been reported in experimentally infected Pacific salmon. The disease is currently diagnosed by microscopic examination of Giemsa-stained blood smears, when darkly stained intracytoplasmic inclusion bodies in erythrocytes and erythroblasts are observed (Figure 4.15). Pyknosis and karyorrhexis can also be seen in affected erythrocytes. Transmission electron microscopy is used to confirm the presence of icosahedral virions in the cytoplasm of affected erythrocytes. The immunofluorescence antibody test can be used, as well. High-throughput sequencing technologies are used for rapid, sensitive, and specific identification, since the virus has not been isolated in cell cultures.
- Differentials: The presence of an iridovirus in the cytoplasm of affected erythrocytes can be used to differentiate from protozoan of blood cells or staining artifacts. Erythrocytic inclusion body syndrome (EIBS) should also be considered a differential diagnosis. It is caused by an RNA virus with icosahedral virions that are 80 nm in diameter. Acridine orange staining provides an indirect differential. With this test, the DNA of erythrocytic necrosis virus emits a green color whereas that of EIBS emits red. Piscine orthoreovirus causes similar lesions with EIBS in experimentally infected fish, and a specific PCR assay is available to differentiate from EIBS.
- Management: There is no effective therapy or vaccine for this disease. Currently, general husbandry (implementing biosecurity measures, minimizing handling/transportation, avoiding adverse environmental conditions such as low dissolved oxygen or low salinity and other stressors), as well as ensuring appropriate diagnosis, treatment, and control can reduce the losses due to viral erythrocytic necrosis. Sustained blood monitoring is an important tool to avoid any possible transmission from broodstock to their offspring. Potential risks related to subclinical infections should be considered (screening with adequate sample size and separation of infected fish from the rest) during international trading.
- For Vacuolating encephalopathy and retinopathy virus/nodavirus disease go online:
- For Heart and Skeletal Muscle Inflammation & Cardiomyopathy Syndrome (CMS) go online:
- For Largemouth bass virus disease go online:

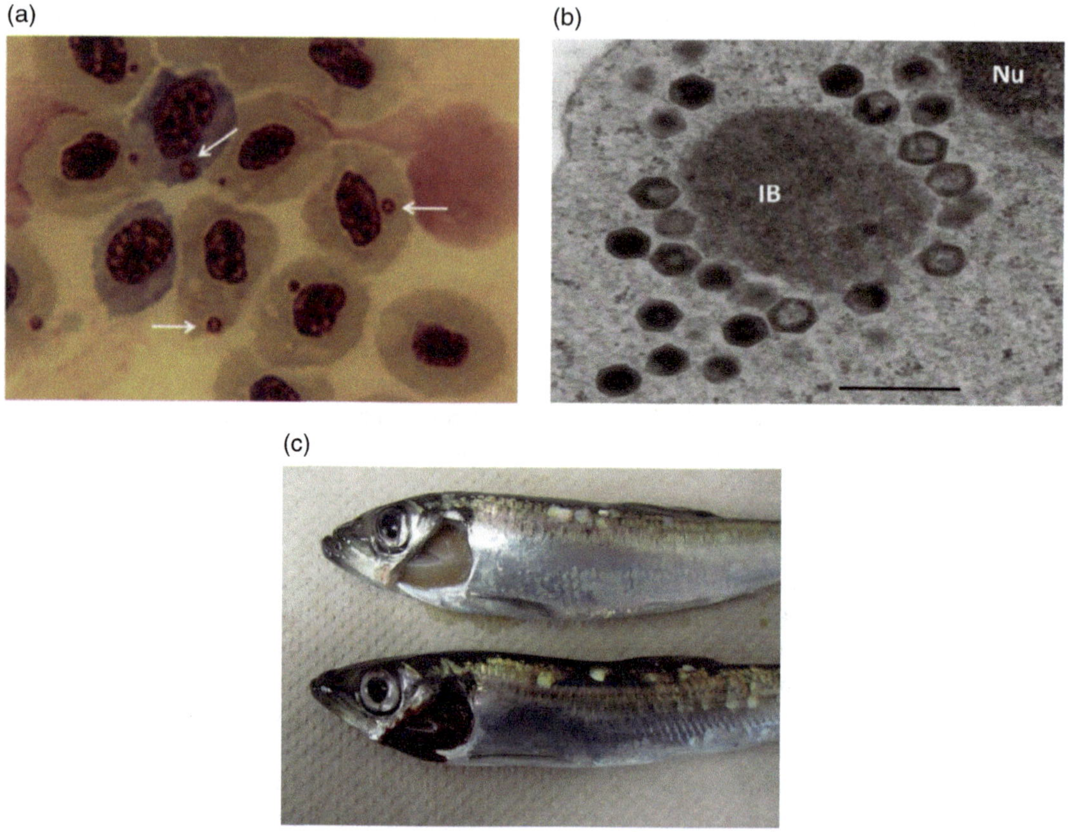

Figure 4.15 Anatomy and histopathology of erythrocytic necrosis virus in a Pacific herring. (a) Giemsa stain. (b) Electron micrograph of a virus inclusion body (IB). (c) *Source:* Glenn *et al.* 2012.

- For Red Sea bream Iridovirus disease go online:
- For Yellowtail Ascites Virus disease go online:

4.2.17 Channel Catfish Virus Disease

- Overview/Etiology: An alphaherpesvirus (*Herpesvirus ictaluri*) that causes severe mortality in juvenile (fry/fingerling) channel catfish above 25°C.
- Host range and transmission: Channel catfish adults can be infected, but typically do not show signs. Blue catfish and channel x blue hybrids are mildly susceptible. Horizontal and vertical transmission. The virus enters through the gills and gut, spreading throughout the body. Virus remains viable in pond water at 25°C for 2 days, but is rapidly inactivated in pond mud and by desiccation.
- Signs/diagnosis: Abdominal distention, exophthalmia, skin and gill hemorrhage, erratic swimming. Visceral hyperemia and hemorrhage and splenomegaly are evident. Kidney culture on channel catfish ovary or brown bullhead cells produces a cytopathic effect; PCR and other methods can confirm.
- Differentials: Enteric septicemia of catfish (edwardsiellosis), aeromonad septicemia, water quality issues, toxicosis.
- Management: Testing of brood stock, use of resistant lines or hybrid catfish are recommended. Quarantine and destruction of infected stock prior to importation is necessary.
- For Grass Carp Haemorrhagic disease go online:

4.2.18 Spinning Tilapia Syndrome

- Etiology: Tilapia syndrome is caused by an iridovirus.
- Host range and transmission: The disease causes high mortality in several tilapia species (especially in young fish), in the Mozambique, blue, Nile and mango tilapias. Transmission is horizontal.
- Signs/diagnosis: Fry swim erratically, sink to the bottom and rise to just below the surface, and gasp for air. Infected fish are anorexic. Spinning fish die within a day, and mortality may be 100% within 60 days. Histology shows renal tubular necrosis and muscle necrosis. Diagnosis is by clinical signs and electron microscopy.
- Differentials: Sepsis, water quality issues, parasites, or other viruses.
- Management: None. Strict quarantine.

4.2.19 Tilapia Lake Virus

- Overview: Tilapia lake virus is an emerging severe viral pathogen of farmed tilapia. The only virus in its family, it is an enveloped RNA virus, discovered in a mass mortality event in Israel, in 2009. There is high mortality (20–90%), peaking in one to two weeks. Other pathogens, including *Aeromonas* spp., are often isolated with the virus.
- Host range and transmission: All species of tilapia, and other species including giant gourami and river barb; all ages. The virus is present throughout southern Asia, India, Lake Victoria, Egypt, Israel, South America, and Mexico.
- Signs/diagnosis: Swimming at the surface. Ascites, exophthalmos, cataracts, lepidorthosis, skin ulcers, hyperemia of fins and skin. Histology shows marked hepatocyte syncytia. Virus is present in many tissues, especially in the cranial kidney and spleen. Viral culture of brain in E-11 cells shows cytopathic effects in 3–5 days. PCR will confirm the infection.
- Differentials: Sepsis, water quality issues, toxicosis, spinning tilapia syndrome.
- Management: Strict biosecurity.

4.2.20 Spring Viremia of Carp

- Brief overview: Spring viremia of carp, also known as infectious ascites or infectious dropsy is a World Organisation for Animal Health reportable disease. It is a rhabdovirus which causes acute severe hemorrhagic disease in carp and cyprinids. There is high mortality from this disease. Disease is related to the immune response of the fish, which is temperature dependent; outbreaks occur at 5–18°C (41–65°F). Outbreaks occur in the spring, tapering off above 20°C. At 25°C and above, the virus cannot be isolated from fish populations.
- Host range and transmission: Many species of carp, including koi, and goldfish, tench, sheatfish, pike, and possibly other species as well can die from natural infection. It has been isolated in penaeid shrimp (rhabdovirus of penaeid shrimp) and has worldwide distribution. All ages are affected, but young fish (less than one year) are more susceptible to disease. The virus enters the gill, and spreads systemically. Virus is shed in the feces.
- Signs/diagnosis: Fish are lethargic. Ascites, skin hemorrhage, exophthalmia (Figure 4.16), gill pallor, visceral petechiation are present. Submit kidney, spleen, gill, and/or brain from fish (or entire fish/visceral mass from smaller specimens) for virus isolation and PCR. Virus often cannot be isolated from survivors of prior outbreaks or in fish at temperatures greater than 20°C. Antibody testing for prior exposure has been reported.
- Differentials: Herpesvirus, viral hemorrhagic septicemia, bacterial sepsis.
- Management: None. Depopulate. Vaccines are not currently available.

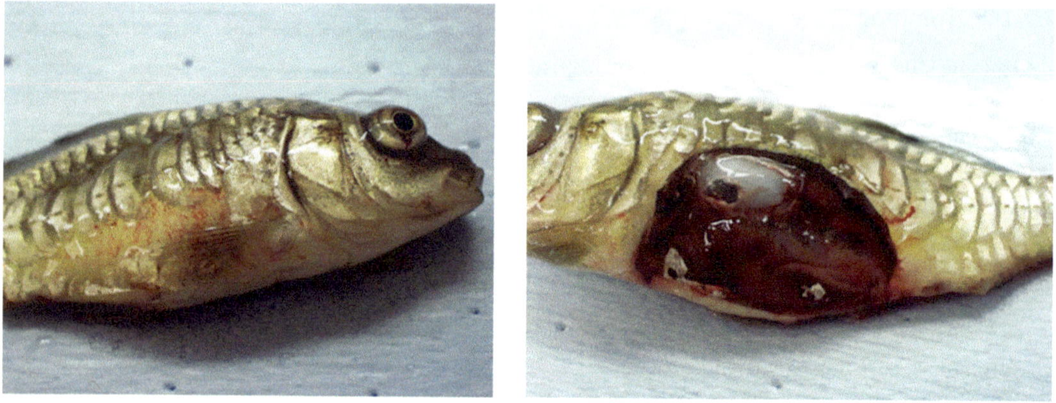

Figure 4.16 Spring viremia of carp, skin hemorrhage and exophthalmos (left), internal hemorrhage (right). *Source:* Andy Goodwin.

4.2.21 Cyprinid Herpesvirus 1

- Brief overview: Cyprinid herpesvirus 1 (also known as herpesviral epidermal hyperplasia, carp pox, or fish papillomavirus) is a mild viral skin infection that causes epidermal hyperplasia.
- Host range and transmission: *Cyprinus carpio* and hybrids can develop disease, but not goldfish. Horizontal spread is highest at 14–18°C (57–64°F), with regression above 20°C (68°F).
- Signs/diagnosis: Smooth, milky, flat lesions (candlewax droplets) develop and may coalesce or become papillomatous (Figure 4.17). They are often seen on the fins. Lesions typically regress and recur and can persist for months. Fatalities in juveniles and adults have been reported in experimental infections, but rarely in nature. Infection in very young fry may cause high mortality. Virus isolation, histopathology for diagnosis.
- Differentials: Neoplasia, granulomatous disease, parasite infection.
- Management: Raise temperatures above 20°C.

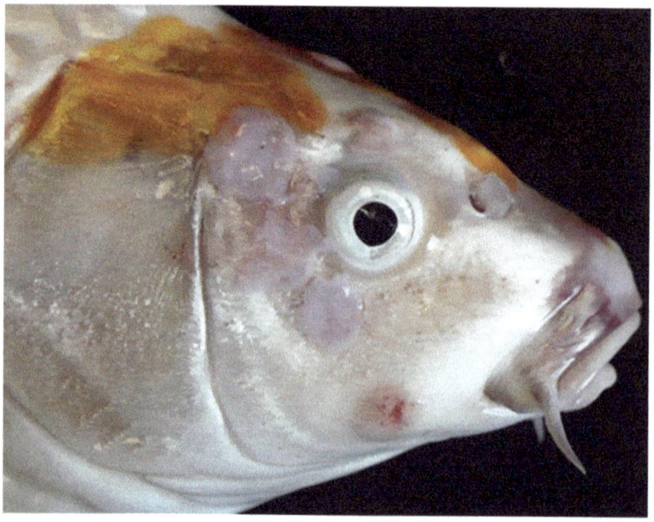

Figure 4.17 Cyprinid herpesvirus 1 (carp pox). *Source:* Andy Goodwin.

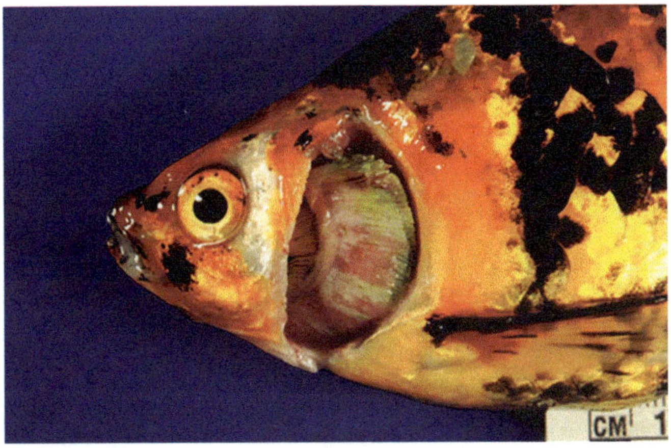

Figure 4.18 Cyprinid herpesvirus 2 gill swelling/necrosis, hyphema. *Source:* Wes Baumgartner.

4.2.22 Cyprinid Herpesvirus 2

- Brief overview: Cyprinid herpesvirus 2 is also known as goldfish herpesvirus, goldfish hematopoietic necrosis virus, and is a severe viral pathogen of *Carassius auratus* (goldfish).
- Host range and transmission: Worldwide, only goldfish and gibel carp are affected. Goldfish–carp hybrids can become infected, but they do not show clinical signs.
- Signs/diagnosis: Fish become lethargic, anorexic, and may die, depending on the temperature. Ascites, pale, swollen gills (Figure 4.18), and splenomegaly have been reported, with high mortality in some cases. Disease occurs at 15–28°C (59–82°F) and regresses above 28°C. Mortalities are highest around 20°C (68°F), and lower at each end of the temperature spectrum. Fish infected at just below 15°C are resistant to disease. Those that recover become carriers to infect naive fish. Histopathology, PCR (kidney/spleen) for diagnosis. Fish that are positive for cyprinid herpesvirus 2 may be merely carriers and are not dying of acute infection; other etiologies/agents need to be ruled out before a confirmed diagnosis is made.
- Differentials: Spring viremia of carp, hemoparasites (*Trypanosoma danilewskyi*), ectoparasites, water quality issues, bacterial sepsis.
- Management: Alter the temperature away from the 20°C zone.

4.2.23 Cyprinid Herpesvirus 3

- Overview: Cyprinid herpesvirus 3, or koi herpesvirus, is a World Organisation for Animal Health reportable disease. It is a highly contagious disease of carp and koi in particular. It has a worldwide distribution but only *C. carpio* develops the disease, which has a high morbidity and mortality. It is a temperature-dependent disease (16–28°C, 60–80°F). Survivors become carriers and are resistant to further disease episodes.
- Host range and transmission: *C. carpio*, goldfish (*Carassius auratus*), and grass carp can harbor the virus. Horizontal transmission is via mucus, feces, and other animals in the pond.
- Signs/diagnosis: Lethargy, gill necrosis, excessive mucus, skin hemorrhage, visceral hemorrhage/necrosis (Figure 4.19). Secondary infection of gills by bacteria and parasites may be evident. Tissue PCR (gill, kidney, spleen). Carrier status may be determined by tissue PCR or serology (UC-Davis VMTH).

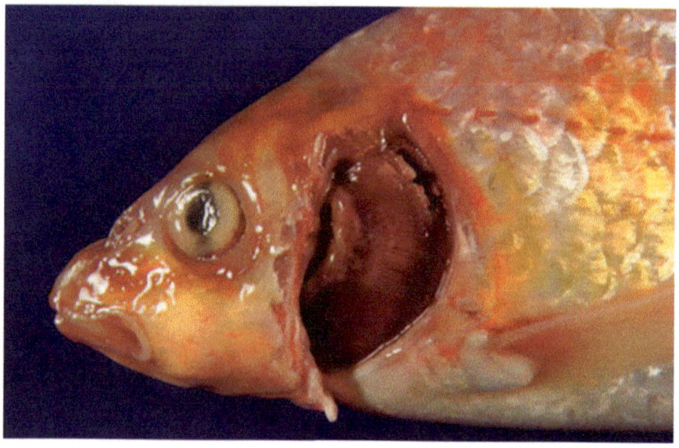

Figure 4.19 Cyprinid herpesvirus 3 gill necrosis (koi herpesvirus). *Source:* Wes Baumgartner.

- Differentials: Spring viremia of carp, *Flavobacterium*, water quality issues, bacterial sepsis, parasites.
- Management: Avoid exposure. Raise water temperature above 28°C to reduce mortality. Saline salt baths (0.1–0.3%) can be used to reduce stress. Depopulate and disinfect the system.

4.3 Parasitic Diseases

4.3.1 Amoebic Gill Disease

- Overview and etiology: Amoebic gill disease, caused by the free-living amphizoic marine amoeba *Neoparamoeba perurans* was first identified in Australia in the mid-1980s, and is the main health issue in a number of aquaculture industries mainly affecting farmed Atlantic salmon (*Salmo salar*) during the marine phase, where it can result in considerable mortalities. It causes grossly visible multifocal gill hyperplasia, which requires multiple treatments. The clinical manifestation, treatment and other consequences, such as reduced food conversion and downgrading, are a considerable burden on economic production and welfare. It is considered one of the main contributors to the recently recognized complex gill disease (Rozas-Serri, 2019).
- Host range and distribution: Amoebic gill disease has been reported from 14 salmon producing countries including Norway, Ireland, France, Scotland, Chile, North America, Canada, and Spain, and it is the most significant health problem in Tasmanian Atlantic salmon culture and possibly in Ireland and Scotland. The disease has affected at least 15 species, including rainbow trout (*Oncorhynchus mykiss*), coho salmon (*O. kisutch*), turbot (*Scophthalmus maximus*), European sea bass (*Dicentrarchus labrax*), halibut (*Hippoglossus hippoglossus*), sharpsnout sea bream (*Diplodus puntazzo*), and more recently, corkwing wrasse (*Symphodus melops*), Ballan wrasse (*Labrus bergylta*) and lumpfish (*Cyclopterus lumpus*), used for controlling the sea lice (*Lepeophtheirus salmonis*) in European salmon culture.
- Signs/diagnosis: The disease initially presents as lethargy, anorexia, congregating near the surface, and increased opercular movements and ventilation. *N. perurans* only colonizes healthy gill tissue and causes a proliferative reaction resulting in grossly visible branchitis characterized by raised, multifocal pale to white mucoid plaques distributed across the gills. These changes can be scored 0–5

(Taylor *et al.*, 2009) to help in determining when to treat the fish. Histopathology is required for definitive diagnosis and reveals minor to severe epithelial hyperplasia of the primary and secondary lamellae, hypertrophy, edema, and secondary lamellar fusion and interlamellar vesicle formation. Gill damage in turn can lead to compromised respiration, osmoregulation, nitrogenous waste excretion, and acid–base balance (Adams *et al.*, 2004). Risk factors may include changes in salinity in the water body, increased stocking density, cage environment (e.g. number of times the nets were changed) and removal of mortalities (*N. perurans* can survive for 30 hours on a dead fish, can replicate and is capable of infecting others during that period). Severely affected fish may also suffer from hypernatremia, and it is possible that vascular hypertension caused by amoebic gill disease may elicit cardiac changes, including ventricular hypertrophy and hyperplasia of the compact layer, suggesting that clinically affected fish may suffer from cardiac pathology (Powell *et al.*, 2002).

- Differentials: Any gill insult causing grossly visible foci of pallor. While history and appearance of white mucoid patches may suggest amoebic gill disease, histopathology or further testing (PCR, in-situ hybridization) is required to confirm.
- Management: The most commercially effective treatment for amoebic gill disease is freshwater bathing, usually for a minimum of two hours, but this is stressful on the fish and, for some, imposes significant cost and management difficulties. The supply of very large volumes of freshwater is problematic. The osmotic difference during bathing removes gill mucus and associated amoeba and promotes rapid healing of gill lesions (Munday *et al.*, 2001). Treatment with fresh water has been reported to have an 86% efficacy and amoeba numbers can recover after approximately 10 days. Amoeba only infect healthy tissue. Other treatments have been trialed with mixed success, including hydrogen peroxide, levamisole and chloramine-T. Water chemistry affects efficacy and some treatments are bactericidal in nature and do not combat the amoeba directly. Managing the problem includes regular prophylactic freshwater baths, which are viewed as being unsustainable in the long term, use of low salinity sites, single age group sites, and reducing stocking density to reduce the number of susceptible hosts.

4.3.2 Dinoflagellate Infestation (*Amyloodinium* spp., *Piscinoodinium* spp.)

- Brief overview: Dinoflagellates are common in aquatic systems and they are largely non-parasitic to fish. Five genera affect fish directly, while others may produce toxins that cause mortalities. *Amyloodinium*, *Piscinoodinium*, *Crepidoodinium*, *Ichthyodinium*, and *Oodinoides* species are known fish parasites.
- Host range and transmission: *A. ocellatum* causes significant disease in brackish and marine warmwater food fish (over 100 species), as well as aquarium fish (including elasmobranchs). *Piscinoodinium* species cause similar disease in tropical freshwater fish. *I. chabelardi* parasitizes the eggs of Atlantic sardines, and it may be an important cause of larval mortality. In all species, the parasitic trophont stage (Figure 4.20) feeds on the skin and gills, causing damage; an encysted tomont stage develops in the environment, producing the free-swimming and infective dinospores, which have flagella.
- Signs/diagnosis: Fish infected with *A. ocellatum* are anorexic, dyspneic, and pruritic. The gills are most heavily infected, but the skin is also affected. In heavy infestations, the skin appears dusty (velvet disease) but fish often die without apparent lesions. *Piscinoodinium* causes freshwater velvet disease, similar to *A. ocellatum*. Diagnosis can be made by examining fish with indirect light in a darkened room to highlight the organisms. Skin and gill wet mounts will show trophonts or tomonts (Figure 4.21), which may congregate in the sediment. Freshwater dips can dislodge them from marine fish, while saltwater baths can dislodge *Piscinoodinium*.

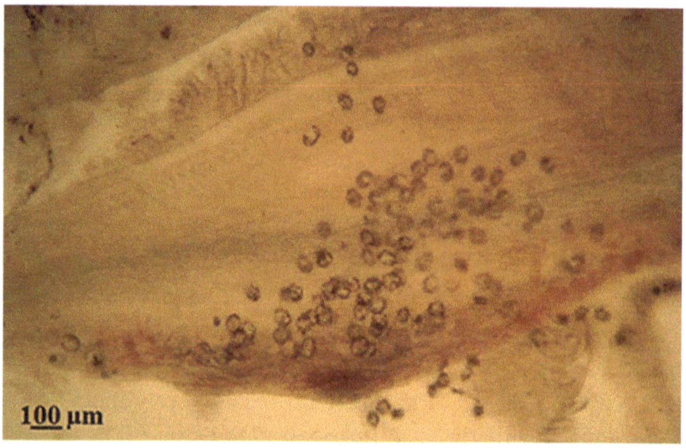

Figure 4.20 Fresh preparation showing trophonts of *Amyloodinium ocellatum* attached to the gills of infected fish. *Source:* Yemmen and Bahri (2017).

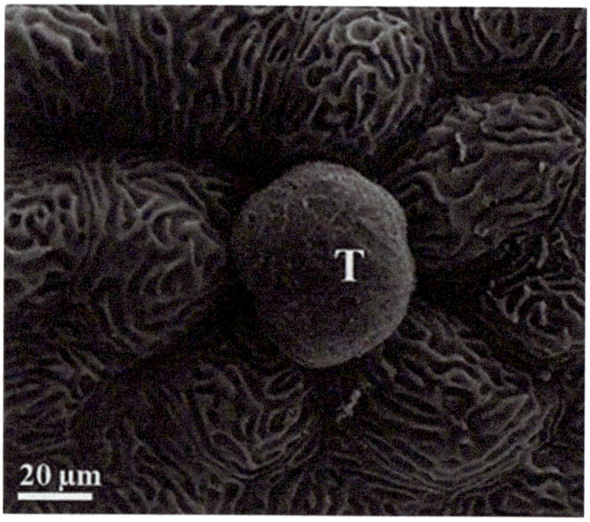

Figure 4.21 Scanning electron microscopy microphotograph showing the location of *Amyloodinium ocellatum* trophont (T) on the gill filaments of *Solea senegalensis*. *Source:* Yemmen and Bahri (2017).

- Differentials: *Ichthyophthirius* (Ich), other external parasites.
- Management: *A. ocellatum*: The dinospore stage is susceptible to treatment. Chloroquine diphosphate is highly effective (10 days' exposure to single water treatment, 5–10 mg/l), but is toxic to invertebrates and cannot be used in reef tanks. Copper is often used to treat, and free copper levels must be maintained at 0.12–0.15 mg/l for 10–14 days. *Piscinoodinium*: salt (1 tsp NaCl/5 gallons) for 10–14 days, or 35 mg/l NaCl dips for one to three minutes can dislodge trophonts.

4.3.3 Diplomonad Infection (*Hexamita/Spironucleus*)

- Brief overview: These flagellated protozoans are found on the skin, gills, digestive tract, and blood of fish (systemic infections). *Hexamita* and *Spironucleus* (hexamitids) are often seen in the gut, and have direct life cycles. They are sometimes associated with disease outbreaks, with mortalities in cyprinids, eels, tropical aquarium fish, and salmon.
- Host range and transmission: Transmission is direct. Distribution is worldwide.

- Signs/diagnosis: Emaciation, weakness, abdominal distension, anemia, fecal casts, ascites, mucoid enteritis. In salmonids, the upper intestine may be severely affected, with spread to other organs, including muscle and skin (ulcers). In aquarium fish, gastroenteritis may develop. Fecal exam or necropsy to examine the upper intestine. Head and lateral line erosion syndrome has been associated with diplomonad infections. Cases with high numbers (15–30 organisms per low power microscope field) in wet mounts may need treatment. Examination of blood and other organs are needed to verify a systemic infection. Hexamitid trophozoites are pyriform and are 5–20 microns wide.
- Differentials: Other parasites, bacterial enteritis.
- Management: Metronidazole baths in aquarium fish. Improve water quality, magnesium sulfate in salmonids.

4.3.4 Diplomonad Infection (*Ichthyobodo*)

- Brief overview: These flagellated protozoans are found on the skin, gills, digestive tract, and blood of fish (systemic infections). *Ichthyobodo necator*, previously known as *Costia necatrix*, is an ectoparasite of freshwater and marine fishes. The organism attaches to skin and gills and, if present in sufficient numbers, can induce mortality. A free-swimming form attaches to fish, where it multiplies by binary fission.
- Host range and transmission: Transmission is direct. Distribution is worldwide.
- Signs/diagnosis: Sudden death, increased mucus, flashing, epithelial hyperplasia (bluish skin; Figure 4.22). Wet mounts of skin and gills will show the attached forms, which are ovoid and flattened with a crescentic curve; they are 5–20 microns wide. Organisms quickly leave dead hosts, so examination of moribund fish is preferable.
- Differentials: Other external parasites, poor water quality, toxin exposure.
- Management: Formalin baths or flush treatment (do not use if fish have bacterial gill disease), copper sulfate. Pond treatments may be necessary, including drainage and liming. The organism dies at temperatures above 30°C.

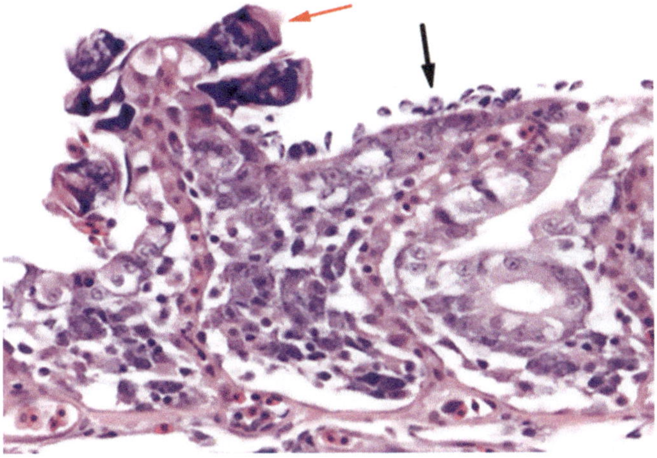

Figure 4.22 Channel catfish gill, hyperplastic branchitis with *Ichthyobodo* (black arrow) and sessile solitary ectocommensal ciliates (red arrow). *Source:* W. Baumgartner.

4.3.5 Diplomonad Infection (*Cryptobia* spp., *Trypanosoma* spp.)

- Brief overview: These flagellated protozoans are found on the skin, gills, and blood of fish (*Trypanosoma*). *Cryptobia* are weak pathogens and are somewhat similar to *Ichthyobodo*. Trypanosomes are common in the wild, but uncommon in farmed fish, and may be associated with mortalities. *C. iubilans* is a common disease of cichlids, causing gastritis (Figures 4.23, 4.24, 4.25).
- Host range and transmission: Transmission is direct for *Cryptobia*, while trypanosomes and some species of *Cryptobia* are spread by leeches. Distribution is worldwide.
- Signs/diagnosis: For skin-infecting species, flashing and increased mucus are evident; wet mounts can diagnose. For hematozoic species, fish exhibit splenomegaly, ascites, anemia; blood smears are used. For cichlids, necropsy and examination of the stomach for granulomatous disease and organisms in the mucus are necessary.
- Differentials: Other parasites (skin infection), causes of anemia, bacterial enteritis (cichlids).
- Management: Vaccines have been developed in salmonids and trout.

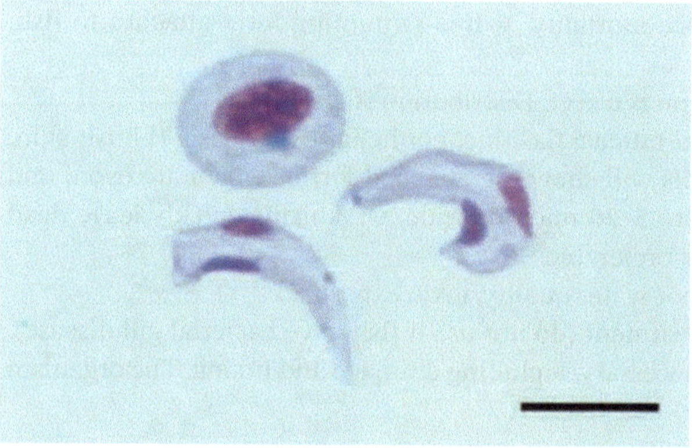

Figure 4.23 *Cryptobia* (*Trypanoplasma*) *salmositica* with red blood cells from an experimentally infected rainbow trout (*Oncorhynchus mykiss*; Giemsa: bar = 10 μm). *Source:* Woo (2003).

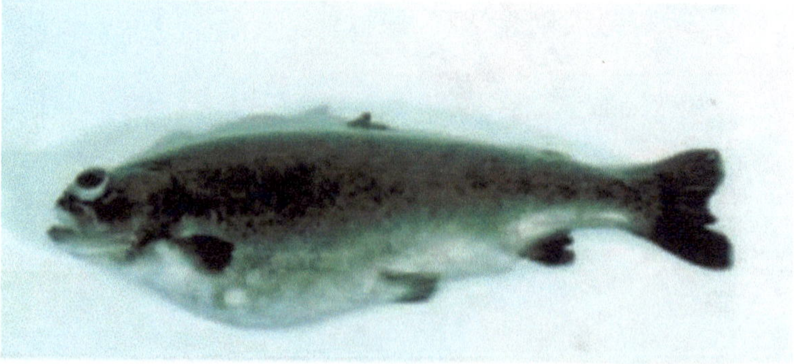

Figure 4.24 General edema with abdominal distension and ascites during acute experimental disease in rainbow trout (*Oncorhynchus mykiss*). *Source:* Woo (2003).

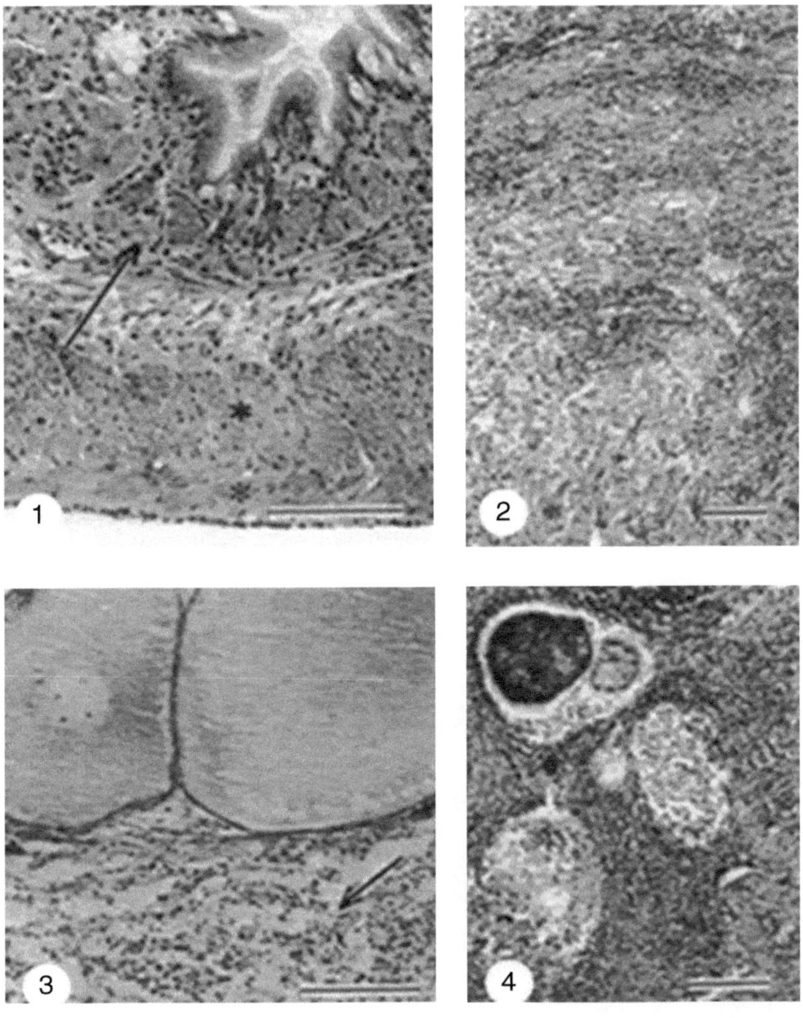

Figure 4.25 Section through the stomach wall of uninfected *Cichlasoma biocellatum*. (1) A layer of gastric glands (arrow) and *lamina muscularis* (asterisk); hematoxylin and eosin (H&E) stain, bar 100 pm. (2) Inflammatory changes in the subepithelial layer and *lamina propria* of a heavily infected specimen of *Cichlasoma meeki*. H&E, bar = 100 pm. (3) A mass of intercellularly occurring cryptobias (arrow) in the *tunica albuginea* covering the ovary. Giemsa stain, bar = 100 pm. (4): Granulomatous inflammatory changes in the intestinal wall reaching as deep as muscularis. H&E stain, bar = 100 pm.

4.3.6 Ciliate Infestation 1: Ich and Marine Ich (*Ichthyophthirius multifiliis*, *Cryptocaryon irritans*)

- Brief overview: *I. multifiliis* (also known as Ich) is one of the most common, well-known, and pathogenic parasites of freshwater fish. The Ich trophozoite/trophont (feeding stage on the fish), after feeding, will escape the fish to form an encapsulated dividing tomont stage, which sticks to environmental substrates. The tomont divides into tomites, which emerge as infectious theronts (20–50 microns wide). Ich is a warmwater disease, with outbreaks often in the 15–25°C (59–77°F) window. Stress can bring about outbreaks, which may occur outside the stated temperature range. Recovering fish have a strong immune response to reinfection.

C. irritans (marine Ich) is a similar pathogen seen in saltwater fish. Infections are most common at 20–25°C. The organism is smaller than Ich and lacks a C-shaped macronucleus. The life cycle is similar to that of Ich. Recovered fish have protective immunity for six months.

- Host range and transmission: All freshwater fish (Ich), Many species of saltwater fish except elasmobranchs (marine Ich); worldwide, horizontal spread.
- Signs/diagnosis: Flashing, respiratory distress (koi), 1–2 mm wide, white, spherical nodules in the skin and gills (Ich; Figure 4.26). Chronic dermatitis with thick skin and excessive mucus. Wet mounts show protozoans covered with fine cilia, and a large C-shaped macronucleus (Ich; Figures 4.27, 4.28 and 4.29). *C. irritans* organisms are less than a 1 mm wide, and scrutiny of the skin may be required for diagnosis.
- Differentials: Other ectoparasites, francisellosis. Ich and marine Ich are highly characteristic.
- Management: Early treatment after diagnosis is critical for control. Affected fish must be quarantined.
- Ich: In aquaria, the theront stage is most susceptible, so tank treatments must continue over the entire life cycle (which varies according to temperature). At 24–26°C (the optimal temperature) the life cycle is three to seven days, but at lower temperatures the life cycle may

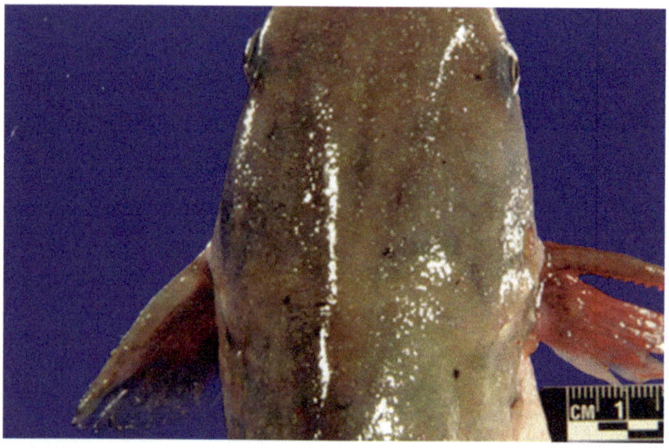

Figure 4.26 *Ichthyophthirius multifiliis* in a channel catfish. *Source:* W. Baumgartner.

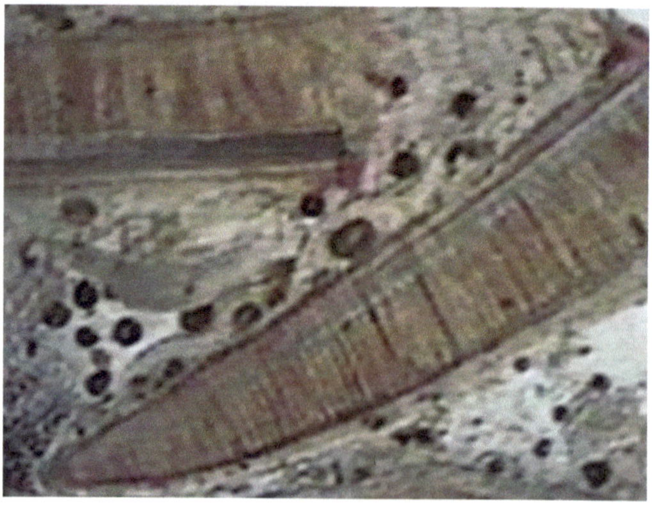

Figure 4.27 Gill wet mount, *Ichthyophthirius ciliates* (low power). *Source:* N. St. Erne.

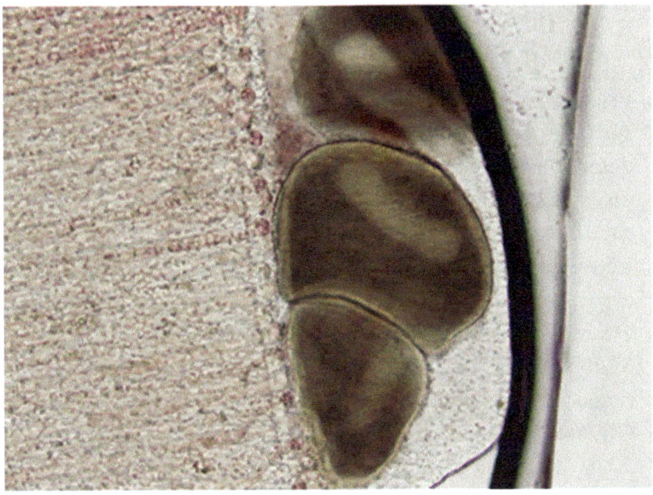

Figure 4.28 Gill wet mount, *Ichthyophthirius ciliates* (high power). *Source:* W. Baumgartner.

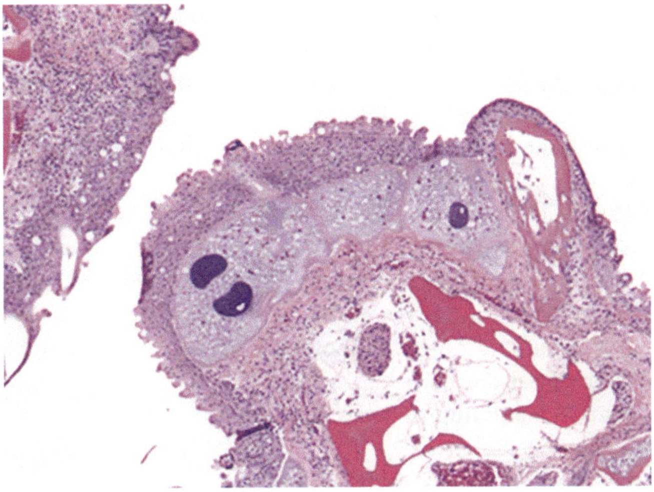

Figure 4.29 Gill bar histopathology, *Ichthyophthirius ciliates* beneath the epithelium. *Source:* W. Baumgartner.

take weeks. Ich cannot complete its life cycle above 30°C; maintaining a tank at this temperature for 10 days will cure. Prolonged formalin immersion treatments every other day, or formalin/malachite green prolonged immersions are effective. Toltrazuril baths (10 μg/ml for four hours every other day for three days) can kill trophozoites on the fish. Ich cannot tolerate salinities greater than 1 ppt, however some isolates can survive; prolonged salt immersions are often used. Ultraviolet light can kill theronts and is effective in preventing spread to other aquaria (not useful to control infections). Removing fish from aquaria for an entire life cycle will remove parasites. Ich cannot tolerate desiccation (all stages). In ponds, copper is effective.

- Marine Ich: Emergence of life stages is circadian, and is often pre-dawn; late-night treatments may be more effective. Hyposalinity works well (16 ppt for 14 days, or 10 ppt for 3 hours every three days, four times). Prolonged copper immersion, prolonged chloroquine immersion. In reef aquaria, sand can be siphoned off every three days (tomont removal) and replaced, four times at three-day intervals.

4.3.7 Other Ciliate Infestations (Genus: *Trichodina, Chilodonella, Brooklynella, Epistylis, Apiosoma, Ambiphrya, Tetrahymena, and Others)*

- Brief overview: This is a highly variable group of organisms that are often found on or in the tissues of normal and diseased fish. The relevance of infestation to disease is often difficult to determine, except where extraordinary numbers are present or they are species known to cause disease. We classify these species into three categories: fish parasites that cause pathology (obligate fish parasites), commensals that cause little if any disease (obligate fish commensals), and free-living organisms that may cause disease (facultative parasites). After death, many of these organisms leave the fish, which will confound gross examination.
- Trichodinids: Discoid ciliated protozoa (30–90 microns wide; Figure 4.30) with a characteristic ring of denticles. Clinically relevant species infect skin and gills, causing mild disease. In severe infections, particularly the young, death may occur. Low numbers in wet mounts are inconsequential.
- Obligate parasites: *Chilodonella* spp. (Figures 4.31, 4.32) are ovoid/discoid organisms, 20–80 microns wide, with two belts of cilia on the ventral surface. Fresh and marine species cause disease. Severe infections cause skin ulcers and ragged skin tags. Gill infection can lead to significant branchitis. Secondary bacterial infections may occur. Outbreaks can occur over a wide range of temperatures. *Brooklynella* is a marine analogue of *Chilodonella*.
- Obligate commensals: Sessile protozoans attach to the skin or gill surfaces, and may be solitary (*Capriniana, Apiosoma, Ambiphrya*) or colonizing (*Epistylis*). They cause little damage.
- Facultative parasites: Tetrahymena (Figure 4.33) are small pyriform ciliates, 30–50 microns wide, that can cause high mortalities. The causative agent of guppy disease, it infects other tropical livebearers, cichlids, and tetras.
- Host range and transmission: Many species, horizontal. Distribution is worldwide.
- Signs/diagnosis: Trichodinids, obligates: flashing, excessive mucus, lethargy. Death in heavy infections. Wet mounts can diagnose. Tetrahymena can infest the skin and invade tissues, producing swellings in the muscle, kidney, and brain. Sudden death. Movement in wet mounts is like a spiraling American football. Tissue invasion is highly diagnostic.
- Differentials: None.
- Management: Improve water quality. Prolonged formalin or copper baths, salt baths for freshwater species.
- For Apicomplexan Infection go online:

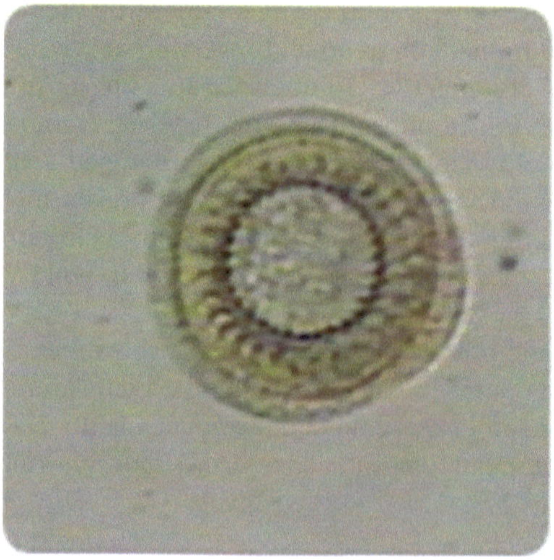

Figure 4.30 *Trichodina* spp. *Source:* N. St. Erne.

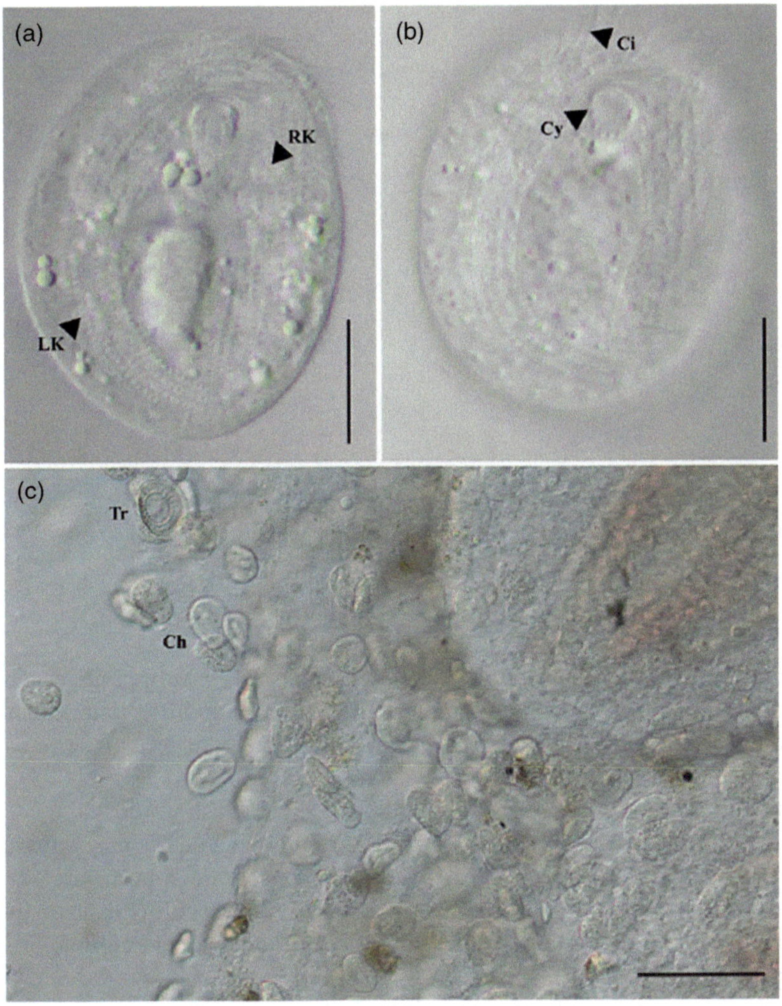

Figure 4.31 *Chilodonella hexasticha* from the gills of farmed barramundi, *Lates calcarifer*, in tropical north Queensland, Australia. (a) Left kinetic bands (LK); right kinetic bands (RK); (b) Cilia (Ci) and morphology of the cytostome (Cy); (c) Infection on gills by *Chilodonella* sp. cells (Ch). Co-infection by *Trichodina* sp. (Tr). Scale bars = 100 μm. *Source:* Gomes *et al.* (2017).

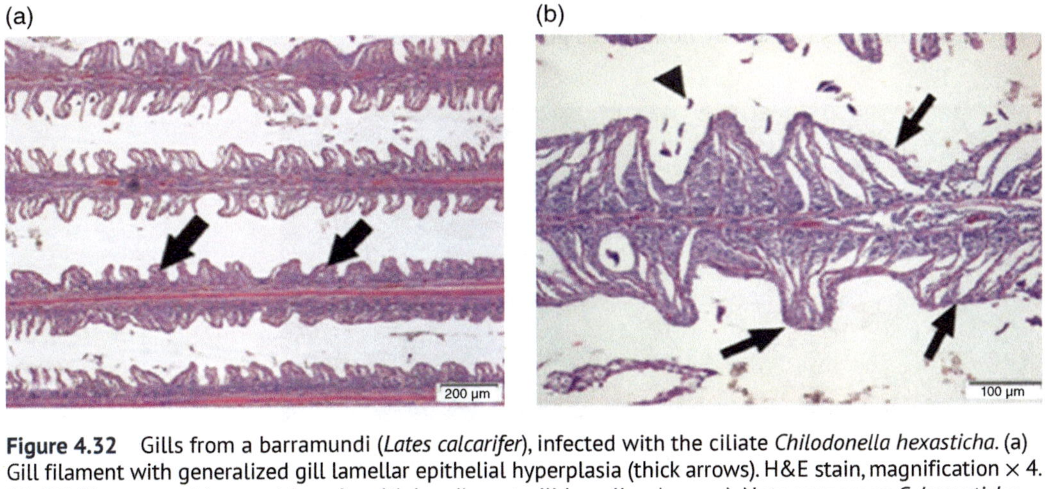

Figure 4.32 Gills from a barramundi (*Lates calcarifer*), infected with the ciliate *Chilodonella hexasticha*. (a) Gill filament with generalized gill lamellar epithelial hyperplasia (thick arrows). H&E stain, magnification × 4. (b) Gill filaments with synechiae of multiple adjacent gill lamellae (arrows). Note numerous *C. hexasticha* parasites (arrowheads). H&E, magnification × 10). *Source:* Bowater and O'Donoghue (2015).

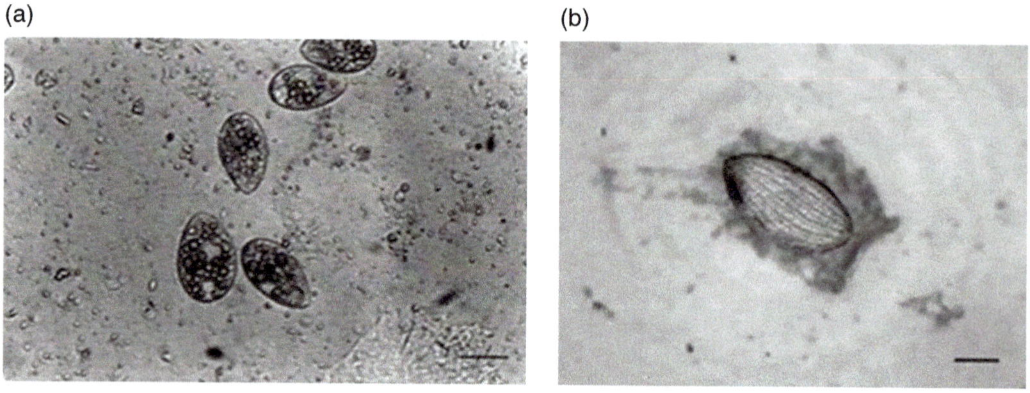

Figure 4.33 Ventral view of *Tetrahymena* sp. (a) From skin scrape of live guppy showing food vacuoles containing pigment (bar = 40 μm). (b) in vitro cultured *Tetrahymena* sp. (Klein silver stain, bar = 16 μm). *Source:* Pimenta Leibowitz *et al.* (2005).

4.3.8 Oomycetes/Water Molds

- Overview/etiology: In addition to *Saprolegnia* spp., *Aphanomyces* spp. and *Achlya* spp., are water molds (not true fungi) that have been associated with mortalities in fresh and fish in brackish water. They are significant skin and gill pathogens, and are generally thought to occur as secondary invaders.
- Host range and transmission: All freshwater fish, and some species in brackish water.
- Signs/diagnosis: Cottony tufts on the skin and gills (Figure 4.34); entrapped debris may impart additional colors. Underlying tissues are necrotic/ulcerated. Organisms are superficial. Wet mounts show branched non-septate, hyphal-like organisms. They may be cultured on malt extract or Sabouraud agar at 20–22°C. Verification can be done by PCR or detailed examination, but is generally not necessary.
- Differentials: *Aphanomyces* (see epizootic ulcerative syndrome), *Achyla* oomycete infection.
- Management: A primary cause for stress and skin or gill disease should be sought. Zoospores (water form) can be treated with formalin, hydrogen peroxide, sodium chloride, potassium permanganate, and iodophors. The vegetative form on the fish is not easily treated, but affected fish can recover if other stressors are removed. Reduce stress and improve water quality.
- For other diseases caused by oomycetes go online:

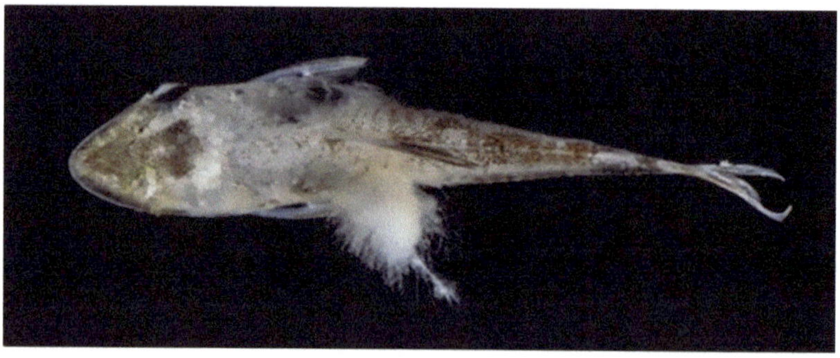

Figure 4.34 Saprolegniasis, cottony growth on the skin of *Otocinclus* sp. *Source:* Ryan Taylor.

4.3.9 Myxozoan Infection (*Myxobolus*)

- Brief overview: Myxozoans are highly specialized metazoan parasites of annelid worms and bryozoans that use vertebrates (mostly fish) as intermediate hosts. They are characterized by multicellular spores that contain polar capsules. They are significant pathogens of many species including salmonids and Ictalurid catfish.

  Myxobolus cerebralis causes whirling disease. Fish in the genus *Oncorhynchus* are susceptible; infection of the axial skeleton leads to neurologic signs and death (see also Chapter 5).
  Further information on salmon whirling disease is available in the website materials accompanying this text and in Chapter 5 - Epidemiology.

  Henneguya spp. cause significant gill disease in channel catfish (proliferative gill disease, Figures 4.35–4.39); transient overwhelming infection of the gills leads to cartilage necrosis, hemorrhage, inflammation, swelling, and respiratory impairment. In later stages, spore cysts appear in the gills, with subsequent rupture and release.

  Tetracapsuloides bryosalmonae causes severe granulomatous nephritis in salmonids (proliferative kidney disease; see also Chapter 5).

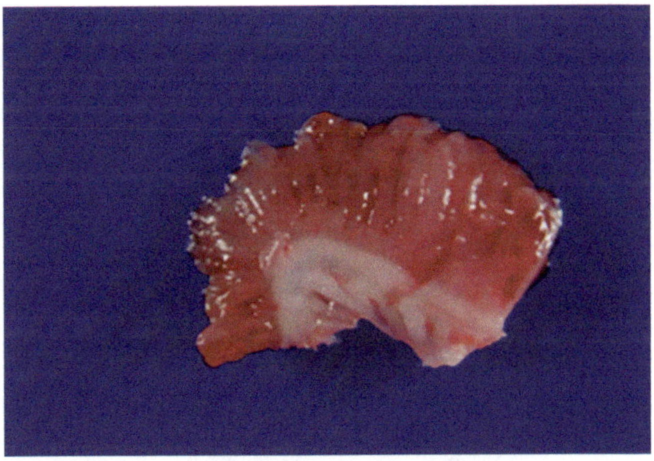

Figure 4.35 Channel catfish gill bar, hemorrhage and necrosis with swelling, *Henneguya ictaluri*, proliferative gill disease. *Source:* W. Baumgartner.

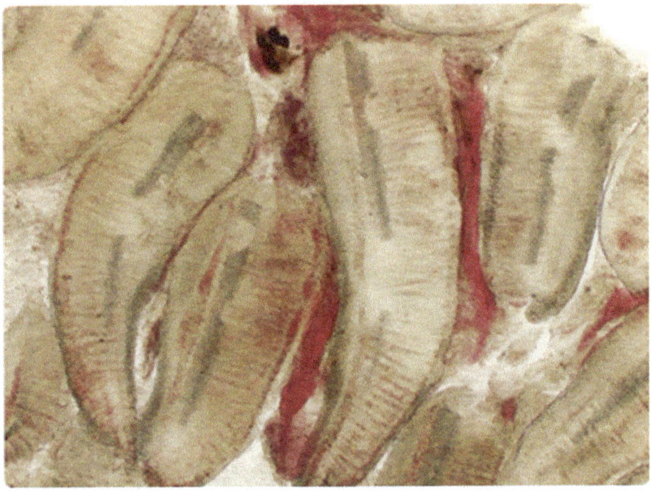

Figure 4.36 Channel catfish gill wet mount, cartilage necrosis, *Henneguya ictaluri*, proliferative gill disease. *Source:* W. Baumgartner.

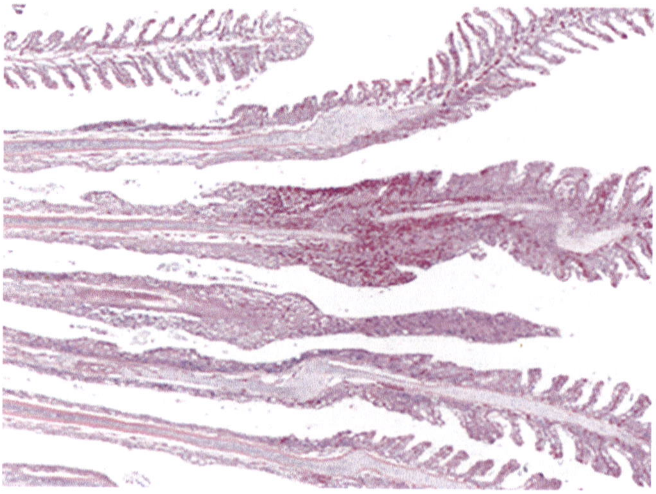

Figure 4.37 Channel catfish gill filaments, hemorrhage and cartilage necrosis, *Henneguya ictaluri*, proliferative gill disease. *Source:* W. Baumgartner.

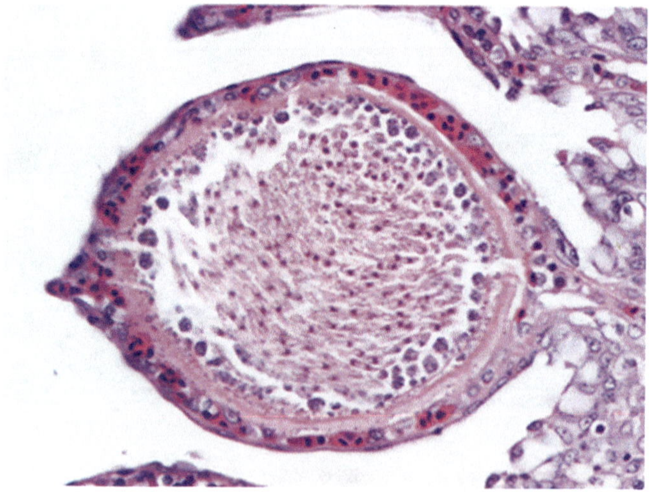

Figure 4.38 Channel catfish gill filament, *Henneguya ictaluri* intralamellar cyst. *Source:* W. Baumgartner.

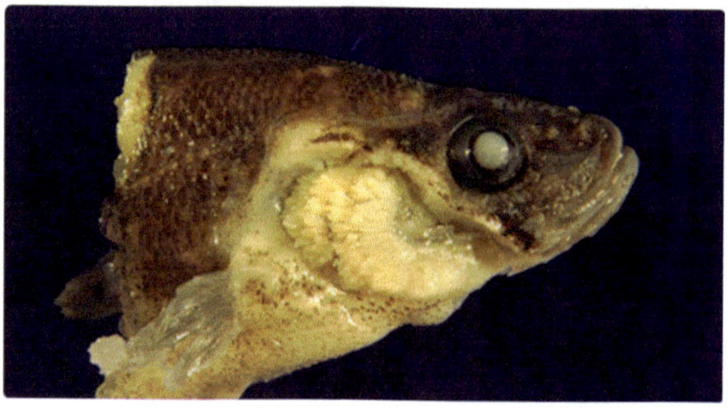

Figure 4.39 Pirate perch gill infection, nodular plasmodia of *Hennegoides flockae* spores. *Source:* W. Baumgartner.

Further information on proliferative kidney disease is available in the website materials accompanying this text.

Hoferellus carassii infects the renal tubule epithelium in goldfish, causing severe cystic enlargement and eventual death (Figures 4.40–4.41).

Ceratomyxa shasta causes severe enteritis in salmonids.

- Host range: Varies, some myxozoans can infect more than one species.
- Signs/diagnosis: Infections in gills, muscle, skeletal tissues, skin, kidneys, viscera leads to plasmodium formation and often granulomatous disease. Skin ulcers, organ failure, neurologic disease, muscle liquefaction; various presentations occur. Wet mounts and histopathology.
- Differentials: Microspora, granulomatous disease, encysted trematodes, neoplasia, sepsis, viral infection.
- Management: None. Disinfect and quarantine.
- For Glochidiodis go online:

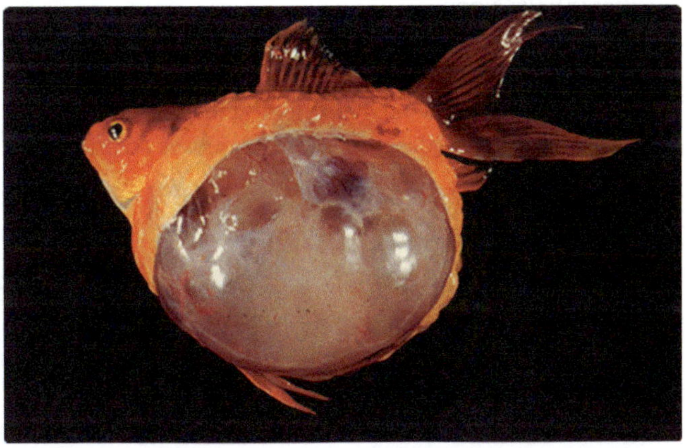

Figure 4.40 Cystic renal hyperplasia (*Hoferellus carassii*, kidney bloater). *Source:* Al Camus, University of Georgia.

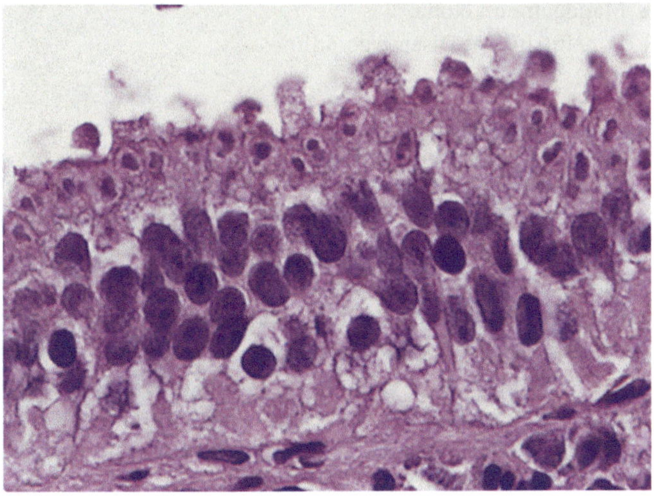

Figure 4.41 Myxozoan infection renal tubule epithelium (*Hoferellus carassii*, kidney bloater). *Source:* Al Camus, University of Georgia.

4.4 Diseases with Multiple Causes

4.4.1 Gas bubble disease

Overview/etiology: Gas supersaturation (ΔP) of the water leads to excess solubilized gas entering the bloodstream, where it comes out of solution leading to gas embolisms. Various causes for supersaturation are reported: small leaks in pipes (venturi effect), waterfalls, pumping water from depths (over 300 feet), rapid increase in water temperature from source to tank, spring water after the thaw, air shipping, heavy macrophyte growth (submerged aquatic plants). The gas may be nitrogen, carbon dioxide, or oxygen. Oxygen levels above 125% saturation are not advisable. Fish able to escape to depth can cope with excess gas. Acute supersaturation ($\Delta P > 50\text{-}200$ mmHg) can cause sudden death while chronic low level supersaturation is associated with low level mortalities, stress related disease.

Host range & transmission: All fish. Fry/young are most susceptible as they cannot escape to deeper water.

Signs/Diagnosis: Gas bubbles in the eyes, gills, tissues. Swimbladder hyperinflation, exophthalmos. Floating fry/eggs. Clipping gills or fins underwater will release gas, confirming the diagnosis. Determination of supersaturation requires measurement of the total gas concentration, via a saturometer; 110% saturation is dangerous for fish.

Differentials: None

Treatment/management: Remove gas source. Aeration of water source, packed column degassers.

For Head and Lateral Line Erosion Syndrome (HLLES) go online:

For Ammonia & Hydrogen Sulfide toxicoses go online:

4.4.2 Nephrocalcinosis

- Overview: The accumulation of hydroxyapatite mineral in the renal tubules. Nephrocalcinosis develops as a consequence of water high in carbon dioxide and phosphates. A debilitating condition rather than a cause of mortalities.
- Host Range and transmission: All fish.
- Signs/diagnosis: Swollen kidneys with white gritty material.
- Differentials: Bacterial kidney disease, proliferative kidney disease.
- Management: None.
- For Nutritional Disease go online:

4.4.3 Neoplasia

- Brief overview: Neoplasia in fish is, in most ways, very similar to that in mammals. It tends to occur in older animals, may be caused by virus infection, and has been associated with environmental pollution. The variety of neoplasms one encounters are familiar to veterinarians who treat mammals. Some of the more common neoplasms are described here.
- Nerve sheath tumors: Certain populations of cyprinids may be predisposed to these skin masses.
- Pigment cell tumors: Fish have, in addition to melanocytes, many other pigment cell types (chromatophores) that can produce neoplasms. They often present as skin masses which have varying colors, and can be malignant (Figure 4.42). Brown bullhead catfish develop a range of pigmented skin lesions from macules to nodules, possibly associated with pollution.
- Lip tumors: Angelfish in particular are prone to nodular lip masses, which can vary from hyperplastic inflammatory reactions to trauma, fibromas, and even odontogenic neoplasms. Typically,

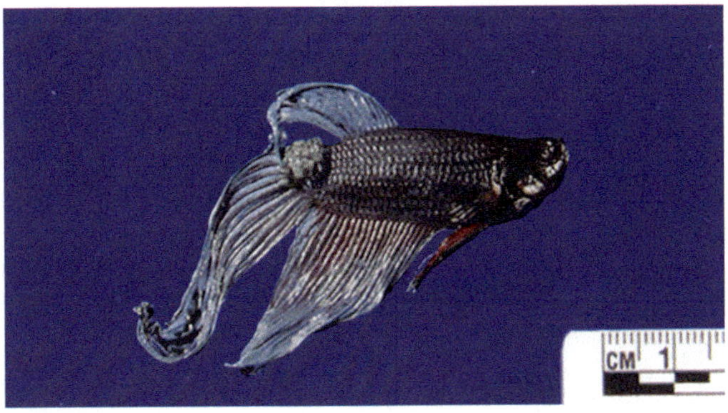

Figure 4.42 Chromatophoroma (mixed melano-iridophoroma), *Betta splendens*. *Source:* Shivley *et al.* 2021.

older fish are affected, and a viral etiology has been proposed, but not proven. European eels develop oral papillomas, which regress; virus and pollution are proposed causes.

- Liver tumors: Tumors are relatively common, both hepatocellular and biliary. Epizootics have been reported in rainbow trout, and are associated with aflatoxin exposure. In the United States, liver tumors are also associated with chlorinated hydrocarbon pollution.
- Papillomas: Foci of skin hyperplasia/neoplasia are common in various species, and may be associated with virus infection, seasonal changes, and environmental pollution. They may reach high prevalence in populations. Carp pox, caused by cyprinid herpesvirus 1, causes candlewax-like areas of epithelial hyperplasia that mimic neoplasia.
- Diagnosis: Histopathology, impression smears, cytology.
- Differentials: Granulomatous inflammation, parasite infection, hyperplastic response.
- Management: Resection/removal.

4.4.4 Cataracts

- Overview: Cataract is defined as opacity or cloudy of the lens; it can affect the vision noticeably or cause complete blindness. It was identified in farmed Atlantic salmon (*Salmo salar*) in Europe in the early 1990s. More than two decades ago, it caused significant economic losses due to increased mortality in affected fish. Ethical concerns also arouse public attention to fish welfare, since it is related to rapid growth and environmental variables. Several etiologies have been reported to cause cataracts in both farmed and wild fish, including dietary factors (related to levels of thiamine, riboflavin, methionine, cysteine, tryptophan and also zinc and vitamin A deficiencies), parasitic infestations (i.e. larval *Diplostomum* spp.), toxic exposure, and trauma, as well as environmental factors (rapid osmotic changes etc.) involved in cataractogenesis. The effect of dietary lipids on cataract development has been studied and and the results are inconclusive. Parr-smolt transformation may be critical in cataract outbreaks. In fish, cataracts are often present as irreversible loss of lens fiber yet osmotic cataracts can be reversible. In wild salmon, cataracts could potentially have negative effects on the population due to reduced feed uptake. Occurrence of cataracts has been used as an indicator factor for evaluate fish health and welfare in aquaculture specially in Atlantic salmon.
- Host range and transmission: All fish species are susceptible to disease and its transmission differs with etiology. Nutritionally linked cataracts are most often seen in trout species. It has been reported that there may be a genetically linked predisposition to cataract formation in different fish species (Atlantic salmon, aquarium-raised tilapia).
- Signs/diagnosis: Clinically, eye opacity gradually changes from contrast sensitivity to complete blindness (Figure 4.43). Affected fish may have displayed behavior alteration such as lack of

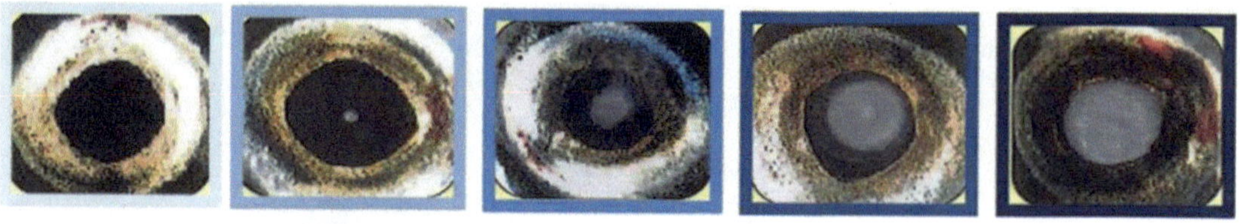

Figure 4.43 Morphological scheme for diagnosing and classifying eye cataracts in Atlantic salmon. *Source:* Noble *et al.* (2018).

response to predator. In addition, fish may lose weight and can be more susceptible to secondary diseases due to decreased feed intake.

- Differentials: Corneal edema or corneal opacity should be distinguished from cataract. Postmortem opacification should be taken into consideration as normal. Trematodes (*Diplostomum* spp.) can infect the eyes and cause cataracts.
- Management: Treatment depends on etiology. Surgical procedures have been used in ornamental fish to remove the lens. In general, the following can be considered for measures to reduce cataracts: elevated dietary composition levels of histidine, antioxidants (vitamins C and E) in feed ingredients, control of environmental conditions (water temperature, oxygen saturation, salinity and stress) and monitoring during periods of excessive growth rates.

4.5 Differential Diagnostics of Diseases in Fish

4.5.1 Salmonids/Coldwater Food Fish

System/symptom	Differential diagnoses
Sudden death	Bacterial septicemia (*Aeromonas, Bacillus, Pseudomonas, Proteus*), water quality issues (ammonia, oxygen, hydrogen sulfide), toxicosis (heavy metal, herbicide, pesticide), trauma, electrocution, botulism, methemoglobinemia/brown blood disease, gas supersaturation, salmonid alphavirus (sleeping disease)
Poor growth	nutritional deficiency, stress/water quality issues, insufficient caloric intake, heavy parasitism (*Chilodonella, Ichthyophthirius*), salmonid alphavirus, *Mycobacterium*
Uncoordinated swimming/nervousness/ buoyancy	generalized infectious disease (virus, fungi, bacteria, myxozoans, microsporidians), electrocution, spinal trauma, toxicosis, central nervous sysytem (CNS) disease, water quality issues, gas bubble disease, Thiamine/ riboflavin/pyridoxine deficiency, botulism, *Ichthyophonus hoferi*, algal blooms, jellyfish
Gasping/asphyxia:	Low dissolved oxygen, high water temperature, high carbon dioxide, toxin exposure/ammonia, organic/inorganic contaminants, suspended sediments, physical impediment/obstruction to gas exchange
Gill disease	Branchiomycosis, *Flavobacterium*, epitheliocystis, parasites
Anemia	Piscirickettsia, salmon leukemia virus, infectious hematopoietic necrosis, hemorrhagic smolt syndrome, zinc toxicosis, lipoid liver disease (rancid feed)

System/symptom	Differential diagnoses
Skin/fins:	
Petechiae	Virus, bacterial septicemia, low pH
Increased mucus	Water quality issues, parasitism
Hemorrhage, necrosis, ulcers	overcrowding (fin-nipping, soreback), improper pH, trauma, sunburn, bacterial infection (*Aeromonas*, *Pseudomonas*, *Moritella*, *Flavobacterium*, *Aliivibrio* (*Vibrio*), *Tenacibaculum*, *Piscirickettsia*, *Mycobacterium*), *Saprolegnia*, *Phialophora*, *Aphanomyces*, infectious hematopoietic necrosis (especially in young fish), spring viremia of carp, rhabdoviruses (including viral hemorrhagic septicemia), herpesvirus, cardiomyopathy syndrome, red mark syndrome (coldwater strawberry disease), gas bubble disease
Parasites	*Monogenea*, ciliates, flagellates, amoeba, copepods, branchiurans, bivalves, leeches, hydroids
Yellow/white flat lesions	*Flavobacterium* infection, necrosis, epidermal hyperplasia, dermal edema, *Saprolegnia*
Depigmentation	Epidermal/dermal injury of any type, toxicosis/environmental
Nodules/lumps	Papillomatosis, neoplasia, granulomatous disease (*Mycobacterium*, other bacteria, fungi), virus (lymphocystis, adenovirus, herpesvirus), *Ichthyophthirius*, foreign body, *Dermocystidium*, furunculosis, encysted trematodes
Segmental darkening	Neurologic disease/infection (*Myxobolus*, *Mycobacterium*, betanodavirus)
Edema/lepidorthosis	Hypoalbuminemia, renal disease, severe skin disease
Red vent	Internal disease (bacterial, viral), *Anisakis* larvae, *Ceratomyxa*
Black spots/nodules	Melanocyte hyperplasia, melanoma, encysted trematodes, microsporidian infection, pigmented fungal granulomas
Gills:	
Hemorrhage/ulcers	Bacterial septicemia, toxins, virus, *Flavobacterium*, *Aerococcus sanguinicola*, diatoms, jellyfish, protozoan parasites
Hyperplasia	gill necrosis virus, water quality issues, dietary imbalance (vitamin B5), chronic inflammation, parasitism (amoeba, flagellates, ciliates)
Necrosis	high/low pH, chlorine, *Flavobacterium*, branchiomycosis, *Saprolegnia*, jellyfish, protozoan parasites
Nodules	encysted trematodes, myxozoan cysts, neoplasia, bacteria (*Nocardia*, *Mycobacterium*), amoebic gill disease, *Dermocystidium*, microsporidian (*Loma*), *Ichthyophthirius*
Pallor	Anemia, salmon leukemia virus, infectious hematopoietic necrosis (especially in young fish), spring viremia of carp, amoebic gill disease
Gas bubbles	Supersaturation of water by gas
Increased mucus	water quality issues, bacterial infection, parasites
Parasites	*Monogenea*, ciliates, flagellates, copepods, branchiurans, bivalves, amoeba
Yellow/white lesions	*Flavobacterium* infection, necrosis, *Saprolegnia*
Pseudobranch:	
Necrosis	*Parvicapsula*, *Flavobacterium*, toxins (herbicides, metals, pesticides)
Swelling	*Xcellia* (X cell disease), *Parvicapsula*
Calcification	Vitamin E deficiency, lipoid liver disease, nephrocalcinosis

(*Continued*)

(*Continued*)

System/symptom	Differential diagnoses
Mouth:	
Gasping/asphyxia	See general comment above, screamer disease (mouth locked open)
Hemorrhage/ulcers	Bacterial septicemia (*Yersinia*, *Flavobacterium*, *Tenacibaculum*, *Vibrio*), parasites (*Metacercariae*, isopods), trauma
Increased mucus/exudate	Bacterial infection (*Flavobacterium*), parasitism
Gas bubbles	Gas supersaturation
Malocclusion	inappropriate food sources, trauma
Nodules	Granulomas, papilloma (*Oncorhynchus masou* virus), dental neoplasia, parasitic cyst, thyroid hyperplasia, thyroid neoplasia, goiter, thymic neoplasia
Eye:	
Exophthalmia	Bacterial septicemia, multiple viral infections (spring viremia of carp), *Mycobacterium*, vitamin A/E/pantothenic acid deficiency, nephrocalcinosis, gas bubble disease/supersaturation, white-eye syndrome (salmon)
Ulcers	Fungus, bacterial septicemia, trauma, blindness
Corneal edema/cloudiness	poor water quality, conspecific aggression, bacterial, viral, fungal, parasitic disease, white-eye syndrome (salmon)
Ophthalmitis	Trauma, hematogenous spread of pathogens, thermal damage, *Piscirickettsia*, *Tenacibaculum*, zinc deficiency, *Diplostomum*, *Tylodelphys*
Cataract	*Diplostomum*, deficiencies (zinc, vitamin A, thiamine, riboflavin, methionine, tryptophan, histidine), rapid osmolar fluctuations, ultraviolet light exposure, temperature fluctuations, gas bubble disease
Gas bubbles	Supersaturation, bacterial infection, corneal perforation
Lens luxation	Trauma
Enucleation	Trauma (predator, stocking density too high, jellyfish), severe ophthalmitis (*Tenacibaculum*)
Muscle:	
Atrophy	Emaciation, denervation, riboflavin deficiency
Liquefaction/necrosis	Microsporidians, myxozoans, bacterial infection
Nodules/swelling	Encysted trematodes, granulomas, microsporidians, myxozoans, emphysematous bacterial infection, *Ichthyophonus hoferi*, neoplasia
Hemorrhage	Viral hemorrhagic septicemia, bacterial sepsis, trauma, vascular disease, myonecrosis
White foci	Magnesium deficiency, other dietary imbalances, necrosis, microsporidians, white-eye syndrome (salmon)
Skeletal deformity	Vitamin A/C/E deficiency, *Myxobolus*, *Mycobacterium*, abnormal egg incubation temperatures, trauma, hereditary, adverse environment conditions, toxicant exposure
Abdomen/celom:	
Enlarged (general)	Neoplasia, overweight, egg binding/dystocia, gastrointestinal impaction, peritonitis, cardiovascular/hepatic disease leading to ascites, renal disease, other causes of hypoproteinemia, parasites
Ascites	Bacterial septicemia, piscine reovirus, cardiomyopathy syndrome, viral hemorrhagic septicemia, vegetative valvular endocarditis

System/symptom	Differential diagnoses
Peritonitis, nodular/ granulomatous	Mycobacteriosis, streptococcosis, *Francisella*, parasites, (including encysted cestodes), fungus, egg binding, *Dermocystidium*, Vaccination, steatitis (sequela to pancreatitis, antioxidant deficiency), neoplasia
Petechiae	Infectious pancreatic necrosis, salmon leukemia virus, viral hemorrhagic septicemia, infectious hematopoietic necrosis (especially in young fish), salmonid alphavirus, *Listonella*
Cysts	polycystic renal disease, blocker ureter
Gas	Swim bladder or gut rupture, body wall perforation, inflammation with gas-producing microbes or fungi
Kidney:	
Diffuse swelling	Virus (salmon leukemia virus), bacterial septicemia, *Sphaerothecum*, immune stimulation, neoplasia
Cystic change	*Hoferellus carassii*, polycystic kidney disease (genetic/environmental), chronic renal disease
Necrosis	Virus, bacterial sepsis, parasite/protozoa (*Spironucleus*), riboflavin deficiency, heavy metals
Granulomas/nodules	Granulomas: bacterial (*Renibacterium*, *Mycobacterium*, *Nocardia*, *Francisella*), fungi, *Ichthyophonus hoferi*, PKD, nephrocalcinosis, neoplasia
Urinary bladder: Stones	Salinity/cation imbalances, renal/gill disease, genetic
Spleen:	
Diffuse swelling	Bacterial septicemia, reovirus, salmon leukemia virus, *Sphaerothecum*, PKD
Nodules	Granulomas: bacterial, fungal, parasitic (*Spironucleus*, *Ichthyophonus hoferi*), neoplasia, *Dermocystidium*, hematoma, cysts (polycystic syndrome)
Liver:	
Necrosis	Virus (infectious pancreatic necrosis, reovirus, others), bacterial sepsis, heavy metals, algal toxin, rancid food, carbohydrates fed to carnivores
Hemorrhage	Infectious pancreatic necrosis, *Listonella*, *Aliivibrio* (*Vibrio*), *Carnobacterium*, infectious salmon anemia (diffuse hemorrhage)
Tan/yellow liver	Fat accumulation: excessive nutrition, toxicosis, choline deficiency, inadequate antioxidants, vitamin E deficiency, lipoid liver disease (rancid feed), seasonal accumulation (especially gadoids)
	Fibrosis/iron accumulation
	Necrosis (see above)
Nodules	*Piscirickettsia*, *Spironucleus*, *Yersinia*, *Renibacterium*, *Mycobacterium*, *Nocardia*, myxozoan infection, encysted parasites (*Anisakis*), fungi, *Ichthyophonus hoferi*, *Dermocystidium*, neoplasia, mineral (biliary lithiasis)
Cysts	Polycystic liver, cestode larvae
Jaundice	Hemolysis, toxins, genetic abnormalities, erythrocytic inclusion body syndrome, infectious hemolytic anemia, erythromycin toxicosis
Stomach:	
Nodules	Granulomas (fungi, *Mycobacteria*), microsporidians, myxozoans, nematodes
Dilation	Gastric dilation and airsacculitis syndrome, foreign bodies

(*Continued*)

(*Continued*)

System/symptom	Differential diagnoses
Intestine:	
Hyperemia/hemorrhage	Rainbow trout gastroenteritis, bacterial enteritis (*Clostridium*), infectious pancreatic necrosis, acanthocephalans
Mucoid feces/casts	Rainbow trout gastroenteritis, infectious pancreatic necrosis, infectious hematopoietic necrosis, parasites (*Spironucleus*), spring viremia of carp, coccidian infection, bacterial enteritis (*Vibrio*), dietary
Nodules	Foreign bodies, granulomas, coccidian cysts, myxozoan cysts, neoplasia, encysted worms
Diffuse thickening	*Piscirickettsia*, *Ceratomyxa*
Swim bladder:	
Enlarged	Hyperinflation: gas supersaturation, torsion, physostome blockage, *Betanodavirus*, acid/base imbalance
	Fluid: exudate (bacteria), protozoa (*Spironucleus*), viral hemorrhagic septicemia
	Fungi: *Isaria farinosa* (*Paecilomyces*), *Phialophora*, *Phoma*, microsporidians, myxozoans
	Thickened wall: nematodes, chronic inflammation
Atrophy	Rupture
Hemorrhage	Virus, bacteria
Reproductive: Nodules/enlarged	*Mycobacterium*, *Ichthyophonus*, egg binding, microsporidians, myxozoans, neoplasia
Heart:	
Pallor	Necrosis, *Aerococcus sanguinicola*, fat deposition
Fibrosis	Reovirus
Inflammation/pericarditis	Bacterial sepsis (*Pseudomonas*, *Renibacterium*, *Piscirickettsia*, *Francisella*, *Lactobacillus*), cardiomyopathy syndrome, *Spironucleus*, *Metacercariae* (*Apatemon*, *Cotylurus*, *Ichthyocotylurus*, *Stephanostomum*)
Hemopericardium	Cardiomyopathy syndrome, heart rupture
Nodules	Granulomas (bacteria, fungus, *Ichthyophonus hoferi*), *Metacercariae*, ventricular aneurysms
Brown/bronze	Lipoid liver disease (rancid feed)

4.5.2 Warmwater Food Fish

System/symptom	Differential diagnoses
Sudden death	Bacterial septicemia (*Aeromonas*), water quality issues (ammonia, oxygen, hydrogen sulfide), toxicosis (heavy metal, herbicide, pesticide), trauma, electrocution, botulism, methemoglobinemia/brown blood disease, gas supersaturation
Poor growth	Nutritional deficiency, stress/water quality issues, insufficient caloric intake, heavy parasitism (*Chilodonella*, *Ichthyophthirius*, *Enteromyxum*, cestodes), *Mycobacterium*

System/symptom	Differential diagnoses
Uncoordinated swimming/nervousness/buoyancy	Generalized infectious disease: virus (*Betanodavirus*), bacteria (*Eubacterium tarantellus*), myxozoans, microsporidians, electrocution, spinal trauma, toxicosis, CNS disease, water quality issues, gas bubble disease, thiamine/riboflavin/pyridoxine deficiency, botulism, *Ichthyophonus hoferi*, fungal infection, algal blooms, parasitism
Gasping/asphyxia:	Low dissolved oxygen, high water temperature, high carbon dioxide, toxin exposure/ammonia, organic/inorganic contaminants, suspended sediments, physical impediment/obstruction to gas exchange
Gill disease	Branchiomycosis, *Flavobacterium*, epitheliocystis, parasites
Anemia	Red sea bream iridovirus, zinc toxicosis
Skin/fins:	
Petechiae	Virus, bacterial septicemia (*Aeromonas*, *Photobacterium*, *Streptococcus*, *Lactococcus*), low pH
Increased mucus	Water quality issues, parasitism (*Cryptobia*, *Ichthyophthirius*, *Amyloodinium* and other dinoflagellates)
Hemorrhage, necrosis, ulcers	overcrowding (fin-nipping, soreback), trauma, improper pH, sunburn, bacterial infection (*Aeromonas*, *Flavobacterium*, *Pseudomonas*, *Mycobacterium*, *Vibrio*, *Edwardsiella*, *Tenacibaculum*, epitheliocystis), *Saprolegnia*, *Aphanomyces*, virus infection (koi herpesvirus, grass carp reovirus, channel catfish virus), gas bubble disease, head and lateral line erosion syndrome
Parasites	*Monogenea*, ciliates, flagellates, amoeba, copepods, branchiurans, bivalves, leeches, hydroids
Yellow/white flat lesions	*Flavobacterium* infection, necrosis, epidermal hyperplasia, dermal edema, *Saprolegnia*
Depigmentation	Epidermal/dermal injury of any type, toxicosis/environmental
Nodules/lumps	Papillomatosis, carp pox, neoplasia, granulomatous disease (*Mycobacterium*, other bacteria, fungi), *Ichthyophthirius*, *Dermocystidium*, encysted trematodes, lymphocystis, foreign body, furuncles (Gram-negative bacteria)
Segmental darkening	Neurologic disease/infection (*Mycobacterium*, *Betanodavirus*)
Edema/lepidorthosis	Hypoalbuminemia, renal disease, severe skin disease
Red vent	Internal disease (bacterial, viral, parasites)
Black spots/nodules	Melanocyte hyperplasia, melanoma, encysted trematodes, microsporidian infection, pigmented fungal granulomas
Gills:	
Hemorrhage/ulcers	Bacterial septicemia, *Flavobacterium*, viral infection (red sea bream iridovirus, koi herpesvirus, channel catfish virus), toxins, diatoms, protozoan parasites
Hyperplasia	water quality issues, dietary imbalance (vitamin B5), chronic inflammation, parasitism (myxozoans, amoeba, flagellates, ciliates)
Necrosis	high/low pH, chlorine, *Flavobacterium*, branchiomycosis, *Streptococcus*, koi herpesvirus, protozoan parasites
Nodules	Encysted trematodes, myxozoan cysts, neoplasia, bacteria (*Nocardia*, *Mycobacterium*), amoebic gill disease, *Dermocystidium*, microsporidians, *Ichthyophthirius*
Pallor	Anemia, viral infection (spring viremia of carp), mild hyperplasia

(*Continued*)

(*Continued*)

System/symptom	Differential diagnoses
Gas bubbles	Supersaturation of water by gas
Increased mucus	Water quality issues, bacterial infection, parasites
Parasites	*Monogenea*, ciliates, flagellates, copepods, branchiurans
Yellow/white lesions	*Flavobacterium* infection, necrosis, *Saprolegnia*
Pseudobranch:	
Necrosis	*Flavobacterium*, toxins (herbicides, metals, pesticides)
Swelling	*Xcellia* (X cell disease)
Calcification	Vitamin E deficiency
Mouth:	
Gasping/asphyxia	See general comment above; screamer disease (mouth locked open)
Hemorrhage/ulcers	Bacterial septicemia (*Yersinia*, *Flavobacterium*), trauma
Increased mucus/ exudate	Bacterial infection (*Flavobacterium*), parasitism
Gas bubbles	Gas supersaturation
Malocclusion	Inappropriate food sources, trauma
Nodules	Granulomas, papilloma, dental neoplasia, parasitic cyst, thyroid hyperplasia, thyroid neoplasia, thymic neoplasia
Eye:	
Exophthalmia	Bacterial septicemia, multiple viral infections (grass carp reovirus, channel catfish virus, golden shiner virus), *Mycobacteria*, vitamin A/E/pantothenic acid deficiency, nephrocalcinosis, gas bubble disease/supersaturation
Ulcers	Fungus, bacterial septicemia, trauma, blindness
Corneal edema/ cloudiness	Poor water quality, conspecific aggression, bacterial, viral, fungal, parasitic disease
Ophthalmitis	Trauma, hematogenous spread of pathogens, thermal damage, zinc deficiency, *Diplostomum*
Cataract	*Diplostomum*, deficiencies (zinc, vitamin A, thiamine, riboflavin, methionine, tryptophan, histidine), rapid osmolar fluctuations, ultraviolet light exposure, temperature fluctuations, gas bubble disease
Gas bubbles	Supersaturation, bacterial infection, corneal perforation
Lens luxation	Trauma
Enucleation	Trauma (predator, stocking density too high, jellyfish), severe ophthalmitis (*Streptococcus*, *Aeromonas*)
Muscle:	
Atrophy	Emaciation, denervation, riboflavin deficiency
Liquefaction/necrosis	Microsporidians, myxozoans, bacterial infection (Gram-negative and anaerobe bacteria)
Nodules/swelling	Encysted trematodes, microsporidians, myxozoans, granulomas, emphysematous bacterial infection, *Ichthyophonus hoferi*, neoplasia
Hemorrhage	Trauma, vascular disease, myonecrosis, viral hemorrhagic septicemia, grass carp reovirus, bacterial sepsis
White foci	Magnesium deficiency, other dietary imbalances, necrosis (winter disease of Mediterranean fishes)

System/symptom	Differential diagnoses
Skeletal Deformity	Vitamin A/C/E deficiency, *Myxobolus*, *Mycobacterium*, abnormal egg incubation temperatures, trauma, hereditary, adverse environment conditions, toxicant exposure
Abdomen/celom:	
Enlarged (general)	Neoplasia, overweight, egg binding/dystocia, gastrointestinal impaction, peritonitis, cardiovascular/hepatic disease leading to ascites, renal disease, other causes of hypoproteinemia, parasites
Ascites	Bacterial septicemia (*Aeromonas*, *Vibrio*, *Edwardsiella*, *Streptococcus*, *Lactococcus*, *Pseudomonas*), viral infection (channel catfish virus, viral hemorrhagic septicemia, spring viremia of carp)
Peritonitis, nodular/ granulomatous	Mycobacteriosis, streptococcosis, *Francisella*, parasites, (including encysted cestodes), virus, fungus, egg binding, vaccination, steatitis (sequela to pancreatitis, antioxidant deficiency), neoplasia
Petechiae	Bacterial septicemia (*Aeromonas*, *Vibrio*, *Edwardsiella*), viral infection (spring viremia of carp)
Cysts	Polycystic renal disease, blocker ureter
Gas	Swim bladder or gut rupture, body wall perforation, inflammation w/ gas producing microbes or fungi
Kidney:	
Diffuse swelling	Virus, bacterial septicemia, immune stimulation, neoplasia
Cystic change	*Hoferellus carassii*, polycystic kidney disease (genetic/environmental), chronic renal disease
Necrosis/hemorrhage	Virus, bacterial sepsis, parasite/protozoa (*Spironucleus*), riboflavin deficiency, heavy metals
Granulomas/nodules	Granulomas: bacterial (*Mycobacterium*, *Nocardia*, *Edwardsiella*, *Francisella*), fungi, *Ichthyophonus hoferi*, nephrocalcinosis, neoplasia, trematode (*Acolpenteron* in bass)
White ureters	Nephrocalcinosis
Urinary bladder stones	Salinity/cation imbalances, renal/gill disease, genetic
Spleen:	
Diffuse swelling	Bacterial septicemia, viral infections (red sea bream iridovirus, grass carp reovirus)
Nodules	Granulomas (bacterial, fungal, parasitic), *Ichthyophonus*, neoplasia, *Dermocystidium*, hematoma
Liver:	
Necrosis	Virus, bacterial sepsis, heavy metals, algal toxin, rancid food, carbohydrates fed to carnivores
Hemorrhage	Virus, bacterial sepsis
Tan/yellow liver	Fat accumulation: excessive nutrition, toxicosis, choline deficiency, inadequate antioxidants, vitamin E deficiency, winter disease of Mediterranean fishes
	Fibrosis/iron accumulation
	Necrosis (see above)
Nodules	Bacteria (*Mycobacterium*, *Nocardia*, *Francisella*, *Pseudomonas*, *Edwardsiella*, among others), myxozoan infection, encysted parasites (*Anisakis*), fungi, *Ichthyophonus hoferi*, *Dermocystidium*, neoplasia, mineral (biliary lithiasis)
Cysts	Polycystic liver, cestode larvae

(*Continued*)

(*Continued*)

System/symptom	Differential diagnoses
Jaundice	Hemolysis, toxins, genetic abnormalities, *Staphylococcus aureus*, rancid feeds
White liver	Necrosis with inflammation (carbohydrate consumption in carnivorous fish)
Stomach:	
Nodules	Granulomas (fungi, *Mycobacteria*), microsporidians, myxozoans, nematodes
Dilation	Ileus, foreign bodies
Intestine:	
Hyperemia/hemorrhage	Bacterial septicemia (*Aeromonas*, *Vibrio*, *Edwardsiella*), viral infections (grass carp reovirus), cestodes, acanthocephalans
Mucoid feces/casts	Parasites, hypothermia, dietary, winter disease of Mediterranean fishes, spring viremia of carp
Nodules	Foreign bodies, granulomas, myxozoan cysts, neoplasia, encysted worms
Swim bladder:	
Enlarged	Hyperinflation: gas supersaturation, torsion, physostome blockage, *Betanodavirus*, acid/base imbalance
	Fluid: exudate (bacteria), protozoa (*Sphaerospora*), viral hemorrhagic septicemia
	Fungi, microsporidians, myxozoans
	Thickened wall: nematodes, chronic inflammation
Atrophy	Rupture
Hemorrhage	Virus (iridovirus), bacteria
Reproductive: Nodules/enlarged	*Mycobacterium*, *Ichthyophonus*, egg binding, microsporidians, myxozoans, neoplasia
Heart:	
Pallor	Amyloid
Inflammation/pericarditis	Bacterial sepsis (*Vagococcus*)
Hemopericardium	Heart rupture, virus
Nodules	Granulomas (bacteria, fungus, *Ichthyophonus hoferi*), *Metacercariae*, ventricular aneurysms

4.5.3 Tropical/Koi/Goldfish

System/symptom	Differential diagnoses
Sudden death	Bacterial septicemia (*Aeromonas*, *Bacillus*, *Pseudomonas*, *Proteus*, others), water quality issues (ammonia, oxygen, hydrogen sulfide, salinity), toxicosis (heavy metal, herbicide, pesticide), trauma, electrocution, botulism, gas supersaturation, vitamin deficiency, cyprinid herpesvirus 2, koi herpes virus, koi ranavirus, carp edema virus, gut torsion, sudden temperature change
Poor growth	Vitamin deficiency, stress, mycobacteriosis, nocardiosis, insufficient nutritional intake, heavy parasitism

System/symptom	Differential diagnoses
Uncoordinated swimming/ nervousness/ buoyancy	Generalized infectious disease: virus (*Betanodavirus*, infectious pancreatic necrosis, angelfish *Rhabdovirus*), fungi, bacteria (mycobacteria), myxozoans, microsporidians (*Pseudoloma neurophila*), electrocution, spinal trauma, toxicosis, CNS disease, swim bladder disease (hyperinflation), gas distention in gut, displacement of swim bladder, swim bladder underinflation/collapse, abdomen neoplasia, water quality issues (ammonia, oxygen, hydrogen sulfide, salinity), gas bubble disease, Flavobacterium neurotoxicosis, thiamine/ riboflavin/pyridoxine deficiency, *Ichthyophonus hoferi*, koi herpes virus, koi ranavirus, carp edema virus
Gasping/asphyxia:	Low dissolved oxygen, high water temperature, high carbon dioxide, toxin exposure/ammonia, organic/inorganic contaminants, suspended sediments
Gill disease	Branchiomycosis, *Flavobacterium*, parasites (*Dactylogyrus*, *Ichthyophthirius*, *Ichthyobodo*, *Chilodonella*, *Trichodina*, others), epitheliocystis, koi herpes virus, spring viremia of carp
Anemia	Pyridoxine deficiency, cyprinid herpes 2, zinc toxicosis
Skin/fins:	
Petechiae	Virus (spring viremia), bacterial septicemia, low pH
Increased mucus	Water quality issues, parasitism (*Ichthyobodo*, *Chilodonella*), koi herpes virus
Reduced mucus	Water quality issues, certain medications
Hemorrhage, necrosis, ulcers	Overcrowding, improper pH, ammonia/nitrite/nitrate, trauma, bacterial infection (*Aeromonas*, *Pseudomonas*, *Flavobacterium*, *Vibrio*, *Mycobacterium*, *Epitheliocystis*), *Saprolegnia*, *Tetrahymena*, *Aphanomyces*, parasites (esp. *Gyrodactylus*, *Ichthyophthirius*, *Ichthyobodo*, *Chilodonella*, *Trichodina*), spring viremia of carp, koi herpes virus, gas bubble disease, head and lateral line erosion syndrome, snakehead ulcerative disease virus, other viruses
Parasites	Ciliates, flagellates, *Monogenea*, turbellarians, copepods, branchiurans, isopods, bivalves, leeches, hydroids
Yellow/white flat lesions	*Flavobacterium*, necrosis, epidermal hyperplasia, edema, excess mucus, *Saprolegnia*, *Epistylis* (*Heteropolaria*)
Depigmentation	Epidermal/dermal injury of any type, neoplasia, vitamin B12 deficiency
Nodules/lumps	Epidermal hyperplasia, neoplasia, granulomatous disease (*Mycobacterium*, other bacteria, fungi), *Ichthyophthirius*, *Dermocystidium*, encysted trematodes, lymphocystis, foreign body, cyprinid herpesvirus 1 (pox), healing fractures
Segmental darkening	Neurologic disease/infection (myxozoans, microsporidians, fungus, bacteria, especially *Mycobacterium*), spinal trauma
Edema/ lepidorthosis	Hypoalbuminemia, renal disease, severe skin disease
Cysts	Breed specific features (goldfish)
Red vent	Internal disease (bacterial, viral), *Hexamita*/*Spironucleus*
Black spots/nodules	Melanocyte hyperplasia, melanoma, encysted trematodes, microsporidian infection (*Pleistophora*), pigmented fungal granulomas
Gills:	
Hemorrhage	Bacterial septicemia, toxins, diatoms, virus, protozoan parasites, spring viremia of carp, koi herpesvirus, chronic ammonia exposure, other viruses
Hyperplasia	Water quality issues, dietary imbalance (vitamin B5), chronic inflammation, parasitism (amoeba, flagellates, ciliates)

(*Continued*)

(*Continued*)

System/symptom	Differential diagnoses
Necrosis	*Flavobacterium*, branchiomycosis, virus (koi herpesvirus), high/low pH, chlorine, protozoan parasites
Nodules	Encysted trematodes, myxozoan cysts, neoplasia, granulomatous disease (*Mycobacterium*, *Nocardia*, other bacteria, fungi), *Ichthyophthirius*, *Dermocystidium*, epitheliocystis
Pallor	Anemia, spring viremia of carp, carp edema virus, other viruses
Gas bubbles	Supersaturation of water by gas
Parasites	*Monogenea*, ciliates, flagellates, copepods, branchiurans, isopods, bivalves, leeches, hydroids
Yellow/white lesions	*Flavobacterium* infection, necrosis, *Saprolegnia*
Mouth:	
Gasping/asphyxia	See general comment above
Hemorrhage/ulcers	Bacterial septicemia (*Flavobacterium*, *Erysipelothrix*), trauma
Increased mucus/exudate	Bacterial infection (*Flavobacterium*), parasitism
Gas bubbles	Gas supersaturation
Malocclusion	Inappropriate food sources, trauma
Nodules	Granulomas, lip papilloma (angelfish fibroma/odontoma), squamous cell carcinomas, dental neoplasia, parasitic cyst, thyroid hyperplasia, thyroid neoplasia, thymic neoplasia
Eye:	
Exophthalmia	Bacterial septicemia, *Mycobacteria*, spring viremia virus/rhabdovirus, vitamin A/E/pantothenic acid deficiency, vitamin A/E/pantothenic acid deficiency, nephrocalcinosis, gas bubble disease/supersaturation, *Tetrahymena*
Ulcers	Fungus, bacterial septicemia, trauma, blindness
Corneal edema/cloudiness	Poor water quality, conspecific aggression, bacterial, viral, fungal, parasitic disease (*Monogenea*, scuticociliates)
Ophthalmitis	Trauma, bacterial sepsis, thermal damage, zinc deficiency, *Diplostomum*
Cataract	*Diplostomum*, deficiencies (zinc, vitamin A, thiamine, riboflavin, methionine, tryptophan, histidine), rapid osmolar fluctuations, ultraviolet light exposure, temperature fluctuations, gas bubble disease
Gas bubbles	Supersaturation, bacterial infection, corneal perforation
Lens luxation	Trauma
Enucleation	Trauma (predator, stocking density too high), severe ophthalmitis
Muscle:	
Atrophy	Emaciation, denervation, riboflavin deficiency
Liquefaction/necrosis	Protozoa (*Kudoa*), microsporidians, myxozoans, bacterial infection
Nodules/swelling	Encysted trematodes, granulomas, microsporidians, myxozoans, emphysematous bacterial infection, *Ichthyophonus hoferi*, neoplasia, *Tetrahymena*
Hemorrhage	Viral hemorrhagic septicemia, bacterial sepsis, trauma, vascular disease, myonecrosis
White foci	Magnesium deficiency, other dietary imbalances, necrosis, microsporidians (*Pleistophora*)

System/symptom	Differential diagnoses
Skeletal deformity	Vitamin A/C/E deficiency, calcium/phosphorus deficiency, *Myxobolus*, *Mycobacterium*, abnormal egg incubation temperatures, trauma, hereditary, adverse environment conditions, toxicant exposure
Abdomen/celom:	
Enlarged (general)	Neoplasia, overweight, egg binding/dystocia, gastrointestinal impaction, peritonitis, cardiovascular/hepatic disease leading to ascites, renal disease, other causes of hypoproteinemia, parasites
Ascites	Bacterial septicemia, spring viremia virus/rhabdovirus, koi herpes virus, other virus
Peritonitis, nodular/ granulomatous	Mycobacteriosis, streptococcosis, parasites (coccidians, amoeba, worms), fungus, egg binding, neoplasia
Petechiae	Viral infection, bacterial infection
Cysts	*Hoferellus carassii*, polycystic renal disease, blocker ureter
Gas	Swim bladder or gut rupture, body wall perforation, inflammation w/ gas producing microbes or fungi
Kidney:	
Diffuse swelling	Virus (spring viremia, cyprinid herpes 2), bacterial septicemia, immune stimulation, necrosis
Cystic change	*Hoferellus carassii*, polycystic kidney disease (genetic/environmental), chronic renal disease
Necrosis	Virus (spring viremia, cyprinid herpesvirus 2, koi herpesvirus), bacterial sepsis, parasite/protozoa, riboflavin deficiency
Granulomas/ nodules	Bacteria (*Mycobacterium*, *Nocardia*, others), amoeba, fungi, myxozoans, microsporidians, nephrocalcinosis, melamine
Urinary bladder: stones	Salinity/cation imbalances, renal/gill disease, genetic
Spleen:	
Diffuse swelling	Bacterial septicemia, cyprinid herpes 2, Ramirez dwarf cichlid virus
Nodules	Granulomas: bacterial (*Mycobacterium*, *Nocardia*, others), fungal, parasitic; hematoma, *Ichthyophonus*
Liver:	
Necrosis	Virus (spring viremia), bacterial sepsis, algal toxins, heavy metal, aflatoxin, rancid food, improper food
Hemorrhage	Bacterial sepsis, virus, necrosis
Tan/yellow liver	Fat accumulation: excessive nutrition, toxicosis, dietary deficiency, inadequate antioxidants/vitamin E deficiency
	Fibrosis/iron accumulation
	Necrosis (see above)
Nodules	bacteria (*Mycobacterium*, *Nocardia*, others), amoeba, fungi, myxozoans, microsporidians
Stomach:	
Nodules	Granulomas (fungi, *Mycobacteria*), microsporidians, myxozoans, *Cryptobia* in cichlids, *Hexamita* in Siamese fighting fish
Dilation	Cichlid bloat, indigestion

(*Continued*)

(*Continued*)

System/symptom	Differential diagnoses
Intestine:	
Hyperemia/ hemorrhage	Bacterial enteritis, viral enteritis, parasitism
Mucoid feces/casts	Spring viremia of carp, Ramirez dwarf cichlid virus, coccidian infection, *Capillaria* infection, bacterial enteritis, dietary, inappetence
Nodules	Foreign bodies, granulomas, coccidian cysts, myxozoan cysts, neoplasia, encysted worms
Torsion	
Swim bladder:	
Enlarged	Hyperinflation: gas supersaturation, torsion, physostome blockage, acid/base imbalance
	Fluid: exudate (bacteria), protozoa
	Fungi, microsporidians, myxozoans
	Thickened wall: nematodes, chronic inflammation
Atrophy	Rupture
Hemorrhage	Virus, bacteria
Reproductive: Nodules/enlarged	*Mycobacterium*, *Ichthyophonus*, egg binding, microsporidians, myxozoans, neoplasia

Supplementary materials available online

Infectious diseases:

- Epitheliocystis
- Francisellosis (*Francisella* spp.)
- Lymphocystis
- *Megalocytivirus*
- Heart and skeletal muscle inflammation
- Cardiomyopathy syndrome
- Largemouth bass virus disease
- Red sea bream iridovirus disease
- Yellowtail ascites virus disease
- Grass carp hemorrhagic disease
- Infectious pancreatic necrosis (further information)
- Salmonid alphavirus (further information)
- Infectious salmon anemia (further information)

Parasitic diseases:

- Apicomplexan infection (*Coccidia,* hemogregarines)
- Salmonid whirling disease
- Proliferative kidney disease
- Glochidiosis

Diseases with multiple causes:

- Head and lateral line erosion syndrome
- Ammonia toxicosis
- Hydrogen sulfide toxicosis
- Nutritional disease (deficiencies, imbalances)

References

Adams, M.J., Lefkowitz, EJ., King, A.M.Q. *et al.* (2017). Change to taxonomy and international code of virus classification and nomenclature ratified by the international committee on taxonomy of viruses. *Archive of Virology* 162: 2505–2538.

Adams, M. B., Ellard, K., and Nowak, B. F. (2004). Gross pathology and its relationship with histopathology of amoebic gill disease (AGD) in farmed Atlantic salmon, *Salmo salar* L. *Journal of Fish Diseases* 27: 151–161.

Ahmadivand, S., Soltani, M., Mardani, K. *et al.* (2016). Isolation and identification of viral hemorrhagic septicemia virus (VHSV) from farmed rainbow trout (*Oncorhynchus mykiss*) in Iran. *Acta Tropica* 156: 30–36.

Ahne, W. and Negele, R.D. (1985). Studies on the transmission of IPNV via eyed eggs and sexual products of salmonid fish. In: *Fish and Shellfish Pathology* (ed. A.E. Ellis), 260–269. London: Academic Press.

Ahne, W., Vestergard-Jorgensen, P.E., Olesen, N.J. *et al.* (1989). Aquatic birnaviruses: virus of the serogroup II isolated from an IPN outbreak in brook trout. *Bulletin of the European Association of Fish Pathologists* 9: 14–16.

Biacchesi, S., Le Berre, M., Le Guillou, S. *et al.* (2007), Fish genotype significantly influences susceptibility of juvenile rainbow trout, *Oncorhynchus mykiss* (Walbaum), to waterborne infection with infectious salmon anaemia virus. *Journal of Fish Diseases* 30: 631–636.

Blake, S., Bouchard, D., Keleher, W. *et al.* (1999). Genomic relationships of the North American isolate of infectious salmon anemia virus (ISAV) to the Norwegian strain of ISAV. *Diseases of Aquatic Organisms* 35: 139–144.

Bootland, L.M. and Leong, J.C. (1999). Infectious hematopoietic necrosis virus. In: *Fish Diseases and Disorders, Volume 3: Viral, Bacterial and Fungal Infections.* (ed. P.T.K. Woo and D.W. Bruno), 57–121. Oxford: CAB International.

Bootland, L.M., Dobos, P. and Stevenson, R.M.W. (1991). The IPNV carrier state and demonstration of vertical transmission in experimentally infected brook trout. *Diseases of Aquatic Organisms* 10: 13–21.

Boucher, P. and Baudin-Laurencin, F. (1996). Sleeping disease and pancreas disease: comparative histopathology and acquired cross-protection. *Journal of Fish Diseases* 19: 303–310.

Bovo, G., Håstein, T., Hill, B. *et al.* (2005). *Fish Egg Trade Work Package 1 Report: Hazard identification for vertical transfer of fish disease agents.* Oslo: VESO.

Bowater, R.O. and O'Donoghue, P.J. (2015). An epizootic of chilodonelliasis in farmed barramundi *Lates calcarifer* (Bloch), a case report. *Journal of Fish Diseases* 38: 931–936.

Bratland, A. and Nylund, A. (2009). Studies on the possibility of vertical transmission of Norwegian salmonid alphavirus in production of Atlantic salmon in Norway. *Journal of Aquatic Animal Health* 21: 73–78.

Bruno, D.W., Noguera, P.A., Black, J. *et al.* (2014). Identification of a wild reservoir of salmonid alphavirus in common dab *Limanda limanda*, with emphasis on virus culture and sequencing. *Diseases of Aquatic Organisms* 5: 89–98.

Castric, J., Baudin-Laurencin, F., Coustans, M.F. and Auffret, M. (1987). Isolation of infectious pancreatic necrosis virus, Ab serotype, from an epizootic in farmed turbot, *Scophthalmus maximus. Aquaculture* 67:117–126.

Christiansen, D.H., Ostergaard, P.S., Snow, M. *et al.* (2011). A low-pathogenic variant of infectious salmon anemia virus (ISAV-HPR0) is highly prevalent and causes a non-clinical transient infection in farmed Atlantic salmon (*Salmo salar* L.) in the Faroe Islands. *Journal of General Virology* 92: 909–918.

Christie, K.E. (1997). Immunization with viral antigens: infectious pancreatic necrosis. *Developments in Biological Standardization* 90: 191–199.

Cunningham, C.O., Gregory, A., Black, J. *et al.* (2002). A novel variant of the infectious salmon anaemia virus (ISAV) haemagglutinin gene suggests mechanisms for virus diversity. *Bulletin of the European Association of Fish Pathologists* 22: 366–374.

Dahle, G., Hjeltnes, B. and Jørstad, K.E. (1996). Infection of Atlantic salmon sibling groups with infectious salmon anaemia (ISA) and furunculosis. *Bulletin of the European Association of Fish Pathologists* 16: 192–195.

Dannevig, B.H., Falk, K. and Namork, E. (1995). Isolation of the causal virus of infectious salmon anaemia (ISA) in a long-term cell line from Atlantic salmon head kidney. *Journal of General Virology* 76: 1353–1359.

Deperasińska, I., Schulz, P. and Siwicki, A.K. (2018). Salmonid alphavirus (SAV). *Journal of Veterinary Research* 62: 1–6.

Desautels, D. and MacKelvie, R.M. (1975). Practical aspects of survival and destruction of infectious pancreatic necrosis virus. *Journal of the Fisheries Research Board of Canada* 32: 523–531.

Dixon, P., Paley, R., Alegria-Moran, R. and Oidtmann, B. (2016). Epidemiological characteristics of infectious hematopoietic necrosis virus (IHNV): a review. *Veterinary Research* 47: 63.

Dobos, P., Hill, B.J., Hallett, R. *et al.* (1979). Biophysical and biochemical characterization of five animal viruses with bisegmented dsRNA genomes. *Journal of Virology* 32: 593–605.

Dorson, M. (1982). Infectious pancreatic necrosis of salmonids: present status of knowledge concerning the viruses and the possibilities of controlling the disease. *Bulletin Français de Pisciculture* 305: 61–66.

Dorson, M. and Torchy, C. (1981). The influence of fish age and water temperature on mortalities of rainbow trout, *Salmo gairdneri* Richardson, caused by a European strain of infectious pancreatic necrosis virus. *Journal of Fish Diseases* 4: 213–221.

Economon, P.P. (1973). Polyvinylpyrrolidone-iodine as a control for infectious pancreatic necrosis (IPN) virus of brook trout. In: *Symposium on the Major Communicable Fish Diseases in Europe and Their Control* (ed. W.A. Dill), 59–66. London: EIFAC.

Eide, G.W. (1992). [A retrospective analysis of outbreaks of infectious salmon anaemia in Sogn and Fjordane in 1985–91.] *Norsk Veterinaertidsskrift* 104: 915–919.

Einer-Jensen, K., Ahrens, P. and Lorenzen, N. (2005). Parallel phylogenetic analyses using the N, G or Nv gene from a fixed group of VHSV isolates reveal the same overall genetic typing. *Diseases of Aquatic Organisms* 67: 39–45.

Einer-Jensen, K., Ahrens, P., Forsberg, R. and Lorenzen, N. (2004). Evolution of the fish rhabdovirus viral haemorrhagic septicaemia virus. *Journal of General Virology* 85: 1167–1179.

Emmenegger, E.J., Glenn, J.A., Winton, J.R. *et al.* (2014). Molecular identification of erythrocytic necrosis virus (ENV) from the blood of Pacific herring (*Clupea pallasii*). *Veterinary Microbiology* 174: 16–26.

Evensen, O., Meier, W., Wahli, T. *et al.* (1994). Comparison of immunohistochemistry and virus cultivation for detection of viral hemarrhagic septicaemia virus in experimentally infected rainbow trout *Oncorhynchus mykiss*. *Diseases of Aquatic Organisms* 20: 101–109.

Evensen, O., Thorud, K.E. and Olsen, Y.A. (1991). A morphological study of the gross and light microscopic lesion of infectious salmon anemia in Atlantic salmon (*Salmo salar* L.) *Research in Veterinary Science* 51: 215–222.

Frantsi, C. and Savan, M. (1971). Infectious pancreatic necrosis virus: comparative frequencies of isolation from feces and organs of brook trout (*Salvelinus fontinalis*). *Journal of the Fisheries Research Board of Canada* 28: 1064–1065.

Fringuelli, E., Rowley, H.M., Wilson, J.C. *et al.* (2008). Phylogenetic analyses and molecular epidemiology of European salmonid alphaviruses (SAV) based on partial E2 and nsP3 gene nucleotide sequences. *Journal of Fish Diseases* 31: 811–823.

Glenn, J.A., Emmenegger, E.J., Grady, C.A. *et al.* (2012). Kinetics of viral load and erythrocytic inclusion body formation in Pacific herring artificially infected with erythrocytic necrosis virus. *Journal of Aquatic Animal Health* 24: 195–200.

Gomes, G.B., Jerry, D.R., Miller, T.L. and Hutson, K.S. (2017). Current status of parasitic ciliates *Chilodonella* spp. (Phyllopharyngea: Chilodonellidae) in freshwater fish aquaculture. *Journal of Fish Diseases* 40: 703–715.

Goodwin, A. E. and Merry, G. E. (2011). Replication and persistence of VHSV IVb in freshwater turtles. *Diseases of Aquatic Organisms* 94:173–177.

Graham, D.A., Fringuelli, E., Rowley, H.M. *et al.* (2012). Geographical distribution of salmonid alphavirus subtypes in marine farmed Atlantic salmon, *Salmo salar* L., in Scotland and Ireland. *Journal of Fish Diseases* 35: 755–765.

Graham, D.A., Rowley, H.M., Fringuelli, E. *et al.* (2007). First laboratory confirmation of salmonid alphavirus infection in Italy and Spain. *Journal of Fish Diseases* 30: 569–572.

Haenen, O.L., Schuetze, H., Cieslak, M. *et al.* (2016). First evidence of infectious hematopoietic necrosis virus (IHNV) in the Netherlands. *Journal of Fish Diseases* 39: 971–979.

Hamor, T. (1996). Practical approach to infectious pancreatic necrosis virus (IPNV) disinfection using gaseous formaldehyde. *Journal of Applied Aquaculture* 6: 1–10.

He, M., Ding, N.Z., He, C.Q. *et al.* (2013). Dating the divergence of the infectious hematopoietic necrosis virus. *Infection, Genetics and Evolution* 18: 145–150.

Hill, B.J. (1994). European community measures for control of fish disease. In: International symposium on aquatic animal health: program and abstracts, 4–8 September 1994, Seattle, WA. Davis, CA: University of California at Davis: VI–5.

Hill, B.J. (1982). Infectious pancreatic necrosis virus and its virulence. In: *Microbial Diseases of Fish* (ed. R.J. Roberts), 91–114. London: Academic Press.

Hill, B.J. and Way, K. (1995). Serological classification of infectious pancreatic necrosis (IPN) virus and other aquatic birnaviruses. *Annual Review of Fish Disease* 5: 55–77.

Hovland, T., Nylund, A., Watanabe, K. and Endresen, C. (1994). Observation of infectious salmon anaemia virus in Atlantic salmon, *Salmo salar* L. *Journal of Fish Diseases* 17, 291–296.

Isshiki, T., Nishizawa, T., Kobayashi, T. *et al.* (2001). An outbreak of VHSV (viral hemorrhagic septicemia virus) infection in farmed Japanese flounder *Paralichthys olivaceus* in Japan. *Diseases of Aquatic Organisms* 47: 87–99.

Jansen, M.D., Bang Jensen, B., McLoughlin, M.F. *et al.* (2017). The epidemiology of pancreas disease in salmonid aquaculture: a summary of the current state of knowledge. *Journal of Fish Diseases* 40: 141–155.

Jansen, M.D., Gjerset, B., Modahl, I. and Bohlin, J. (2010). Molecular epidemiology of salmonid alphavirus (SAV) subtype 3 in Norway. *Virology Journal* 7: 188.

Jarp, J. and Karlsen, E. (1997). Infectious salmon anaemia (ISA) risk factors in sea-cultured Atlantic salmon *Salmo salar*. *Diseases of Aquatic Organisms* 28: 79–86.

Jørgensen, P.E.V. and Kehlet, N.P. (1971). Infectious pancreatic necrosis (IPN) viruses in Danish rainbow trout: their serological and pathogenic properties. *Nordisk Veterinaermedicin* 23: 568–575.

Kerbart Boscher, S.K., McLoughlin, M., Le Ven, A. *et al.* (2006). Experimental transmission of sleeping disease in one-year-old rainbow trout, *Oncorhynchus mykiss* (Walbaum), induced by sleeping disease virus. *Journal of Fish Diseases* 29: 263–273.

Kibenge, F.S., Gárate, O.N., Johnson, G. *et al.* (2001). Isolation and identification of infectious salmon anaemia virus (ISAV) from Coho salmon in Chile. *Diseases of Aquatic Organisms* 45: 9–18.

Kibenge, F.S.B., Godoy, M.G., Wang, Y. *et al.* (2009). Infectious salmon anaemia virus (ISAV) isolated from the ISA disease outbreaks in Chile diverged from ISAV isolates from Norway around 1996 and was disseminated around 2005, based on surface glycoprotein gene sequences. *Virology Journal* 6: 88.

Kibenge, F.S.B., Kibenge, M.J.T., Wang, Y. *et al.* (2007). Mapping of putative virulence motifs on infectious salmon anaemia virus surface glycoprotein genes. *Journal of General Virology* 88: 3100–3111.

Kibenge, F.S.B., Kibenge, M.J.T., Groman, D. and McGeachy, S. (2006). in vivo correlates of infectious salmon anemia virus pathogenesis in fish. *Journal of General Virology* 87: 2645–2652.

Kongtorp, R.T., Stene, A., Andreassen, P.A. *et al.* (2010). Lack of evidence for vertical transmission of SAV 3 using gametes of Atlantic salmon, *Salmo salar* L., exposed by natural and experimental routes. *Journal of Fish Diseases* 33: 879–888.

Kristoffersen, A.B., Viljugrein, H., Kongtorp, R.T. *et al.* (2009). Risk factors for pancreas disease (PD) outbreaks in farmed Atlantic salmon and rainbow trout in Norway during 2003–2007. *Preventive Veterinary Medicine* 90: 127–136.

Kurath, G. and Leong, J.C. (1985). Characterization of infectious hematopoietic necrosis virus mRNA species reveals a nonvirion rhabdovirus protein. *Journal of Virology* 53: 462–468.

Kurath, G. and Winton, J. R. (2011). Complex dynamics at the interface between wild and domestic viruses of finfish. *Current Opinion in Virology* 1: 73–80.

Kurath, G., Garver, K.A., LaPatra, S.E. and Purcell, M.K. (2010). Resistance and protective immunity in Redfish Lake sockeye salmon exposed to M type infectious hematopoietic necrosis virus (IHNV). *Journal of Aquatic Animal Health* 22: 129–139.

Kurath, G., Garver, K.A., Troyer, R.M. *et al.* (2003). Phylogeography of infectious haematopoietic necrosis virus in North America. *Journal of General Virology* 84: 803–814.

Laird, M. and Bullock, W. (1969) Marine fish haematozoa from New Brunswick and New England. *Journal of the Fisheries Research Board of Canada* 26: 1075–1102.

Lewisch, E., Frank, T., Soliman, H. *et al.* (2018). First confirmation of salmonid alphavirus infection in Arctic char Salvelinus alpinus and in Austria. *Diseases of Aquatic Organisms* 130: 71–76.

Liltvedt, H., Hektoen, H. and Efraimsen, H. (1995). Inactivation of bacterial and viral fish pathogens by ozonation or UV irradiation in water of different salinity. *Aquacultural Engineering* 14: 107–122.

Lo, C.F., Hong, Y.W., Huang, S.Y. and Wang, C.H. (1998). The characteristics of the virus isolated from the gill of clam, *Meretrix lusoria*. *Fish Pathology* 23: 147–154.

Lyngstad, T.M., Kristoffersen, A.B., Hjortaas, M.J. *et al.* (2012). Low virulent infectious salmon anaemia virus (ISAV-HPR0) is prevalent and geographically structured in Norwegian salmon farming. *Diseases of Aquatic Organisms* 101: 197–206.

McAllister, P.E. (1990). *Viral Haemorrhagic Septicaemia of Fish*. Fish Disease Leaflet 73. Kearneysville, WV: Fish and Wildlife Service, US Department of the Interior.

McAllister, P. E., and Owens, W. J. (1992). Recovery of infectious pancreatic necrosis virus from the faeces of wild piscivorous birds. *Aquaculture* 106: 227–232.

McBeath, A.J., Bain, N. and Snow, M. (2009). Surveillance for infectious salmon anaemia virus HPR0 in marine Atlantic salmon farms across Scotland. *Diseases of Aquatic Organisms* 87: 161–169.

McLoughlin, M.F., and Graham, D.A. (2007). Alphavirus infections in salmonids: a review. *Journal of Fish Diseases* 30: 511–531.

McLoughlin, M.F., Nelson R.N., McCormick J.I. *et al.* (2002). Clinical and histopathological features of naturally occurring pancreas disease in farmed Atlantic salmon, *Salmo salar* L. *Journal of Fish Diseases* 25: 33–43.

McVicar, A.H. (1990). Infection as a primary cause of pancreas disease in farmed Atlantic salmon. *Bulletin of the European Association of Fish Pathologists* 10: 84–87.

Melville, K.J. and Griffiths, S.G. (1999). Absence of vertical transmission of infectious salmon anemia virus (ISAV) from individually infected Atlantic salmon *Salmo salar*. *Diseases of Aquatic Organisms* 38: 231–234.

Mjaaland, S., Rimstad, E., Falk, K. and, Dannevig, B.H. (1997). Genomic characterisation of the virus causing infectious salmon anemia in Atlantic salmon (*Salmo salar* L.): an orthomyxo-like virus in a teleost. *Journal of Virology* 71: 7681–7686.

Mortensen, S.H., Nilsen, R.K. and Hjeltnes, B. (1998). Stability of an infectious pancreatic necrosis virus (IPNV) isolate stored under different laboratory conditions. *Diseases of Aquatic Organisms* 33: 67–71.

Mortensen, S.H., Hjeltnes, B., Rødseth, O. *et al.* (1990). Infectious pancreatic necrosis virus, serotype N1, isolated from Norwegian halibut (*Hippoglossus hippoglossus*), turbot (*Scophthalmus maximus*) and scallops (*Pecten maximus*). *Bulletin of the European Association of Fish Pathologists* 10: 42–43.

Mullins, J. (1998). Infectious salmon anemia management and control in New Brunswick. Abstract. In: 6th annual New England farmed fish health workshop, 3 April 1998, Eastport, ME, Marine Technology Center. Orono, ME: University of Maine Cooperative Extension: 13.

Munday, B.L., Zilberg, D. and Findlay, V. (2001). Gill disease of marine fish caused by infection with *Neoparamoeba pemaquidensis*. *Journal of Fish Diseases*, 24: 497–507.

Murray, A.G. (2001). Modeling epidemic spread of two emerging diseases: Pilchard herpesvirus, Australia, and infectious salmon anaemia, Scotland. Abstract. In: Proceedings of the 10th international conference of the European Association of Fish Pathologists, 9–14 September 2001, Dublin, Trinity College (ed. M.H. Hiney), O10. Dublin: European Association of Fish Pathologists.

Murray, A.G., Smith, R.J. and Stagg, R M. (2002). Shipping and the spread of infectious salmon anemia in Scottish aquaculture. *Emerging Infectious Diseases* 8: 1–5.

Nakajima, K., Maeno, Y., Arimoto, M. *et al.* (1993). Viral deformity of yellowtail fingerlings. *Gyobyo Kenkyu* 28: 125–129.

Neukirch, M. (1985). Uptake, multiplication and excretion of viral hemorrhagic septicemia virus in trout (*Salmo gairdneri*). In: *Fish and Shellfish Pathology* (ed. A.E. Ellis), 295–300. London: Academic Press.

Noble, C., Gismervik, K., Iversen, M.H. *et al.* (eds.) (2018). *Welfare Indicators for farmed Atlantic salmon: Tools for assessing fish welfare*. Tromsø, Norway: Nofima.

Novoa, B., Figueras, A., Puentes, C.F. *et al.* (1993). Characterization of a birnavirus isolated from diseased turbot cultured in Spain. *Diseases of Aquatic Organisms* 15: 163–169.

Nylund, A., Plarre, H., Karlsen, M. *et al.* (2007). Transmission of infectious salmon anaemia virus (ISAV) in farmed populations of Atlantic salmon (*Salmo salar*). *Archive of Virology* 152: 151–179.

Nylund, A., Devold, M., Plarre, H. *et al.* (2003). Emergence and maintenance of infectious salmon anaemia virus (ISAV) in Europe: a new hypothesis. *Diseases of Aquatic Organisms* 56: 11–24.

Nylund, A., Kvenseth, A.M., Krossoy, B. and Hodneland, K. (1997). Replication of the infectious salmon anaemia virus (ISAV) in rainbow trout, *Oncorhynchus mykiss* (Walbaum). *Journal of Fish Diseases* 20: 275–279.

Nylund, A., Alexandersen, S., Rolland, J. B. and Jakobsen, P. (1995a). Infectious salmon anemia virus (ISAV) in brown trout. *Journal of Aquatic Animal Health* 7: 236–240.

Nylund, A., Kevenseth, A. M. and Krossøy, B. (1995b). Susceptibility of wild salmon (*Salmo salar* L.) to infectious salmon anaemia (ISA). *Bulletin of the European Association of Fish Pathologists* 15: 152–155.

Nylund, A., Hovland, T., Hodneland, K. *et al.* (1994). Mechanisms for transmission of infectious salmon anemia (ISA). *Diseases of Aquatic Organisms* 19: 95–100.

Olesen, N.J. and Skall, H.F. (2013). Viral haemorrhagic septicaemia virus. In: *Mononegaviruses of Veterinary Importance Vol I: Pathobiology and molecular diagnosis* (ed. M. Munir), 323–336. Wallingford, UK: CABI International.

Olesen, N. J., Jørgensen, P.E.V., Bloch, B. and Mellergaard, S. (1988). Isolation of an IPN-like virus belonging to the serogroup II of the aquatic birnaviruses from dab, *Limanda limanda* L. *Journal of Fish Diseases* 11: 449–451.

Øye, A.K. and Rimstad, E. (2001). Inactivation of infectious salmon anaemia virus, viral haemorrhagic septicaemia virus and infectious pancreatic necrosis virus in water using UVC irradiation. *Diseases of Aquatic Organisms* 48: 1–5.

Penaranda, M.M., Lapatra, S.E. and Kurath, G. (2011). Specificity of DNA vaccines against the U and M genogroups of infectious hematopoietic necrosis virus (IHNV) in rainbow trout (*Oncorhynchus mykiss*). *Fish and Shellfish Immunology* 31: 43–51.

Peters, F. and Neukirch, M. (1986). Transmission of some fish pathogenic viruses by the heron, *Ardea cinerea*. *Journal of Fish Diseases* 9: 539–544.

Pimenta Leibowitz, M., Ariav, R. and Zilberg, D. (2005). Environmental and physiological conditions affecting *Tetrahymena* sp. infection in guppies, *Poecilia reticulata* Peters. *Journal of Fish Diseases* 28: 539–547.

Powell, M.D., Nowak, B.F. and Adams, M.B. (2002). Cardiac morphology in relation to amoebic gill disease history in Atlantic salmon, *Salmo salar* L. *Journal of Fish Diseases*, 25: 209–215.

Powers A.M., Brault A.C., Shirako Y. *et al.* (2001). Evolutionary relationships and systematics of the alphaviruses. *Virology* 75: 10118–10131.

Reno, P.W. (1999). Infectious pancreatic necrosis virus and its virulence. In: *Fish Diseases and Disorders. Volume 3: Viral, Bacterial and Fungal Infections* (ed. P.T.K. Woo and D.W. Bruno), 1–55. Wallingford, UK: CABI Publishing.

Rimstad, E., Dale, O.B., Dannevig, B. H. and Falk, K. (2011). Infectious Salmon Anaemia. In: *Fish Diseases and Disorders, Volume 3: Viral, Bacterial and Fungal Infections* (ed. P.T.K. Woo and D.W. Bruno), 143–165. Wallingford, UK: CAB International.

Rodger, H.D. and Frerichs, G.N. (1997). Clinical infectious pancreatic necrosis virus infection in farmed halibut in the United Kingdom. *Veterinary Record* 140: 401–402.

Rodger H. and Mitchell S. (2007). Epidemiological observations of pancreas disease of farmed Atlantic salmon *Salmo salar* L., in Ireland. *Journal of Fish Diseases* 30, 157–168.

Rolland, J.B. and Nylund, A. (1999). Sea running brown trout: carrier and transmitter of the infectious salmon anemia virus (ISAV). *Bulletin of the European Association of Fish Pathologists* 18: 50–55.

Rolland, J.B. and Nylund, A. (1998). Infectiousness of organic materials originating in ISA-infected fish and transmission of the disease via salmon lice (*Lepeophtheirus salmonis*). *Bulletin of the European Association of Fish Pathologists* 18: 173–180.

Ross, K.U., McCarthy, P.J., Huntly, B.P. *et al.* (1994). An outbreak of viral haemorrhagic septicaemia (VHS) in turbot (*Scophthalmus maximus*) in Scotland. *Bulletin of the European Association of Fish Pathologists* 14: 213–214.

Rozas-Serri, M. (2019). Gill diseases in marine salmon aquaculture with an emphasis on amoebic gill disease. *CAB Reviews Perspectives in Agriculture Veterinary Science* 14: 1–15.

Saint-Jean, S.R., Borrego, J.J. and Perez-Prieto, S.I. (2003). Infectious pancreatic necrosis virus: biology, pathogenesis, and diagnostic methods. *Advances in Virus Research* 62: 113–165.

Shivley, J.M., Brookshire, W.C. and Baumgartner, W.A. (2021). Mixed chromatophoroma (benign irido-melanocytoma) in a male Siamese fighting fish, *Betta splendens*, Regan. *Journal of Fish Diseases 2021*; 44: 351–354.

Schönherz, A.A., Lorenzen, N. and Einer-Jensen, K. (2013). Inter-species transmission of viral hemorrhagic septicemia virus (VHSV) from turbot (*Scophthalmus maximus*) to rainbow trout (*Oncorhynchus mykiss*). *Journal of General Virology* 94: 869–875.

Shannon, D. (1998). ISA hits Shetland: minister links spread with wellboats. *Fish Farming International* 25: 4.

Smail, D.A. (1999). Viral Haemorrhagic Septicaemia. In: *Fish Diseases and Disorders, Volume 3: Viral, Bacterial and Fungal infection* (ed. P.T.K. Woo and D.W. Bruno), 123–147. Wallingford, UK: CABI International.

Smail, D.A. and Snow, M. (2011). Viral Haemorrhagic septicaemia. In: *Fish Diseases and Disorders, Volume 3: Viral, Bacterial and Fungal Infections*, 2e (ed. P.T.K Woo and D.W. Bruno), 110–142. Wallingford, UK: CABI International.

Smail, D.A. and Munro, A. L. S. (1989). Infectious pancreatic necrosis virus in Atlantic salmon: transmission via the sexual products? In: *Viruses of Lower Vertebrates* (ed. W. Ahne and Kurstask, E.), 292–301. New York, NY: Springer.

Smail, D.A., Grant, R., Rain, N. and Hastings, T S. (2001). Veridical effects of iodophors, chloramine T and chlorine doxide against cultured infectious salmon anaemia (ISA) virus. (Abstract) In: *Proceedings of the 10th International Conference of the European Association of Fish Pathologists, 9–14 September 2001, Dublin (Trinity College)*. (ed. M.H. Hiney), O–10. Dublin: European Association of Fish Pathologists.

Snow, M., Bain, N., Black, J. *et al.* (2004). Genetic population structure of marine viral haemorrhagic septicaemia virus (VHSV). *Diseases of Aquatic Organisms* 61: 11–21.

Snow, M., Cunningham, C.O., Melvin, W.T. and Kurath, G. (1999). Analysis of the nucleoprotein identifies distinct lineages of viral haemorrhagic septicaemia virus within the European marine environment. *Virus Research* 63: 35–44.

Strauss, J.H. and Strauss, E.G. (1994). The alphaviruses: gene expression, replication, and evolution. *Microbiological Reviews* 58: 491–562.

Taylor, R.S., Muller, W.J., Cook, M.T. *et al.* (2009). Gill observations in Atlantic salmon (*Salmo salar*, L.) during repeated amoebic gill disease (AGD) field exposure and survival challenge. *Aquaculture* 290: 1–8.

Thorud, K.E. (1991). *Infectious Salmon Anemia*. DSc. dissertation, Norwegian College of Veterinary Medicine.

Thorud, K.E. and Djupvik, H. O. (1988). Infectious salmon anaemia in Atlantic salmon (*Salmo salar* L.). *Bulletin of the European Association of Fish Pathologists* 8: 109–111.

Tordo, N., Benmansour, A., Calisher, C. *et al.* (2005). "Rhabdoviridae". In: *Virus Taxonomy. Eighth Report of the International Committee on Taxonomy of Viruses* (ed. C.M. Fauquet, M.A. Mayo, J. Maniloff *et al.*), 623–644. London, UK: Elsevier Academic Press.

Totland, G.K., Hjeltnes, B.K. and Flood, P.R. (1996). Transmission of infectious salmon anemia (ISA) through natural secretions and excretions from infected smolts of Atlantic salmon *Salmo salar*. *Diseases of Aquatic Organisms* 26: 25–31.

Underwood, B.O., Smale, C.J., Brown, F. and Hill, B.J. (1977). Relationship of a virus from Tellina tenuis to infectious pancreatic necrosis virus. *Journal of General Virology* 36: 93–109.

Vagsholm, I., Djupvik, H.O., Willumsen, F.V. *et al.* (1994). Infectious salmon anaemia (ISA) epidemiology in Norway. *Preventive Veterinary Medicine* 19: 277–290.

Viljugrein, H., Staalstrøm, A., Molvær, J. *et al.* (2009). Integration of hydrodynamics into a statistical model on the spread of pancreas disease (PD) in salmon farming. *Diseases of Aquatic Organisms* 88: 35–44.

Walker, P.J. and Winton, J.R. (2010). Emerging viral diseases of fish and shrimp. *Veterinary Research* 41: 51.

Walker, P. J., Benmansour, A., Dietzgen, R. *et al.* (2000). Family Rhabdoviridae. In: *Virus Taxonomy: Classification and nomenclature of viruses. Seventh Report of the International Committee on Taxonomy of Viruses* (ed. M.H.V. van Regenmortel, C.M. Fauquet, D.H.L. Bishopet al.), 563–583. San Diego, CA: Academic Press.

Weston, J.H., Welsh, M.D., McLoughlin, M.F. and Todd, D. (1999). Salmon pancreas disease virus, an alphavirus infecting farmed Atlantic salmon, *Salmo salar* L. *Virology* 256: 188–195.

Winton, J.R. (1991). Recent advances in the detection and control of infectious hematopoietic necrosis virus (IHNV) in aquaculture. *Annual Review of Fish Diseases* 1: 83–93.

Wolf, K. (1988). *Fish Viruses and Fish Viral Diseases*. Ithaca, NY: Cornell University Press.

Wolf, K. and Quimby, M. (1971). Salmonid viruses: Infectious pancreatic necrosis virus. *Archiv für die gesamte Virusforschung* 34: 144–156.

Wolf, K. and Quimby, M. (1962). Established eurythermic cell line of fish cells in vitro. *Science* 135: 1065–1066.

Woo, P.T.K. (2003). *Cryptobia* (*Trypanoplasma*) *salmositica* and salmonid cryptobiosis. *Journal of Fish Diseases* 26: 627–646.

Wood, E.M., Snieszko, S.F. and Yasutake, W.T. (1955). Infectious pancreatic necrosis of brook trout. *American Medical Association Archives of Pathology* 60: 26–28.

World Organisation for Animal Health. (2019). Infection with haematopoietic necrosis virus. Chapter 2.3.4. In: *Manual of Diagnostic Tests for Aquatic Animals*, Chapter 2.3.4. https://www.oie.int/en/what-we-do/standards/codes-and-manuals/aquatic-manual-online-access/?id=169&L=1&htmfile=chapitre_ihn.htm (accessed 4 May 2021).

Yasutake, W.T. and Mead, R.W. (1969). A hematopoietic virus disease of rainbow trout and sockeye salmon. *Transactions of the American Fisheries Society* 98: 796–804.

Yemmen, C. and Bahri, S. (2017). Seasonality of *Amyloodinium ocellatum* Brown 1931 (Dinophyceae) infesting the Senegalese sole *Solea senegalensis* from Bizerte lagoon, Tunisia. *Journal of Fish Diseases* 40: 853–857.

Zhu, L., Wang, X., Wang K. *et al.* (2017). Outbreak of infectious pancreatic necrosis virus (IPN) in farmed rainbow trout in China. *Acta Tropica* 170: 63–69.

5

Epidemiology of Aquatic Animal Diseases

Leo Foyle

Learning Objectives

- Gain a working understanding of the lymphoid system in fish, including the role of the various tissues.
- Understand the role of the pronephros in the immune system.
- Be able to conduct a basic comparison of fish with mammals.
- Describe the main elements of the innate and adaptive systems in fish.
- Discuss the types of vaccine available in aquaculture.
- Discuss how vaccines are administered in aquaculture.
- Recognize and grade the main sequalae from vaccinating fish.
- Know how to assess vaccination success such as the relative percent survival.

5.1 Introduction

The principles of epidemiology are used regularly in population medicine to examine rates of morbidity and mortality on a very broad scale. These principles include attributes of disease as they relate to the host, the pathogen of interest, and the environment. A Venn diagram is commonly used to describe how these attributes relate to each other and lead to disease when out of equilibrium.

Understanding the interrelationships of factors associated with the agent, host, and environment in the initiation, propagation, treatment, and control of disease is of paramount importance for an efficient control or constraint of the disease. Prevention and control of diseases in aquatic animal populations is crucial to ensuring a sustainable development of aquatic animal populations. Emerging diseases and diseases of public health concern merit consideration because of hazards they pose to animal, human, and environmental health. To monitor and control such diseases, surveillance systems are established at national and/or regional levels. These systems include evidence-based epidemiological data referring to identification of pathogens, susceptible species, sources, reservoirs. Disease testing and clinical assessments are used to determine the presence or absence of a particular disease within an epidemiological unit. Pathogen identification and characterization, as well as pathogenesis of a disease, are of paramount importance in testing and diagnosis of a disease, allowing for effective prevention and management if such diseases occur.

Fundamentals of Aquatic Veterinary Medicine, First Edition. Edited by Laura Urdes, Chris Walster, and Julius Tepper.

Companion website: www.wiley.com/go/urdes/aquatic-veterinary-medicine

Based on the widespread distribution of aquatic birds, in addition to their high degree of mobility (i.e., flight), disease control and prevention of large or widespread disease outbreaks is often challenging. In some cases, collection and removal of infected carcasses is practiced and may reduce environmental contamination. Remaining healthy birds may be dispersed or relocated to non-outbreak areas and if species are of conservation concern, rehabilitation may be attempted. If these methods are employed, timely response is critical (United States Geological Survey, 1999d). Land management practices, such as reducing the output of potentially toxic chemicals and organic compounds, especially into water sources or into run-off, may help in the management of some of the diseases listed in Chapter 4 (e.g., botulism, numerous toxicoses; United States Geological Survey, 1999c). Although vaccines for some pathogens have been established for use in poultry and may be used in valued zoo collections and other captive settings (e.g., West Nile virus), they are generally not used in free-ranging birds. West Nile fever and eastern equine encephalitis are World Organisation for Animal Health (OIE; 2020) listed notifiable diseases under the "Multiple species diseases, infections and infestations" category. Under the "Avian diseases and infections" category, avian chlamydiosis, Newcastle disease (avian paramyxovirus-1), fowl typhoid (*Salmonella gallinarum* and *S. pullorum*), avian influenza viruses, and influenza A viruses of high pathogenicity (World Organisation for Animal Health, 2020).

Migratory aquatic birds provide unique epidemiological challenges in tracking disease maintenance and spread, as well as potential management, because some species (e.g., waterfowl) travel long distances and congregate at high densities on water bodies at stopover, breeding, or overwintering sites. Such a scenario provides abundant opportunities for sharing of infectious agents and toxins, especially because birds are often immunosuppressed and energetically challenged (e.g., avian influenza viruses, avian paramyxoviruses, *Pasteurella multocida*, *Clostridium botulinum* toxin; Stallknecht *et al.*, 2007).

Examination of mortality data in a population can be useful in early detection and initial diagnosis of disease, especially in production settings. Daily mortality, when routinely recorded, can be graphed, and trendlines can be used to identify any increases early on. The rate of increase in mortality can be used to distinguish among commonly known pathogens for a group of production animals; for example, mortality in young rainbow trout fry due to infectious hematopoietic necrosis virus (IHNV) will often show a very rapid, exponential rate of growth over a period of even just a few days, whereas mortality due to other husbandry-related issues, such as poor water quality or poor feed intake, may have a more gradual rate of increase over a longer period of a week or more.

Management of chronic, persistent disease over a long period is aided by a multi-year analysis of morbidity and mortality indicators. For example, management of bacterial kidney disease in a hatchery population of spring chinook salmon in Washington State, where it is enzootic, can be approached from this angle. A comparison of the results of enzyme-linked immunosorbent assays (ELISA) in female broodstock over multiple years can be conducted to identify increasing or decreasing trends of bacterial loads in a stock, and can be used to indicate whether changes in husbandry have been successful over time.

5.2 Basic Principles of Aquatic Epidemiology

Epidemiology is normally understood to be the study of patterns of disease in populations, although it can also refer to other aspects of population dynamics (Loeber and Farrington, 2001). The term "epidemiology" originally referred to humans but is now widely used in place of the more animal-focused "epizootiology" (Turnbull *et al.*, 2011). Similarly, "epidemic" and "endemic" tend to be used rather than "epizootic" and "enzootic", although these terms may still be in use. When studying such patterns, the population must be broken into units. These patterns can be individual animals or groups of ponds, farms, water catchment areas, bays, or tidal excursions at sea. Apart from obvious differences between terrestrial and aquatic animals, there are also differences in some basic concepts. According to European Union legislation, for example, "zone" for terrestrial animals means a precise geographical delimitation, containing an animal subpopulation with a distinct health status with respect to a specific disease or specific diseases subject to appropriate surveillance, disease control, and biosecurity measures. For aquatic animals, "zone" is taken as a contiguous hydrological system with a distinct health status with respect to a specific disease or specific diseases that forms an area that is referred to in one of the following ways:

- An entire water catchment from the source of a waterway to the estuary or lake.
- More than one water catchment.
- Part of a water catchment from the source of a waterway to a barrier that prevents the introduction of a specific disease or diseases.
- Part of a coastal area with a precise geographical delimitation.
- An estuary with a precise geographical delimitation.

Epidemiology can focus on individual pathological changes or can delve even further into molecular structure, and its main aim is to improve outcomes for health, welfare and productivity by understanding the determinants of their occurrence, and sometimes their costs (Turnbull *et al.*, 2011). While epidemiology often deals with infectious agents, the same approach can be used for non-infectious agents. Importantly, there remains a need to be pragmatic, despite any findings. Being familiar with aquaculture farming techniques and production systems allows epidemiological findings to be translated into meaningful strategies.

Unlike terrestrial animal populations, aquaculture species have some common characteristics (Turnbull *et al.*, 2011). With the exception perhaps of some poultry units, farmed aquaculture stock numbers can be much higher, in the order of hundreds of thousands and even millions of individuals. A typical sea cage can hold 50 000–80 000 salmon, with multiple cages per sea site and 1 meter-deep, hectare-sized shrimp ponds can hold over a million *Litopenaeus vannamei* (based on Briggs *et al.*, 2004). Many aquaculture populations depend on water supplies that are subject to natural processes like currents, tides, water catchment, and run-off, meaning that water quality, pathogen load, and sometimes wild fish incursion can be difficult for the farmer to control. Finally, aquaculture animals can be hard to view and inspect without handling them. Obtaining a random sample is challenging and not always possible, and depth and turbidity render routine observations less than ideal.

Epidemiology can be used to identify risk factors, but identifying them alone does not always allow control to be established. Smoking was identified to be a risk factor for cardiovascular disease but smoking remains a problem long after the risk factor was identified (Burns, 2003). However, there are many instances where identification of risk factors can lead to control. Important work established fish processing plants (gutting, filleting and packaging) and live fish transport in well-boats as risk factors for infectious salmon anemia. This has helped with control of the virus (Amundrud and Murray, 2009). Of course, the challenge when identifying risk factors is to determine cause. Risk factors may mask other factors. Turnbull *et al.* (2011) reported that it is difficult to investigate the association between sea lice (*Lepeophtheirus salmonis*) on farmed and wild salmon because of the distance between populations confounded by currents that change with the wind. Recognizing and assessing confounding factors, even if they appear statistically significant, is important to differentiate between real risk factors and those factors simply associated with the cause. This applies to cause and effect in disease assessments but also to other assessments such as aquatic ecotoxicology, where naturally occurring pH fluctuations may be responsible for observed toxicity and not the actual test conditions (Postma *et al.*, 2002). In some cases, ruling risk factors out, rather than identifying them, can be useful in establishing control.

Simply identifying risk factors is not always the answer. As with other livestock industries, it is important for veterinarians and other aquatic animal health experts to be very familiar with how to farm and how to rear aquatic organisms, since effective control usually requires attention to best practices – good farming and hygiene practices among others, which involve changes in management and husbandry. Cause and effect is usually multifactorial, with primary and secondary determinants of disease. A simple explanation is rarely forthcoming, and aquatic animal health practitioners should avoid the temptation to jump to conclusions based on simple, rapidly acquired evidence. In addition to veterinary science, understanding how to produce, and using epidemiological evidence judiciously, will foster long-term success.

Further information on the basic principles of aquatic epidemiology is available in the website materials accompanying this text.

5.3 Disease Reporting

With increasing globalization of trade, the risk of importing an exotic disease is very real. Approximately 34 alien fish species have established populations in Australian freshwaters, with a further 53 native fish species translocated within the country (Lintermans, 2004). Of the 34 species established, 22 are thought to have been introduced via the ornamental fish trade. It is clear that some animal diseases, terrestrial and aquatic, are significant enough to be reported as soon as possible. Depending on the jurisdiction, these diseases are typically known as reportable or notifiable diseases. Official notification allows serious and often exotic pathogens to be confirmed and contained as early as possible to minimize widespread and detrimental effects on industries (not just the immediate livestock industry), the economy and the natural environment. In many countries, veterinarians and anyone with responsibility for aquatic animals, such as producers, are usually obliged by law to be aware of the list of notifiable diseases or biosecurity risks, and are then required to report suspicions or diagnostic evidence, and to take reasonable and practical measures to minimize the risk. Importantly, the reporting mechanism does not always require conclusive evidence of a definite organism but rather reporting of the suspicion of the organism or of unusual patterns and events. National lists of notifiable animal diseases are based on the list of diseases notifiable to the OIE (2020) and disease information is available through the World Animal Health Information System. Regional bodies also collect and publish data (the Network of Aquaculture Centres in Asia-Pacific). Many countries also include endemic diseases over and above those reportable to the OIE, for surveillance purposes, to detect unusual events involving mortality or sickness of animals, including aquatic animals, and diseases of public health significance. In the United States, the Animal and Plant Health Inspection Service (2021) delivers programs such as veterinary services and plant protection and quarantine to help protect aquatic animal and plant health. In Europe, the European Commission Decision 2005/176/EC lays down conditions for the notification of certain contagious animal diseases, including aquatic diseases, and relevant persons must, as a precaution, report any suspected serious disease, even if they are uncertain what infectious disease it is (European Commission, 2005).

Further details on the notification of aquatic animal diseases are available in the website materials accompanying this text.

5.4 Control and Eradication of Disease

Control is essentially reduction of the morbidity and mortality from disease; it is a general term covering all measures intended to interfere with the unrestrained occurrence of disease, whatever its cause, and is a continuing process. Control can be achieved by treating (reducing prevalence) or by preventing (reducing incidence and prevalence). The individual is the foundation of medicine but, increasingly, prevention is recognized as better than cure. Prevention avoids failures in diagnostics and treatments, and avoids the potential development of antimicrobial resistance. Prevention can also have positive welfare and economic benefits.

One form of preventing spread and aiding containment is eradication, which has a number of meanings (Dowdle, 1998). One meaning relates to extinction of an infectious agent completely, with no single agent left. This is more accurately called elimination: the complete and permanent reduction of disease to zero, with eradication referring to a defined geographical area, although there can be some differences in terminology (Miller *et al.*, 2006). Elimination of a disease agent has not yet deliberately occurred but it has nearly been achieved for smallpox and, more recently, rinderpest. Virus stocks are maintained in at least 2 and approximately 20 laboratories, respectively. This might be better described as a second form of eradication, which is the reduction of infectious disease prevalence in a specified area to a level at which transmission does not occur.

In parts of Nigeria, trypanosomiasis, the cause of sleeping sickness can be "eradicated" by clearing the vector, the tsetse fly, and various success has been achieved eradicating malaria and yellow fever in the Caribbean by targeting *Aedes aegypti*. A third interpretation of eradication can be the reduction of infectious disease prevalence to levels at which the disease ceases to be a major health problem, although some transmission may still occur. Most commonly in veterinary and animal health contexts, eradication refers to regional extinction of an infectious agent such has been seen in a number of responses to infectious salmon anemia; for example, the 1998–99 and 2008–09 Scottish outbreaks. Importantly, eradication is a time-limited campaign, meant to have an achievable deadline and outcome, rather than a protracted affair with no end in sight. Before undertaking control and eradication programs, the following must be considered:

- Knowledge about the cause, distribution, transmission (if infectious), maintenance, host range and nature of the host/infectious agent relationship.
- The veterinary infrastructure, including official veterinary services.
- Diagnostic feasibility.
- Adequate surveillance.
- Availability of replacement stock.
- Producers' and society's views.
- The public health significance of the disease, if any.
- The existence of suitable legislation with provision for compensation.
- The possible ecological consequences.
- Economic costs and availability of funds for the program.

Quarantine is used as one of a number of tools to prevent incursion of exotic agents and involves isolation of infected or suspected, or of non-infected but at-risk, stock. Other valuable imports such as fertilized eggs may have to be isolated until confirmation of infection status can be achieved one way or the other. Usually, quarantine will be used when an infectious agent is exotic or introduced, is not spreading through a population, and ultimate eradication can be achieved. The period of quarantine depends on the infectious period, the time taken for the infection to be confirmed and the time taken for individuals to become non-infectious. Slaughter may have to be used as a form of control. Productivity can be reduced through disease, or individuals can act as a source of infection. In some cases, emergency harvesting might allow the farmer to recoup some of the production costs and Atlantic salmon experiencing cardiomyopathy syndrome may be sent to slaughter at the first signs of an outbreak. This might even occur as a result of poor environmental conditions such as harmful algal blooms and even construction work (Chase, 2020). Preemptive slaughter is usually conducted during epidemics, to remove animals that may have been exposed and therefore may be at risk of developing the disease. This is done in the face of many notifiable disease outbreaks. Blanket culling of animals on premises immediately surrounding (contiguous culling) an infected premise is often required – a particular category of preemptive slaughter. With terrestrial animals in particular, this is contentious; slaughtering a large proportion of healthy animals such as pigs, chickens and cattle to control African swine fever, avian influenza and foot and mouth disease, for example, can be justified by mathematical models but, depending on the context, seems to be rarely justified in the public mind. Animal slaughter in epidemics is usually accompanied by other procedures to reduce transmission and control zones in surrounding areas limit movement and transmission. Entire areas of New South Wales and South Eastern Queensland are restricted zones due to ostreid herpesvirus type 1 microvariant and white spot syndrome virus respectively. Stamping out is another form of control with disinfection and destruction of carcasses by burning and burial, a very laborious and time-consuming process fraught with difficulties such as avoiding water tables, cost, transport of carcasses, and avoidance of predators (piscivorous birds, seals).

Further information on the control and eradication of diseases is available in the website materials accompanying this text.

5.5 Vaccination

Vaccination is a well-known tool if suitable candidates for antigens can be found and various platforms are available. Fish vaccines are typically oil or water based, and oil adjuvants usually elicit a more pronounced immune reaction, and are more common as a result. Vaccination is a major growth area in aquaculture, with approximately two vaccines licensed in 1982 compared with over 27 in 2016. Their importance has grown over residue level concerns, environmental impacts, and the need to reduce antibiotics and chemicals and associated problems with antibiotic resistance. In addition, vaccination saves on the cost associated with morbidity and mortality (treatments, disposals, loss of income, and other tangible and intangible costs). Vaccination is used to control significant diseases and appropriate vaccination has resulted in dramatic reduction in the volume of antimicrobials needed to farm fish (McLoughlin, 2005). Time of vaccination varies between species and between vaccines.

While less employed in aquatic medicine, in countries that do not routinely vaccinate against an organism, strategic vaccination aims to prevent incursion from endemic areas and spread during epidemics. In the face of an outbreak, strategies include ring vaccination of animals in properties circumjacent to an infected property or infected area. Barrier vaccination, which is not completely circumjacent, in terrestrial veterinary medicine, could involve vaccination of animals in border regions of Europe to prevent foot and mouth entry from Asia. Another form involves suppressive or dampening-down vaccination, both within and around a region where an outbreak occurs. Vaccination can also be used in countries that do routinely vaccinate to boost immunity following an outbreak or to protect against new serotypes.

Vaccination is the best method to increase survival rate and profitability in aquaculture when used in combination with several factors that are necessary to guarantee the highest possible survival rate.

No mortality is typically associated with the vaccination process itself, although some weak fish may die due to the handling process, and some vaccines can cause debilitating viscera adhesions. A number of prerequisites represent best practice prior to vaccination. Fish stock must already have been provided with good nutrition, and fingerlings must be of high quality. Good farming and husbandry practices must be in place with appropriate and continuous health management. The vaccine used is species dependent, and ultimate success will depend on the status of the immune system, production cycle and life history, and what diseases need to be controlled. Success will also be influenced by when the diseases occur. Will vaccination occur with cooling or warming waters, and what sizes are the stock? Will their immune system respond sufficiently? Decreasing stress prior to, during, and after vaccination is also critical, and this will be influenced by farming technology, handling, mechanization and environment (temperature, salinity, dissolved oxygen, and potentially rising ammonia in the sedative bath water). Ultimately, there needs to be a cost benefit in the vaccination. It is very important that fish vaccination principles be adhered to, and vaccination can only be recommended for healthy fish – do not vaccinate sick or stressed fish. It should be a main objective of consulting clinicians to assess stock health prior to vaccination. Fish subjected to a dry curfew, deprived of food prior to vaccination, suffer less handling stress and respond better to anesthetics; the smaller the fish size and the higher the water temperature, the shorter the required fasting interval; a disease-free environment must be present and maintained prior to and during the vaccination period. Vaccination must precede exposure to disease or transfer to a disease prone site by the relevant or appropriate time, taking into account any lag phase when immunity is developing.

5.5.1 Vaccine Delivery

Delivery by injection is the most effective route but fish need to be anesthetized and handled. Immersion vaccination is practical for mass vaccination of small fish, but does not work for all vaccines. Oral delivery is most suitable for mass vaccination, but dosage is uncertain and sometimes there is poor potency.

Injectable vaccines can be multivalent and easy to store (attention to the cold chain is usually required), but they require sedation, involve stress, accidental trauma and can be labor intensive, and are potentially a human health and safety concern (furunculosis vaccine adjuvant intraperitoneal vaccine). Many injectable vaccines are licensed internationally, including intramuscular (vibriosis in salmonids, grouper, yellowtail, cod, and halibut) and intraperitoneal (bacterial kidney disease, enteric septicemia of catfish, motile aeromonas septicemia in striped catfish and furunculosis and marine aeromonas disease in salmonids) vaccines. Injection can be intraperitoneal or intramuscular, with intraperitoneal being the most common form in aquaculture.

Injectables can potentially cause stress resulting from the handling and injection of the fish. Stock are sedated and netted onto smooth tables, typically stainless steel or equivalent, with a very low level of running water. Fish are supported on the table in dorsal recumbancy with the head away from the operator's body, or are lifted up, and the needle is inserted into the coelomic cavity at a 90–45-degree angle to a depth of approximately 0.5 cm and approximately 0.05–0.1 ml of vaccine is injected at the correct midline site. Landmarks such as one and a half times the length of the pelvic fin may be used to guide the vaccinator. Automatic injection guns with a position guard are typically used to avoid incorrect placement. Vaccination will fail if the operator injects into the pelvic girdle, into the lumen of the gut, or into the liver. Depending on how visible the vaccine or adjuvant is, operator accuracy can be assessed by sacrificing 100 fish to determine the presence of a free drop of vaccine in the celom. A team of four people can vaccinate approximately 5000 salmon per hour, but accuracy must be maintained. Fish are often graded at the same time.

Injectables can provide a long duration of protection (over one year) sufficient to get over the risk period. Multiple antigens can be combined in a single vaccine and, therefore, in a single administration, and every fish in the population will receive the correct dose. Up to 10 000 fish can be vaccinated per liter via the intraperitoneal route (>25 g). Injections are in general superior to any other vaccine application method; however, from a practical point of view, they can only be applied to fish of 10 g or more (usually larger). They usually include adjuvants to stimulate non-specific defense mechanisms and enhance the specific immune response. Injectables should have good efficiency, low levels of adverse effects, and easy handling. Initial short-term protection may be provided due to non-specific defense factors, while the adjuvants can result in release of interleukins which, in turn, results in non-specific activation of macrophages. Some adjuvants, particularly oil-based examples, can cause a strong inflammatory reaction (depending on conditions) including adhesions as a sequela of vaccination (Poppe and Breck, 1997). In addition, autoimmune disease has been described with marked glomerulonephritis and characteristic Splendore–Hoeppli lesions seen on histopathology (Figure 5.1; Foyle, 2001).

Adhesion severity can be a welfare issue following intraperitoneal vaccination with multivalent, oil-adjuvanted vaccines, and subsequent inflammatory response can lead to focal or diffuse peritonitis with adhesions between viscera and the abdominal wall. Adhesions become organized with invasion of fibroblasts, macrophages, and lymphocytes, and a large number of melanomacrophages, resulting in multiple granulomas. Adhesion severity can be assessed using the Spielberg or Midtlyng scale (0 = no reaction and 6 = very severe) based on macroscopic pathology (McLoughlin, 2005). At water temperatures of 10–12°C, the progression of injection site reactions in Atlantic salmon may take 6–12 months and a score of ≤ 2.5 can be considered acceptable. Adhesions will cause only slight reduction in growth rates when injection site lesions are moderate but overall reduction in growth may increase beyond 10% among fish showing Spielberg scores of 3 or higher; scores ≥ 4 can expect 20–25% growth reduction. A score of 5 indicates severe fusing and melanization. The scoring scale is subjective and does require training, standardization and checking. Distribution of scores is more important than mean, and a minimum of 30 fish per group should be examined at least three times during the production cycle.

Adhesions are often organized and fibrosed with visible melanin deposition that can also be scored. The melanization scores are:

0 No melanin.
1 Small amount on viscera.

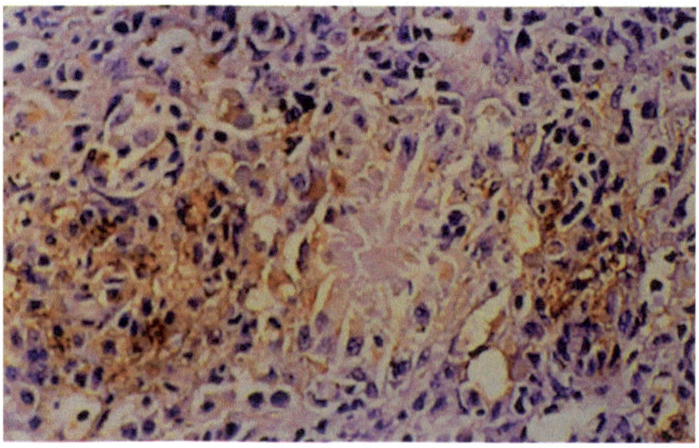

Figure 5.1 Splendore–Hoeppli reaction. Immunohistochemistry using rabbit anti-*Pasteurella salmonicida* serum of fixed tissue in the spleen of a naturally infected Atlantic salmon; Splendore–Hoeppli reaction is described as a volcanic rim and is seen to be free of bacterial antigen (brown staining). *Source:* Foyle (2001).

2 Highly visible melanin and/or slight pigmentation of abdominal wall which is easily removed.
3 Melanization of the abdominal wall and fillet; removal results in damage and downgrading.

Other influences that need to be considered are the size and condition of the fish at vaccination, with smaller fish representing an increased risk of higher local reactions, and the temperature at vaccination, with higher temperatures increasing the probability of higher local reactions (Berg *et al.*, 2006); onset of immunity is also temperature dependent. Berg *et al.* (2006) also reported a possible association between vaccination, growth rates and vertebral malformation.

Immersion vaccination is fast, effective, low stress, easy and economical; however, it can be time consuming and relatively expensive for larger fish, and cannot be used with adjuvants and other immunostimulants. There are typically two application methods: dip and bath. Dip vaccination is more widely used. Small fish are immersed for very short durations, perhaps 30 seconds, in a highly concentrated vaccine solution (one part vaccine to nine parts water). Dip vaccination allows rapid vaccination of large numbers of fish (up to 100 kg of fish per liter of vaccine), and is widely used for vaccination of fry weighing 1–5 g. It provides relatively good protection but the duration of immunity is not very long and a booster vaccination is required when the disease prevails over longer periods. Dip vaccination is impractical for larger fish due to cost effectiveness and the stress that could be induced by vaccination. In fish smaller than 1 g, the immune system might still be immature and vaccine efficacy may be reduced.

Bath vaccination is useful for larger fish. Stock are exposed for a longer period, usually from one to several hours, in a lower concentration of vaccine. Large groups of fish are partitioned off from the rest in a cage, and usually a low dose of diluted anesthetic is added. Air or oxygen is continuously pumped in to avoid anoxia.

Suspended antigens are adsorbed by skin and gills, and lymphocytes in the skin and gill epithelium are activated and protect the fish when they are exposed to the live pathogen at a later stage. Other cells in the epithelium of skin and gills, such as antigen presenting cells (e.g., macrophages), also absorb vaccine antigens and transport them to specialized tissues where the systemic immune response builds up.

Delivery of antigen to the gut-associated lymphoid tissue can be achieved by oral vaccination, a technique most suitable for mass vaccination; however, dosage is uncertain and sometimes there is poor potency. Oral vaccines, including DNA vaccines, are low stress, of moderate cost, and are safe to administer to fish of all sizes, but stability may be a problem. There are few on the market and usually only as boosters. Vaccine is either mixed with the feed, coated on top of the feed (top dressed) or bioencapsulated. Bioencapsulation is used where fry are to be vaccinated. Live feed, such as *Artemia nauplii*, copepods or rotifers, are incubated in a vaccine suspension or altered bacteria, after which they are fed to the fry. Since these live organisms are non-selective filter feeders, they will accumulate the antigen in their digestive tract and transform themselves into living microcapsules. The p57 protein of *Renibacterium salmoninarum* has been delivered in *Chlamydomonas* algae and has resulted in systemic protection (Dadar *et al.*, 2017). When antigens are to be incorporated in feed, the heat sensitivity of the antigen has to be considered, and when vaccines are used as top dressing in feed, a coating agent is usually applied, either to prevent leaching of the antigen from the pellets or to prevent breakdown of the antigen in the acidic environment of the stomach. Micro- or nanoparticles such as alginates, chitosan and poly lactide coglycolide can be used as encapsulating agents.

Three criteria can be used to assess vaccine efficacy: the rate at which protection is achieved, the final degree of protection (relative percent survival) and duration of immunity.

$$\text{Relative percent survival (RPS)} = (1 - \%\ \text{mortality in vaccinated} \,/\, \%\ \text{mortality in control}) \times 100.$$

Improved uptake is influenced by the disease status and degree of risk, the size of the fish, and the temperature of the water. The effect of temperature can be put to good use during vaccination. For example, an increasing water temperature can result in an effective antibody response being mounted, with long-term memory that would not occur at low temperatures for salmonids, or alternatively fish can be successfully vaccinated in the autumn with the acquired immunity surviving the drop in temperature over the winter, then being effective the following spring when water temperatures rise, as do the number of disease outbreaks. A drop in subsequent temperature might also help to reduce adhesions if they are an issue.

Immune response can be measured by assessing blood parameters, identification of cell types and how these populations change, and simple functional assays like ELISA (although the immunoglobulin IgM may be easy to measure by ELISA but not IgT; i.e., mucosal antibody). Gene expression of cytokines and IgT can also be assessed.

Vaccine types include inactivated and live, with the former using alkylating agents for example, to inactivate and render nucleic acid incapable of replication. Rainbow trout (*Oncorhynchus mykiss*) can be vaccinated against IHNV by inactivating the virus using beta-propiolactone, while formalin is used to inactivate iridovirus causing red sea bream iridoviral disease, and *Pseudomonas anguilliseptica* in olive flounder (*Paralichthys olivaceus*). These vaccines are typically safe, and produced quickly, but can be expensive and stimulate a lower response, requiring boosters, although in aquaculture, lifelong cover may not be required; it may be sufficient to cover fish for the period of main risk only. Other inactivated vaccines are available against infectious salmon anemia virus, infectious pancreatic necrosis virus, pancreas disease virus, *Pasteurella piscicida* in sea bass (*Dicentrarchus labrax*) and sea bream (*Sparus aurata*) and a bivalent *Streptococcus* spp. vaccine in tilapia (*Oreochromis* sp.). See Dadar *et al.* (2017) and Ma *et al.* (2019) for reviews of advances in fish vaccines and development strategies.

Live attenuated vaccines provide better immunity but may revert to virulence and are usually slower to produce. They are chemically or genetically weakened and stimulate cellular, humoral and mucosal immunity. In some cases, particularly with terrestrial viruses, they may be difficult to distinguish from field strains (usually therefore precluding their use in notifiable diseases). Attenuated *Cryptobia salmositica* vaccine is available for rainbow trout, and koi herpesvirus is available as an immersion or injectable attenuated vaccine. Natural vaccination by exposure to low levels of challenge from agents in the environment such as "feedback" of transmissible gastroenteritis virus and parvovirus in feces to pregnant sows is not a common vaccine technology in aquaculture. New technology such as recombinant vaccines that express genes of interest through vectors like *Escherichia coli*, yeasts, baculovirus and DNA vaccines are increasingly available. DNA vaccines, which stimulate both arms of the immune system, are cheap, stable, and easy to transport and store. G glycoprotein IHNV subunit vaccine expressed in *E. coli* is an option for rainbow trout, and identifying the virulence factor of *Vibrio anguillarum* may be a good DNA vaccine candidate in orange spotted grouper (*Epinephelus coioides*). Autogenous vaccines that involve isolating an agent from affected fish in a production site, and creating a custom-made killed vaccine are commonly used in many forms of aquaculture, though with breakdowns in protection and mixed success a continuing problem (Agnew and Barnes, 2007; Heath, 2016). This is a main method used to control streptococcosis in barramundi in Australia.

Other control techniques include therapeutic and prophylactic chemotherapy. Antibiotics, anthelminthics, and hyperimmune serum are used therapeutically and prophylactically at times of high risk, to increase productivity. Use of antimicrobials for prophylaxis should be discouraged and every attempt should be made to identify any underlying cause, otherwise undesirable consequences such as antimicrobial resistance, including horizontal transfer between bacteria, can occur.

Movement of hosts between regions and from high-risk areas must be tightly controlled. Movement is restricted by government authorities during epidemics and eradication (e.g., white spot syndrome and ostreid herpesvirus protection zones in Australia).

In aquatic species, avoiding the use of "trash" fish or other forms of by-catch will reduce transmission of fish pathogens and zoonotic agents. This is a continuing problem in Asian sea bass (barramundi) culture in parts of South East Asia. Fish-borne zoonotic trematodes representing a zoonotic risk to consumers can be avoided by feeding pelleted feed, and keeping fish in cages above the substrate of the pond to reduce the number of intermediate snail hosts consumed. The latter is a form of control by avoidance of biological vectors. Control of mechanical vectors such as *Lepeophtheirus salmonis* can reduce the transmission of a number of infectious agents, including infectious salmon anemia. People and their equipment must also be controlled routinely and during epidemics. Disinfection of fomites – cars, equipment, nets, clothing, scuba gear, wellboats and the like – must be given proper attention, and prevention of iatrogenic transfer by veterinary and other personnel is key to prevention and containment. Biosecurity is the application of management practices that reduce the opportunities for infectious agents to gain access to, or spread within, an animal or food animal production unit. Practices include cleanliness, disinfection, reduction of exposure (e.g., maintenance of perimeter fencing and netting), testing of new animals, isolation, waste management), and management of personnel (limiting visitors and adequate training of staff). Biosecurity is also important at the national level, and most countries have dedicated government units to deal with biosecurity and import and export. Biosecurity is sometimes described as the "application of informed common sense".

5.6 The Immune Response to Infectious Diseases in Fish

Fish are thought to display an apparent intersection between the innate (non-specific) immune response and the emergence of the adaptive (acquired) immune response. See Magnadóttir (2006), Uribe *et al.* (2011), Salinas (2015), and Noguera *et al.* (2015) for more discussion of innate and adaptive teleost immunity, and fish endocrinology.

Acquired immunity is mediated by lymphocytes and affected mainly through antibodies. Fish antigen-specific responses are different from mouse and human models; memory is less widely known. The role of fish antibodies in the recovery from disease has not been studied thoroughly; however, high activities of neutralizing antibodies are often induced by vaccination and provide complete protection against infections. Lymphocyte proliferation and antibody titers in fish take longer times to reach a peak, once challenged with a pathogen, and antibody titers in the secondary response are smaller with respect to the primary response than in mammals. Acquired immunity in fish seems to be of transient nature, however, it could persist well over one year once vaccinated, and probably longer following acute disease – probably long enough to get stock over the relevant risk period.

Similar immune organs to those of the mammalian immune system are found in fish, but the functioning of the immune system of fish is not only conditioned by the particular environment, but also by their poikilothermic nature. In comparative immunology, invertebrates possess natural, non-adaptive, innate, non-clonal responses, whereas those of vertebrates are induced, adaptive, acquired, clonal, and anticipatory. This is important when shrimp/prawn "vaccination" is considered. Fin fish possess both innate immunity as well as adaptive immunity; however, innate immunity is stronger than adaptive immunity. There are differences in body compartments and cell organization, but most of the secondary lymphoid organs present in mammals are also found in fish, except for the absence of lymph nodes and hematopoietic bone marrow. The entire kidney contains immune cells: the anterior kidney (head kidney or pronephros) has the highest concentration of developing B lymphoid cells, is aglomerular and assumes haemopoietic functions, similar in function and often in consistency, to mammalian bone marrow.

The head kidney, unlike in higher vertebrates, is the principal immune organ responsible for phagocytosis, antigen processing and formation of IgM and immune memory through melanomacrophage centers. It is typically formed by two Y arms that spread cranially underneath the gills. In fish, the head kidney is a well innervated organ and also serves as an important endocrine organ, homologous to mammalian adrenal glands, releasing corticosteroids and other hormones. Thus, the head kidney is an important organ with key regulatory functions and the central organ for immune–endocrine interactions and neuroimmunoendocrine connections. Furthermore, it is also the major site of antibody production. In contrast, the posterior kidney possesses both renal and immune tissues.

The spleen functions as the major secondary immune organ, as found in mammalian species, with abundant IgM+ mature B cells. It also plays a major role in the clearance of bloodborne antigens and immune complexes in the splenic ellipsoids, and in antigen presentation and initiation of the adaptive immune response. The fish spleen as a secondary lymphatic and scavenging organ, plays a vital role in hematopoiesis, antigen degradation, and antibody production processing. Since fish have no lymph nodes, the spleen plays an essential role in antigen trapping. The spleen size of fish is widely used as a simple measurable immune parameter with a potential role in immune response against parasite infections (Lefebvre *et al.*, 2004).

The thymus is a subepithelial organ in the upper quadrant of each opercular cavity (organ's position can vary) typically covered by a connective tissue capsule. The main cellular components are lymphoid (thymocytes, lymphocytes, and macrophages). The thymus only produces T lymphocytes, and these are involved in stimulation of phagocytosis, allograft rejection, and antibody production by B cells. Much like the mammalian immune system, teleost erythrocytes, neutrophils, and granulocytes are believed to be present in the spleen, whereas lymphocytes are the major cell type found in the thymus. The thymus of some species has a cortex and medulla, as well as corpuscles comparable to Hassall's corpuscles in mammals. The involution of thymus in fish is more dependent on hormonal cycles and seasonal variations than on age, and depending on the species, it can disappear in adulthood or be retained; it may also regress during spawning. There is little information on any pathology associated with it. A lymphatic system with similarities to the mammalian system has been described in zebrafish (*Danio* spp.; Küchler *et al.*, 2006).

The gut-associated lymphoid tissue of teleosts consists principally of different sized lymphocytes, plasma cells, and macrophages, as well as several types of granulocytes and eosinophil granular cells. In teleosts, gut intraepithelial lymphocytes are largely considered T cells, whereas lymphoid cells present in the lamina propria are mainly B lymphocytes. In bony fish, a very early (prethymic) appearance of T-like cells occurs in the gut similar to the extrathymic origin of some T cells in mammals. There are many mammalian leukocyte cell types also found in teleost fish, including neutrophils, monocytes, thrombocytes, plasma cells, B cells, T cells, natural killer cells, and eosinophilic granular cells. Certain leukocytes also act as antigen-presenting or dendritic-like cells, however, fish leukocytes are still poorly characterized owing to the lack of specific tools. Leydig and epigonal organs also play a role in the immune response in elasmobranchs.

Non-specific immune elements not only act as a first line of defense against all pathogens, but also play an instructive role in the development of the acquired immune response. Elements of non-specific immune components include antibacterial peptides, lysozyme, lectins, acute phase protein, and the complement system.

Lysozyme is synthesized in the liver and extra hepatic sites and acts on bacterial cell walls resulting in lysis of the bacterium. It is involved in many defense mechanisms, such as bacteriolysis, opsonization, as well as restricted antiviral and antineoplastic activity. Lysozyme is present in mucus, lymphoid tissue, plasma, and other fluids, and is also expressed in a wide variety of tissues. Lectins (hemagglutinins) are proteins of non-immune origin which agglutinate cells and precipitate glycol conjugates. These proteins are able to bind certain sugars and have been reported in larvae and eggs, ova and mucus, and in the serum of many fish. Lectins could act as opsonin for phagocytosis of bacteria and are also involved in activation of the complement system (one of the three pathways: classical, alternative and lectin).

C-reactive protein is a highly conserved acute-phase protein which participates in the systemic response to inflammation. It reacts with phosphorylcholine, a widespread component of surface structures of bacteria, fungi, and parasites. These acute phase proteins function in a variety of defense-related activities such as limiting the dispersal of infectious agents, inactivation of proteases, killing of microbes, and repair of tissue damage. They also play an active role in the immune system, activating the classical complement pathway, enhancing phagocytosis and removal of apoptotic cells. C-reactive protein is present in quite high concentrations in the normal serum of many fish species (about 50 μg/ml), which increases up to 20-fold following high temperature shock or administration of inflammatory agents. Many acute phase proteins, such as serum amyloid, transferrin, and thrombin, are well characterized in fish.

The complement system links the innate and adaptive immune responses; it "complements" the ability of antibodies and phagocytic cells to clear pathogens and consists of a system of over 30 serum proteins, which remain inactive until an infection or other trigger activates them. The bactericidal activity of complement has been reported in many fishes. Both marine and freshwater bony fish have the alternative complement pathway (ACP) and classical complement pathway of activation, directly comparable to those of mammals. The ACP activity, which is antibody independent, is very prominent in fish serum compared with mammalian serum, suggesting that this pathway is more important in fish than in mammals. Besides other functions in innate response and in its connection with adaptive response, complement plays important roles in the killing of pathogens through opsonization and activation of phagocytes. Lipopolysaccharide in the cell walls of Gram-negative bacteria directly activates ACP and can result in lysis of the bacterial cell.

The innate and adaptive immune responses are closely related, as the innate immune responses play an instructive role in the development of acquired immune response. These two components are connected in many ways. The elements involved in such connections are lymphocytes, natural killer cells, and the major histocompatibility complex (MHC) receptors, among others. The basic principle of innate control of adaptive immunity is based on establishing an association between the antigen recognition by lymphocytes and pathogen-associated molecular patterns. Non-specific cytotoxic cells, a type of killer cell, have also been found in many teleost species, and this may represent an evolutionary precursor of mammalian NK cells. Non-specific cytotoxic cells are very potent immune elements, as they participate in the immune response against protozoan parasites and a role in induction of apoptosis. In addition, they also possess cytotoxic activities. The MHC receptors are immunoglobulin proteins that interact with T-cells through a specific T-cell receptor, to initiate immune responses and their role in the integration of innate and adaptive responses. These MHC molecules are highly polymorphic in nature, both types of major histocompatibility receptors (i.e. class I, for intracellular pathogens, and class II, for extracellular pathogens) are present in teleosts. There is still much to be learned and there are significant differences between species. The Atlantic cod (*Gadus morhua*) has developed many changes to its immunity, such as lacking MHC II and CD4+ T cells. They only make IgM, which is present in its blood in concentrations approximately 10 times more than that found in other examined species (Parham, 2016). Atlantic cod do not mount an antibody response to pathogens or immunization, and the fish are able to develop immunity to pathogens that is not antibody mediated.

Fish are the most primitive vertebrates to possess an adaptive immune system that includes lymphocytes, immunoglobulins, T cell receptors, and products of MHC to allow the clonal selection of B and T cells. Both B and T lymphocytes have diverse rearranging and adapting antigen receptors and can survive as long-lived memory cells. The overall shape of the specific immune elements and the recombination mechanisms (the cause of diversity in T cell receptors and immunoglobulins) are similar in fish and mammals. While fish have been shown to have lymphocyte subpopulations analogous to the mammalian B and T cells, the antibody representative in teleosts is more limited to that seen in mammals, being IgM tetramer in the most prevalent form (produced by B cells) rather than the pentameric structure of mammalian IgM. Two heavy chain isotypes IgD and IgT have been identified, although they have not been completely functionally characterized. IgD is thought to be located in the cell membrane of B cells, where it might act as a receptor. The other Ig class IgZ (or IgT) has also been reported in fish. This latter IgZ/IgT isotype has also recently been found in stickleback and carp, and appears to be a unique heavy-chain isotype restricted to bony fish.

The occurrence of fish IgM is not limited to the serum: antibodies are also found in the fish epithelial mucus. Mucus IgM may be of local origin rather than derived from the serum which suggests that fish immune systems may have systemic and mucosal parts.

Lymphocytes mediate the acquired immunity to reinfection and functions mainly through antibodies that can neutralize viruses, facilitate phagocytosis of pathogens through opsonization, and activate classical complement. T cells release factors to coordinate responses of other immune cells or cytotoxic factors to directly kill infected or abnormal cells. Numerous genes associated with T cell functioning and signaling have been identified in fish, but understanding the correlation between (presumed) T cell-associated genes and T cell activity in adaptive immunity in fish has yet to be fully elucidated. The presence of T cells and T cell markers in teleosts have been demonstrated. Other putative T cell markers in fish, such as CD3, CD4 and CD8, have been reported in a few species.

B cells are characterized by the expression of surface immunoglobulin receptors: B cell receptors. The immunoglobulins (or antibodies), which are the principal indicators of acquired immunity to pathogens, have evolved toward producing highly diversified molecules that recognize a very large number of different antigens. As with mammals, resistance to and recovery from infections are the result of complex interactions between non-specific and specific defense mechanisms. Other immune elements include cytokines which act as modulators of the immune responses and are related to both innate and adaptive responses. In particular, proinflammatory cytokines, including interleukin 1 beta (IL-1β) and IL-6 are commonly used immune regulatory genes in fish.

Interleukin-1β, mainly produced by macrophages, has been characterized in bony fish and cartilaginous fish. It is an important mediator of inflammation in response to infection and recently it has been reported to directly affect hypothalamic–pituitary–interrenal axis function and to stimulate cortisol secretion in trout. This suggests the possibility of autocrine regulatory circuits within the composite immunoendocrine organ, the head kidney, which may affect hematopoiesis as well as immune functions, apart from affecting cortisol secretion. Another important cytokine, tumor necrosis factor alpha (TNFα) has also been cloned and characterized in various fish species. Furthermore, TNF-like protein activity has been shown to induce apoptosis, enhance neutrophil migration and macrophage respiratory burst activity.

Further information on the epidemiology of common diseases of fish is available in the website materials accompanying this text.

Bibliographic references for this chapter are available in the website materials accompanying this text.

Supplementary materials

- Basic principles of aquatic epidemiology.
- Control and eradication of diseases.
- Epidemiology of common diseases of fish:
  - Viral hemorrhagic septicemia
  - Infectious hematopoietic necrosis
  - Infectious salmon anemia
  - Salmonid alphavirus
  - Infectious pancreatic necrosis
  - Proliferative kidney disease
  - Salmonid whirling disease
- Bibliography

References

Agnew, W. and Barnes, A.C. (2007). *Streptococcus iniae*: an aquatic pathogen of global veterinary significance and a challenging candidate for reliable vaccination. *Veterinary Microbiology* 122: 1–15.

Amundrud, T.L. and Murray, A.G. (2009). Modelling sea lice dispersion under varying environmental forcing in a Scottish sea loch. *Journal of Fish Diseases* 32: 27–44.

Berg, A., Rødseth, O.M., Tangerås, A. and Hansen, T. (2006). Time of vaccination influences development of adhesions, growth and spinal deformities in Atlantic salmon *Salmo salar*. *Diseases of Aquatic Organisms* 69: 239–248.

Briggs, M., Funge-Smith, S., Subasinghe, R. and Phillips, M. (2004). *Introductions and Movement of* Penaeus vannamei *and* Penaeus stylirostris *in Asia and the Pacific*. RAP publication, 10. Bankok: Food and Agriculture Organization of the United States, Regional Office for Asia and the Pacific.

Burns, D.M. (2003). Epidemiology of smoking-induced cardiovascular disease. *Progress in Cardiovascular Diseases* 46: 11–29.

Chase, C. (2020). Atlantic Sapphire forced to "initiate emergency harvest" of 200,000 fish. *SeaFoodSource* 29 July. https://www.seafoodsource.com/news/aquaculture/atlantic-sapphire-forced-to-initiate-emergency-harvest-of-200-000-fish (accessed 7 May 2021).

Dadar, M., Dhama, K., Vakharia, V.N. *et al.* (2017). Advances in aquaculture vaccines against fish pathogens: global status and current trends. *Reviews in Fisheries Science and Aquaculture* 25: 184–217.

Dowdle, W.R. (1998). The principles of disease elimination and eradication. *Bulletin of the World Health Organization* 76(Suppl 2): 22.

European Commission. (2005). 2005/176/EC: Commission Decision of 1 March 2005. Eur-Lex. https://eur-lex.europa.eu/legal-content/EN/ALL/?uri=CELEX%3A32005D0176 (accessed 7 May 2021).

Foyle, L. (2001). *The Experimental Reproduction and Pathology of Pasteurella salmonicida: A new pathogen of farmed salmonids*. Master's thesis, Institute of Aquaculture, University of Stirling.

Heath, C. (2016). Evolution of *Streptococcus iniae* after Vaccination and Molecular Uunderpinnings of Capsular Antigenicity. D Phil. thesis, School of Biological Sciences, University of Queensland.

Küchler, A.M., Gjini, E., Peterson-Maduro, J. *et al.* (2006). Development of the zebrafish lymphatic system requires VEGFC signaling. *Current Biology* 16: 1244–1248.

Lefebvre, F., Mounaix, B., Poizat, G. and Crivelli, A.J. (2004). Impacts of the swimbladder nematode Anguillicola crassus on *Anguilla anguilla*: variations in liver and spleen masses. *Journal of Fish Biology* 64: 435–447.

Lintermans, M. (2004). Human-assisted dispersal of alien freshwater fish in Australia. *New Zealand Journal of Marine and Freshwater Research* 38: 481–501.

Loeber, R. and Farrington, D.P. (2001). Young children who commit crime: epidemiology, developmental origins, risk factors, early interventions, and policy implications. *Development and Psychopathology* 12: 737–762.

Ma, J., Bruce, T.J., Jones, E.M. and Cain, K.D. (2019). A review of fish vaccine development strategies: Conventional methods and modern biotechnological approaches. *Microorganisms* 7: 569.

McLoughlin, M. (2005). Fish vaccination: a brief overview. https://www.hpra.ie/docs/default-source/default-document-library/fish-vaccine-overview.pdf?sfvrsn=0 (accessed 7 May 2021).

Magnadóttir, B. (2006). Innate immunity of fish (overview). *Fish and Shellfish Immunology* 20: 137–151.

Miller, M., Barrett, S. and Henderson, D.A. (2006). Control and eradication. In: *Disease Control Priorities in Developing Countries*. 2e. (ed. D.T. Jamison, J.G. Breman, A.R. Measham *et al.*), chapter 62. New York, NY: International Bank for Reconstruction and Development/World Bank; Oxford University Press.

Noguera, P., Ubeda, C., Bruno, D. and Semenas, L. (2015). *The Fish Necropsy Manual*. European Association of Fish Biologists. http://www.necropsymanual.net/en (accessed 7 May 2021).

Parham, P. (2016). How the codfish changed its immune system. *Nature Genetics* 48: 1103–1104.

Poppe, T.T. and Breck, O. (1997). Pathology of Atlantic salmon *Salmo salar* intraperitoneally immunized with oil-adjuvanted vaccine: a case report. *Diseases of Aquatic Organisms* 29: 219–226.

Postma, J.F., De Valk, S., Dubbeldam, M. *et al.* (2002). Confounding factors in bioassays with freshwater and marine organisms. *Ecotoxicology and Environmental Safety* 53: 226–237.

Salinas, I. (2015). The mucosal immune system of teleost fish. *Biology* 4: 525–539.

Stallknecht, D.E., Nagy, E., Hunter, D.B. *et al.* 2007. Avian influenza. In: *Infectious Disease of Wild Birds* (ed. N.J. Thomas, D.B. Hunter, and C.T. Atkinson), 108–130 Ames, IA: Blackwell Publishing.

Turnbull, J.F., Berrill, I.K., Green, D.M. *et al.* (2011). Applied epidemiology with examples from UK aquaculture. *Aquaculture Research* 42: 21–27.

United States Animal and Plant Health Inspection Service. (2021). Animal health. https://www.aphis.usda.gov/aphis/ourfocus/animalhealth (accessed 7 May 2021).

United States Geological Survey. (1999c). Avian botulism. In *Field Manual of Wildlife Diseases: : General field procedures and diseases of birds*. (ed. M. Friend and J.C. Franson), 271–282. Information and Technology Report 1999-001. Madison, WI: Biological Resources Division.

United States Geological Survey. (1999d). Disease control operations. In: *Field Manual of Wildlife Diseases: General field procedures and diseases of birds*. (ed. M. Friend and J.C. Franson), 19–48. Information and Technology Report 1999-001. Madison, WI: Biological Resources Division.

Uribe, C., Folch, H., Enríquez, R. and Moran, G. (2011). Innate and adaptive immunity in teleost fish: a review. *Veterinarni Medicina* 56: 486–503.

World Organisation for Animal Health (2020). Animal diseases. https://www.oie.int/en/what-we-do/animal-health-and-welfare/animal-diseases (accessed 6 May 2021).

6

Diagnostics and Treatment of Aquatic Animal Diseases

Richmond Loh, James E. Bogan, Jr, Mansour El-Matbouli, Soliman Hatem, Jack Kottwitz, Nicholas Saint-Erne, Mona Saleh, and Vasile Vulpe

Learning Objectives
The student should be familiar with various sampling techniques, other diagnostic procedures and the administration of therapeutics and surgical interventions.

6.1 Introduction

Diagnosis can be seen as a Bayesian process. There is an *a priori* probability of diagnosis based on history, clinical symptoms, species, sex, age, and management system. There is an *a posteriori* probability based on the clinical examination, which may lead to a presumptive diagnosis. Diagnostic tests are used to confirm this diagnosis.

With many aquatic species, pathognomonic clinical signs are limited and can be similar across multiple diseases. Diagnostic tests are an essential part of the clinical examination (which is a diagnostic test in itself) to distinguish between diseases in aquatic species. Water testing, skin scrapes, and gill snips, imaging, and exploratory surgery are often part of the clinical examination.

Treatment considerations are also slightly different in aquatic species, owing to a limited number of licensed products, greater consideration of environmental effects, particularly on surrounding free-living species, and the methodology of treating perhaps tens of thousands of animals or multiple species at the same time.

This chapter discusses these differences and highlights differences in techniques used between species. It further discusses molecular diagnosis of World Organisation for Animal Health listed diseases.

6.2 Diagnostics

6.2.1 Basic Sampling

- Cytology: Wet mount preparations should be examined immediately to detect motile parasites. Air-dried smears need to be dried immediately to prevent post-sampling bacterial overgrowth artifact.

Fundamentals of Aquatic Veterinary Medicine, First Edition. Edited by Laura Urdes, Chris Walster, and Julius Tepper.

Companion website: www.wiley.com/go/urdes/aquatic-veterinary-medicine

- Bacteriology and mycology: Sample fresh tissue aseptically into separate bottles, or take swabs into Amies transport media.
- Virology: Preserve samples in virus transport media that contains antibiotics and antimycotic agents suitable for viral culture and molecular testing of target organs such as liver, kidney, spleen, heart, brain.
- Histopathology: Samples are generally preserved less than 10 mm wide into 10% neutral-buffered formalin. Crustacea are preserved into Davidson's solution, while marine mollusks, into seawater formalin.
- Electron microscopy: Preserve tissue samples less than 1 mm into glutaraldehyde.
- Toxicology: Sample materials that either contain or store toxins or their metabolites, such as liver, kidney, gut contents, brain and fat into separate inert containers.
- Molecular testing: Aseptically sample into molecular grade ethanol.

6.3 Diagnostic Techniques

Students are expected to be aware of diverse diagnostic techniques. There are many good online resources. An example is the Webinars for Global Aquatic Veterinary Education (wavma.org). Start with a good resource, then use the references provided in that resource to build up good knowledge of procedures.

6.3.1 Phlebotomy

- Crustaceans (crabs, shrimp): Collection of hemolymph. In animals with a carapace greater than 15 mm in length, hemolymph can be collected from the arthrodial membranes of the leg joints or from the junction of the carapace and abdomen.
- Fish: Ventral tail vein, using ventral midline or lateral approach.
- Amphibians: Ventral tail vein (Caudata), saphenous vein (Anura), cardiocentesis – research animals only. Phlebotomy is best performed in animals that are lightly to moderately sedated.
- Reptiles: Ventral tail vein (Squamata and Crocodilia), dorsal tail vein (Chelonia), jugular vein, occipital sinus (Chelonia and Crocodilia), subcarapacial sinus (Chelonia), cardiocentesis (Ophidia) – a controversial method, palatine vein (Ophidia).
- Birds: Jugular – right jugular vein tends to be larger, ulnar vein, tarsal vein.
- Mammals: For cetaceans, Barco *et al.* (2016) provides information on many techniques, although it focuses primarily on euthanasia.

6.3.2 Biopsy

- Fish: Gill biopsy of distal 1/10th of 3–5 filaments per fish.
- Birds: Similar techniques to those used for land-based birds.
- Mammals: In free-living whales, often used for skin and blubber samples. Sample can provide information on genetics, diet, contaminants, and physiological processes.

6.4 Diagnostic Imaging

Fish can be restrained in a plastic bag filled with water, which is an excellent conductor for ultrasound. This technique is useful for identifying swim-bladder lesions and tumoral abdominal masses, and to assess the general state of reproductive organs.

6.4.1 Imaging Methods Used in the Examination of Fish

6.4.1.1 Radiography

The radiological examination may be carried out on fish using direct radiography or with the aid of contrast media (contrast agent solution or air; Figures 6.1–6.5). There are several steps specific to any radiological examination procedure:

- Place the fish on the table in the required position.
- Place markers (right, left).
- Place the radiography cassette under the patient or inside the radiography table.
- Diaphragm collimation of the x-ray beam, adjusting radiological parameters.
- The actual exposure.
- Developing or recording the digital image on the computer.
- Image interpretation.

Proper positioning for radiography usually requires anesthesia, using tricaine methanesulfonate (MS222), clove oil (eugenol solution; see also Treatment) and/or special bands for restraining the fish and maintaining it in the desired position (with fast action). The position is chosen depending on the anatomical region and the shape of the fish body (spindle-shaped, flat); the position may be lateral (often, horizontal beam lateral), dorsoventral or ventrodorsal. Depending on the size of the fish and the thickness of the body region of interest, the values of the x-ray parameters (tension and intensity) are established.

The radiography of the cranium, spine and fins serves to highlight changes in direction and position (kyphosis, lordosis, scoliosis, subluxation, luxation, medullar compression), in continuity (fractures), in radiodensity (osteolysis, osteitis, bone tumors). The celomic cavity can exhibit fluid (ascites), leading to general increased radio-opacity (intra-abdominally), sometimes containing gas bubbles that may originate from bacterial infection; the swim bladder is easily visible on the film due to its gaseous content (Figures 6.1, 6.5). Radio-opacity can be locally increased as a result of organ hypertrophy or tumors.

A technical description of the radiological examination in fish is available in the website materials accompanying this text.

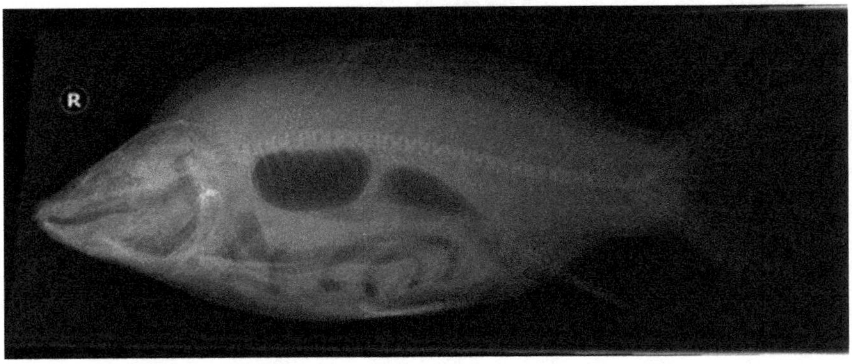

Figure 6.1 Common carp, whole body radiography, lateral view. Good image for observing the skeleton (including the fins), gills, swim bladder and the intestines, that contain a slight increased amount of gas.

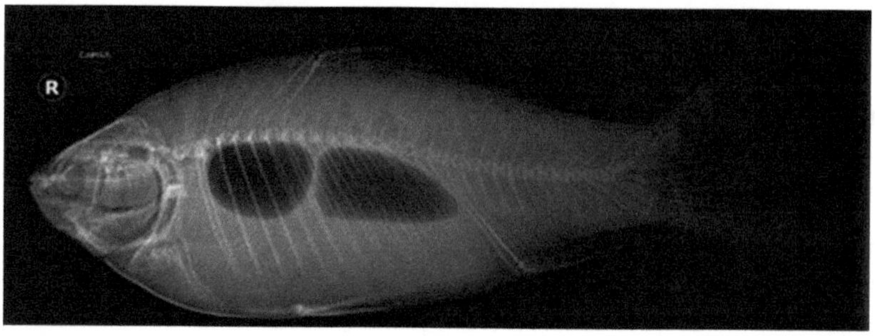

Figure 6.2 Crucian carp, whole body radiography, lateral view. Good image for observing the skeleton (including the fins), gills, swim bladder; the intestines are not radiologically visible.

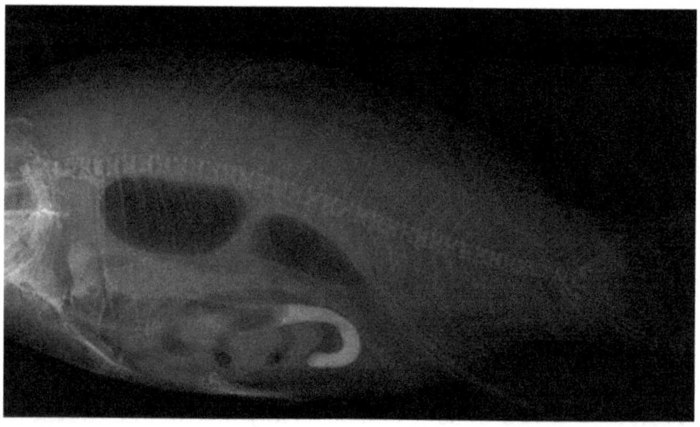

Figure 6.3 Carp, x-ray, lateral view. Enterography (contrast study); observing the probe reaching the esophagus, contrast solution can be seen in the first part of the intestine.

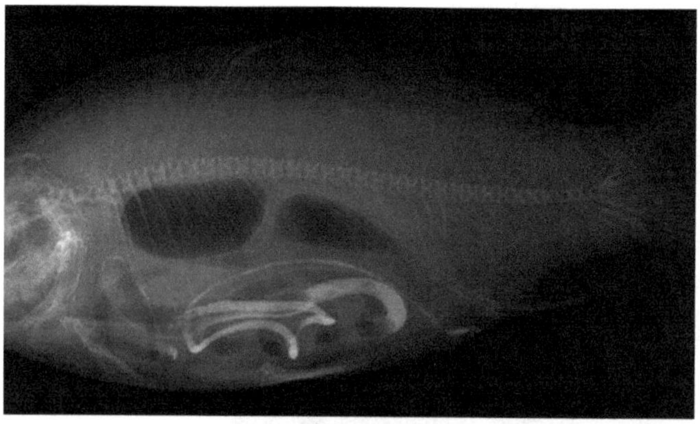

Figure 6.4 Carp, x-ray, lateral view. Enterography (contrast study); the contrast solution is introduced through the anus and reaches the middle of the intestine.

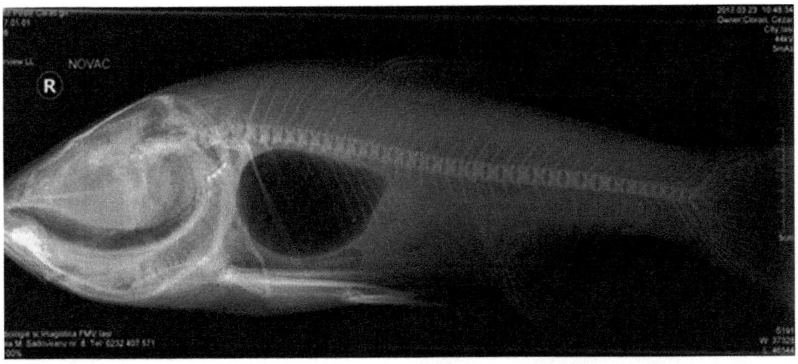

Figure 6.5 Bighead carp, whole body radiography, lateral view. High visibility of the bone structure, including fins, and the cartilaginous base of the gill lamellae. The swim bladder is easily visible as a result of the gaseous content; only the anterior of the swim bladder is visible – a possible abnormality.

6.4.2 Ultrasound

Ultrasonography (echotomography) is a non-invasive diagnostic imaging technique that relies on the echoes caused by an ultrasound beam upon passing through an organ or tissue. Ultrasound is used on a regular basis in imaging, internal medicine, surgery, and obstetrics. Its use is widespread due to its innocuous nature, affordability, and diagnostic sensitivity in diseases of soft-tissue organs.

Sounds or sound waves are mechanical radiations, which is why they require a propagation environment. Ultrasound is sound with a frequency above the 20 000 Hz threshold, inaudible to the human ear. Ultrasound propagation is produced through compression and rarefaction of the molecules constituting the environment. A sound wave (including ultrasound) is defined by frequency (measured in Hertz), wavelength (distance in meters between two compression peaks or rarefaction troughs), propagation speed (frequency × wavelength = meters/second), intensity (wave amplitude, expressed as watts/cm^2, pascal, or more commonly, decibels) and period (time occurred between the passing of two wavefronts in the same point).

A technical description of the ultrasound examination in fish is available in the website materials accompanying this text.

Clinically, ultrasound is used in fish to detect ascites and masses in the internal organs, to assess the development of the gonads and the liver (Figure 6.6). Basically, a continuous water current must pass through the gill cavity of the fish examined by ultrasound, to ensure survival. Depending on the fish size and the depth of the organ, various ultrasound probes (microconvex, linear) can be used with a frequency margin between 3 and 12 MHz. Depending on the position of the probe in contact with the fish, the images obtained will be in sagittal or transverse section (Novelo, 2012).

Ultrasound can also be applied to the abdomen and to the heart (echocardiography; Figures 6.7, 6.8), enabling the clinician to view the proper cardiac chambers (atrium and ventricle; Figures 6.9, 6.10) and the accessory chambers (venous sinus, arterial bulb). The B mode is used in the examination of the internal appearance of the chambers (endocardium) and valves (sinoatrial, atrioventricular, bulboventricular, semilunar); the TM mode is used to assess the myocardium volume and contractility, and the state of openness of the valves; the Doppler mode is used to assess blood flow motion, turbulence, blood flow velocity, and the pressure in cardiac structures (Sande, 1995). Echocardiography can also be used to identify large blood vessels (including with Doppler mode) possibly for puncture, respectively for blood collection (Figures 6.11).

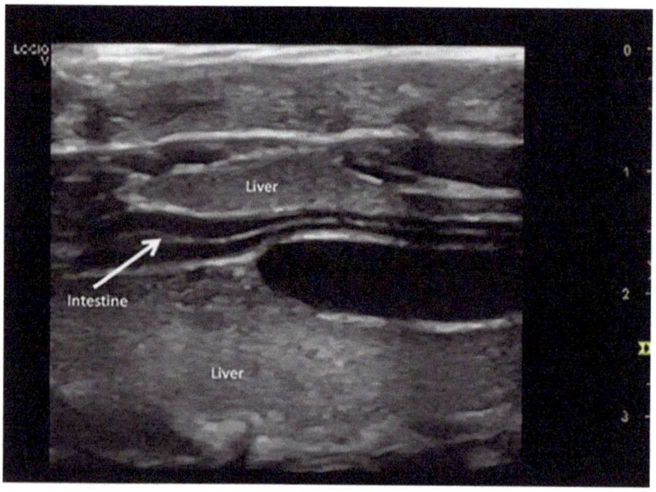

Figure 6.6 Common carp, abdominal ultrasound. Intestine with stratified wall, flanked above and below by the liver, with specific echogenicity.

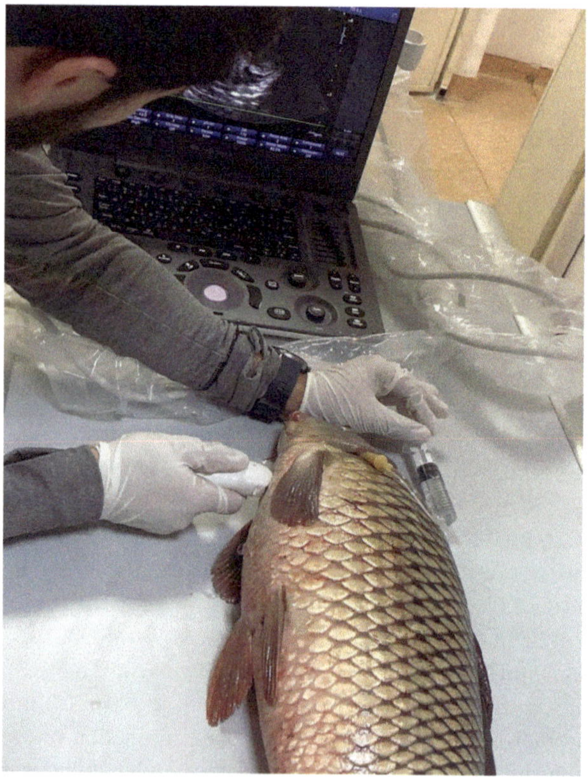

Figure 6.7 Common carp, abdominal ultrasound. Puncture of caudal vein (CV) for blood collection.

For radiography or ultrasonography examinations, amphibians can be restrained by placing them into sealed plastic bags with small amounts of fluid (dechlorinated water or amphibian Ringer's solution).

In reptiles, radiography can be performed on horizontal or vertical projections. For latero-lateral views horizontal projections are preferred over vertical projections.

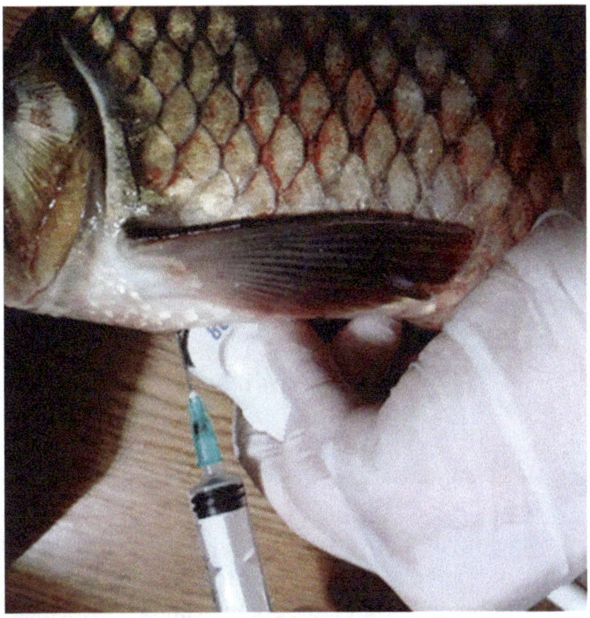

Figure 6.8 Common carp, echocardiography. Eco-assisted heart puncture.

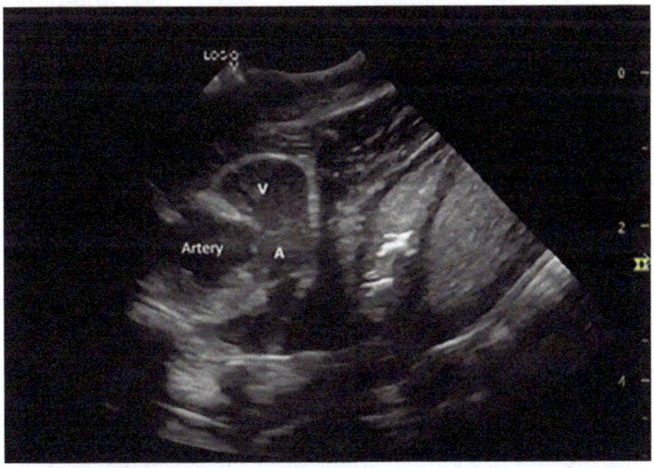

Figure 6.9 Common carp, abdomen ultrasound. Cardiac chambers are visible: V - ventricle, A - atria

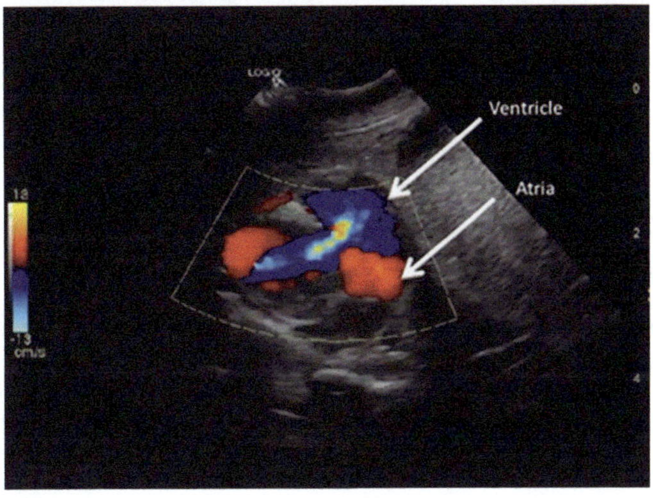

Figure 6.10 Common carp, abdominal ultrasound in Doppler mode.

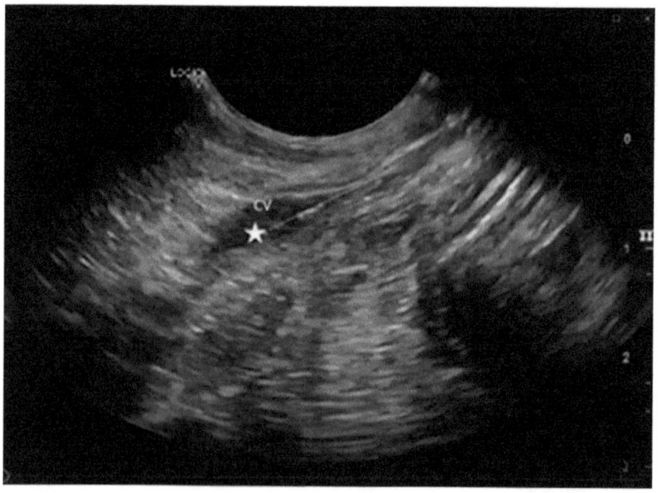

Figure 6.11 Common carp, abdominal ultrasound. Puncture of the caudal vein (CV) for blood collection.

In chelonians, dorsoventral, laterolateral (horizontal beam), and craniocaudal (horizontal beam), radiography can be performed to thoroughly evaluate celomic contents and lung fields.

In snakes (Ophidia), radiography can be performed by placing the animal in an acrylic tube to prevent coiling. This maneuver allows for proper positioning and diagnostic images.

Aquatic birds are approached in the same manner as terrestrial birds.

Aquatic mammals are examined in the water and can be trained to present the appropriate side for ultrasonography.

6.4.3 Necropsy

Most aquatic animals will start decomposition more rapidly compared with terrestrial animals. The sooner the necropsy can be performed following death, the lower the degree of confounding artifacts. A duplicate set of tissues should be saved in a freezer for potential molecular diagnostics. If histology of formalin fixed tissues suggests a potential infectious agent, frozen tissues can yield better results on polymerase chain reaction analyses than tissues fixed in formalin.

In fish, necropsy starts with a ventral midline approach entering via the thoracic inlet, and extending the incision just cranial to the vent, to prevent fecal contamination. Aseptic samples from the anterior kidney are taken for bacteriology examinations. For small fish (less than 5 cm body length), one operculum and one side of the coelomic wall should be sampled for fixation. For larger fish, internal organs are sampled individually for fixation.

Aquatic birds are approached in the same manner as terrestrial birds.

6.5 Exploratory Surgery

The detailed protocol for anesthesia and presurgery in fish can be found in the Treatment section 6.6.

In fish, a ventral midline approach is used. Closure can be made with 3-0, non-absorbable, monofilament, swaged-on, reverse-cutting needle, using a simple interrupted pattern, at a maximum of 5 mm apart. Some fish surgeons recommend that sutures should be retained at least three to four weeks. Others have recommended that, ideally, one should remove skin sutures when the incision is healed, usually in 10–14 days, depending on the degree of healing. Fish may not readily absorb nominally absorbable sutures, because of lower temperatures inhibiting hydrolysis (Cannizzo *et al.*, 2016). Healing rate can be temperature and/or species dependent. The removal of sutures eliminates a potential risk for inflammation and can speed the final stages of incision healing. Cyanoacrylate should be avoided in fish. Possible complications include celomitis or wound dehiscence, especially in females, during oogenesis (spring time).

Anesthesia and analgesia agents used in amphibians: MS222, alfaxalone, opioids, non-steroidal anti-inflammatory drugs (NSAIDs), ketamine, dexmedetomidine and isoflurane. In amphibians, it is required to prepare the skin aseptically with diluted povidone-iodine solution (1 : 10) or diluted chlorhexidine solution (0.75%). The skin of amphibian patients must remain moist throughout the procedure. For this purpose, dechlorinated water must be used. Celiotomy incisions are closed in two layers: a simple continuous pattern for muscle with celomic membrane, and a simple interrupted everting pattern for skin.

- Anesthesia and analgesia agents used in reptiles: NSAIDs, opioids (pure mu agonists only; butorphanol and buprenorphine do not provide analgesia in reptiles), propofol, alfaxalone, ketamine, dexmedetomidine, midazolam, lidocaine (for local anesthesia). An everting pattern is commonly used to close the skin. If the suture placement is proper, the skin can be closed with an intradermal pattern.
- Sauria: Caution on ventral midline approach to avoid ventral abdominal vein. Alternately, use paramedian approach for dorsally compressed lizards (e.g., bearded dragons) or flank approach for laterally compressed lizards (e.g., chameleons).
- Ophidia: Entry into celom by incising skin between the ventral two rows of scales along the lateral aspect and reflecting the skin ventrally to enter the celom just ventral to the rib margin. Do not incise through ventral scales.
- Chelonia: Entry through skin of prefemoral fossa. The advantage is that it allows for quicker healing than plastronotomy. However, this approach may limit visualization, it requires endoscopic assistance. One advantage of plastronotomy is greater visualization over prefemoral fossa entry; disadvantages include prolonged healing of incision site. Thorough cleansing of the shell prior to aseptic surgical preparation is imperative.
- Crocodilia: there are multiple membranous septations within the celom which make exploratory surgery difficult.

6.5.1 Endoscopy

To perform celioscopy in fish enter via ventral midline incision, caudal to pelvic girdle. Insufflate with sterile saline rather than gas, to prevent postoperative positive buoyancy. Complications may include hemorrhage, the rupture of the gonadal capsule or the formation of visceral adhesions. Instruments should be sterilized after usage. Residual chemicals should be removed with sterile water rinsing before usage.

Endoscopy in amphibians can be performed through multiple procedures. See recommended resources at the end of this chapter (Chai, 2015).

Endoscopy in reptiles can be performed through multiple procedures. See recommended resources at the end of this chapter (Divers, 2010; Martínez-Silvestre, 2015).

Endoscopy equipment should be sterilized following each use. Preferred sterilization techniques are ethylene oxide or steam autoclave. Some endoscopic equipment cannot be steam autoclaved;

refer to the manufacturer's instructions. Alternatively, endoscopic equipment may by sterilized with glutaraldehyde or ortho-phthalaldehyde, but this is inferior to autoclave or ethylene oxide, as some pathogens are resistant to glutaraldehyde and ortho-phthalaldehyde (e.g., *Cryptosporidium*).

Information on molecular diagnosis of some fish diseases is available in the website materials accompanying this text.

6.6 Treatment

6.6.1 Management Strategies

Drug therapy of fish and aquatic invertebrates generally involves treating all organisms in a given volume of water or treating the patient individually. The vast differences in species treated and environments housing fish means that the specific method of drug therapy often becomes the attending veterinarians' choice. While management practices differ between commercial fisheries and ornamental fish aquarists, the principles of drug therapy apply to all fish and aquatic invertebrate species.

Generally speaking, drugs or other chemicals (such as formalin or copper sulfate) are used in the following ways:

- To treat bacterial or fungal infection of fish or aquatic organisms in the water.
- To treat free-living or transmissible parasites.
- To immobilize or sedate fish to allow for transport, surgery, or other therapeutic interventions such as examination, and specimen collection.

Traditionally, captive fish and aquatic invertebrates have received pharmaceutical therapies by adding drugs directly to the water of their tank, pond, or habitat. This may be the addition of drugs to a community tank or a specified hospital tank or holding pond or a larger body of water, depending upon the species and the specific disease being treated. Treating the individual fish involves the same methods as drug administration to land animals, in that drugs can be administered via injection (intramuscularly, subcutaneous, or intracelomically; Figure 6.12) or orally, via gavage tube (Figure 6.13) or mixed with food.

Topical administration of drugs is possible with fish, but may require general anesthesia to apply the drug. The intravenous route of drug delivery may be used in larger fish, but generally is not used in smaller fish because of size constraints and volume of drug administered. Instead, the gills provide a potential means of administering drugs in a manner that is rapidly absorbed into the blood stream. Invertebrates have anatomical differences, such as a chitinous exoskeleton, which may complicate drug administration, although it is possible to administer drugs via injection. The pharmacokinetics of a drug are primarily dependent upon the method of administration of that specific drug and water temperature. This must be considered as drugs administered parenterally or orally to a fish may have different doses and dosing intervals than drugs administered by adding the drug to the water the fish is in.

Individual drug administration methods can be stressful to aquatic organisms, so care must be taken when administering drugs individually to consider the stress of being handled (typically with a net and/or by hand) and the stress of being out of the water while drugs are administered. It may be possible to decrease stress by administering drugs requiring injection or gavage with at least half of the fish, ideally including the gills, submerged in well-oxygenated water. If the fish or

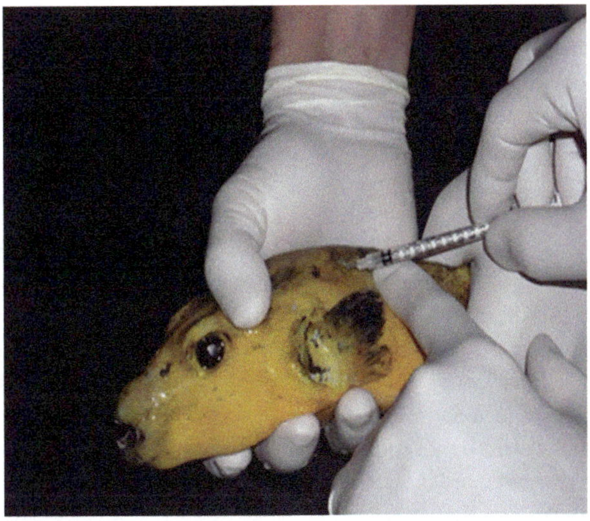

Figure 6.12 Intramuscular injection of antimicrobial drugs administered to epaxial muscles of puffer fish (*Arothron meleagri*).

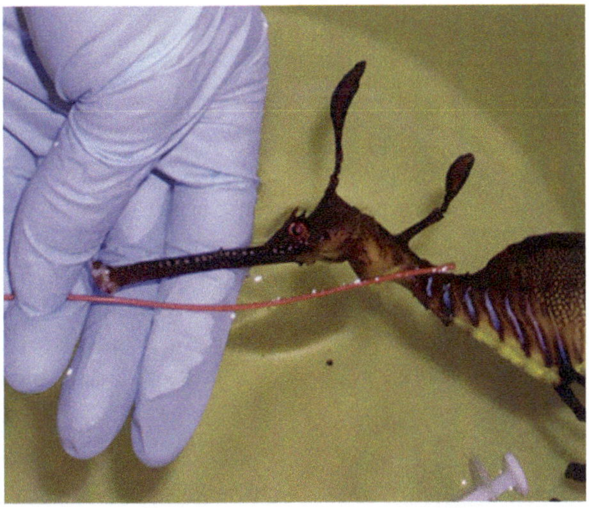

Figure 6.13 Determination of red-rubber tube length for gavage administration of antimicrobial drugs and food slurry to a sedated weedy sea dragon (*Phyllopteryx taeniolatus*).

invertebrate must be removed from the water to administer drugs, every effort should be made to minimize that time out of the water.

Adding drugs directly to the water where a fish or invertebrate is kept has traditionally been the most widely used method of drug administration. Depending on the species, fish skin may be permeable to water soluble non-polarized drugs or chemicals. The salinity of the water can impact transdermal absorption of drugs. Freshwater fish and aquatic organisms have physiological systems that excrete water to maintain homeostasis. Conversely, marine and brackish water organisms have physiological mechanisms to conserve water while excreting electrolytes. These intrinsic physiological systems must be considered when choosing medications, as these environmental adaptations may impact drug clearance and excretion.

Absorption of drugs dissolved in the water also varies depending upon other environmental factors such as water alkalinity, salinity, and temperature. In addition to the limited transcutaneous absorption of drugs, administration of a drug into the water also allows for drug absorption through the gills. In general, the gills should be considered the primary site of drug absorption for drugs administered through the water. Generally, lipophilic drugs will diffuse across gill membranes, but this varies between species of fish. This interspecies variation means that clinicians treating fish by adding drugs directly into the water must consider the species treated and whether the drug is actually absorbed in that species.

The physical properties of some drugs may make their administration in the water impractical. If the disease condition being treated disrupts normal gill structure and circulation, as in damage to the gill arches or via formation of plaques or mucous that may coat the gills, there may be substantial limitations to the absorption of drugs administered into the water. Gill health and function must be considered for water administration of drugs to be successful.

The advantage of administering drugs in the water is that large numbers of fish or fish that are too small for individual therapy can be treated. The ability to treat multiple patients at one time makes these methods of drug delivery desirable for larger systems, such as pet stores, fish hatcheries, ponds, or lakes. The disadvantages to treating disease by adding drugs to the water the fish are in are as follows:

- Species variation in drug absorption and resultant variation in pharmacokinetics may alter desired drug efficacy.
- The waste of unabsorbed drug in the water results in an unnecessary therapeutic expense.
- The impact of drugs on biological filters in enclosed environments and any discharge to the environment.

Clinicians should specifically determine the potential effects on biological filters of enclosed systems prior to adding antimicrobials or chemicals to avoid damaging them. As a general rule, antimicrobials such as erythromycin or chemicals such as methylene blue can result in rapid death of beneficial bacteria in the biological filter, subsequent collapse of biological filtration, and death of fish secondary to a rapid rise in ammonia. Immersion therapy or adding antimicrobials directly into the water works best in smaller enclosed systems such as a hospital aquarium, raceways, or controlled environments such as dipping tanks (Figure 6.14).

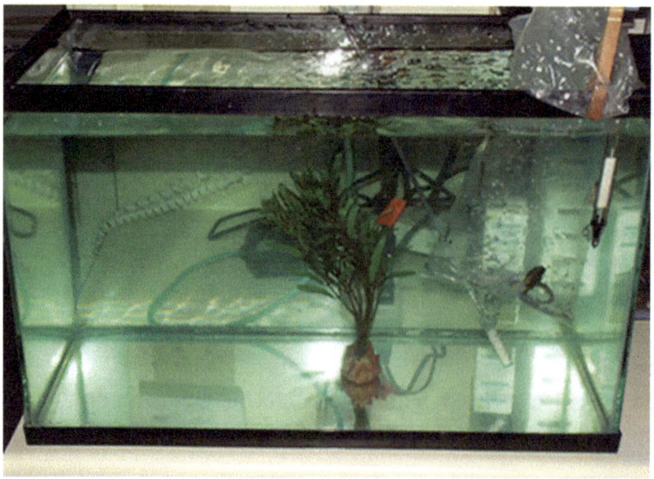

Figure 6.14 An example of a hospital aquarium, composed of an aquarium with minimal substrate and limited filtration. Water parameters are maintained by a simplistic filter system (bubble filter or sponge filter) or frequent water changes.

Flushing and bath methods of drug therapy are more focused methods of administering drugs to fish when adding the drug directly into the water. Flushing is a specialized form of drug immersion therapy used in specific aquatic environments consisting of running water which is not recirculated. This water can be drained from an enclosed system or can be managed as a continuous flow as in a raceway at a fish hatchery. This method is employed in fish hatcheries for the control of fungal organisms, or in the event of potential contamination of a fish farm's water supply. The procedure involves removing affected fish from the main pond or holding area and placing them in a raceway or trough system that normally receives continuously flowing water from the same source as the pond. Water input and output flows are temporarily stopped before appropriate medication is added to the raceway water containing the fish. There may initially be an uneven distribution of the drug in the water, depending upon the size and shape of the area used for drug administration. Circulation of water within the now temporarily enclosed environment may be accomplished by aeration or use of specific recirculating pumps to facilitate even drug distribution. Then, after an appropriate treatment interval, as indicated by the drug or chemical used, the water flow is restarted. This results in a rapid rise in drug concentration to a maximum desired concentration in the water, then a slower fall over time as the drug is flushed from the system.

Obviously, this method of drug delivery is more environmentally contaminating than other methods, with initial efflux potentially containing high concentrations of drug or therapeutic chemicals (such as copper sulfate). Care must be taken in therapeutic drug or chemical choices as potential deleterious effects from the waste water may occur downstream. For fish, short exposure times are typically needed for drugs in the water to reach maximum plasma concentrations, ranging from 30 seconds to 30 minutes. Depending on the number and size of fish being treated, in addition to the disease condition, the placing of fish in this smaller than normal aquatic environment may dictate the need to aggressively aerate the water to prevent hypoxia and/or associated pH changes due to carbon dioxide accumulation in the water as the fish are being treated. Alternately, a flushing system can be built as a small aquasystem or a sump unit adjacent to larger aquariums, with water overflow to the system and return to the aquarium or to a drain independent of the main aquarium. The treatment system is then flushed with water drained from the main system as part of a routine water change (Figure 6.15).

The practice of immersion or "dipping" affected fish in a medicated tank or trough for a specific amount of time then returning them to their original area is another method of administering

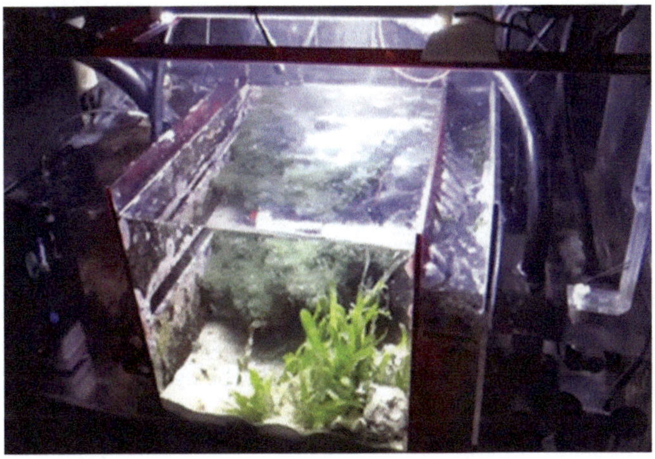

Figure 6.15 A flushing tank that is part of a larger interconnected marine aquarium system. This specific tank is built much like a sump and serves as such when not used to treat affected fish or invertebrates.

drugs through the water. This is a simple method that requires only a five-gallon bucket and a means of capturing the fish, typically a net. It may be difficult to dip larger fish. The amount of time the fish stays within the dipping container is dictated by individual species and drugs administered. Dipping the fish in medicated water for a brief period has the advantage of minimizing antimicrobial and chemical effects on the biological filter of enclosed systems as minimal antimicrobials may enter that water to alter the biological filter. Removing water from the normal environment and adding it to the dipping container, then adding antimicrobials to that water has the added advantage of minimizing stress associated with changes in temperature, pH, or salinity. The disadvantage to this method of drug therapy is creating drug or chemical exposure sufficient to provide therapeutic results. Often this method may use drugs at very high water concentrations or chemicals such as copper sulfate or formalin, which may be toxic with prolonged exposure.

Unfortunately, veterinary literature is lacking in controlled pharmacokinetic studies to determine the specifics of drugs for each of these methods of drug delivery. Many published pharmacokinetic studies are derived from the aquaculture industry and extrapolated to ornamental fish, although this is changing. Specific drug and drug information is becoming more readily available for multiple species.

6.6.2 Drug Therapy: Selection and Use of Drugs

When treating aquatic animals like fish, and in particular food species, the veterinarian has limited choices. For ornamental fish (and other non-food species), the veterinarian can use medications off label, provided that they are not contraindicated or banned for use in that species. Generally, for food producing species, a veterinarian may use a medicine off label, provided that it is registered for use in another food species, as long as it is not contraindicated or banned for use in that species. Some medicines such as hormones, may only be permissible for non-food individuals of a food species (Peter Scott, personal communication). The veterinarian must ascertain that there is sufficient data on which to base a treatment regimen and must establish withholding periods when treating an animal whose tissues or products have the potential to enter the human food chain. Where no minimum withdrawal period is specified for a pharmaceutical then the veterinarian should refer to their local jurisdiction legislation. Within the European Union, this period is 500 degree days (e.g. if water temperature is 20°C then withdrawal is 25 days).

If treating farmed species, drug selection can be further complicated by the necessity to obtain discharge consents prior to the usage. This consent can take several months to obtain. Even where the necessary discharge consents are in place, you are not allowed to exceed the permitted frequency or volume of discharge.

6.7 Anesthetics and Analgesics

6.7.1 Terminology

- Sedation is the administering of a sedative drug to produce a state of calm or sleepiness.
- Tranquilization is the use of a sedative/tranquilizer for aiding in handling, examination, and transportation. Tranquilizing fish makes them easier to handle for physical examinations and diagnostic tests. Tranquilization may be used for taking external tissue (fin and gill) biopsies and for ova/milt stripping during breeding.

- Analgesia is insensibility to pain without loss of consciousness. It is useful to provide postoperative or post-injury pain relief.
- Anesthesia is loss of sensation (with or without loss of consciousness) artificially produced by the administration of drugs that block the impulses along nerve pathways to the brain.
- General anesthesia is the loss of sensation and the loss of consciousness for invasive procedures and surgery. Anesthetizing fish prior to any surgical procedure is essential, especially with large species such as koi or fish in a public aquarium.
- Euthanasia is derived from the Greek terms *eu* meaning good and *thanatos* meaning death. The term is used to describe ending the life of an animal in a way that minimizes or eliminates pain and distress. Euthanasia differs from slaughter or depopulation (Saint-Erne, 2016).

6.7.2 Methods of Delivering Anesthesia in Fish

The most common method of administering anesthesia to fish is by adding the drug directly to a container of water. Fish rapidly absorb many chemicals through the gill membranes into the blood stream. With this method, it is important to accurately measure the volume of water that is being medicated so that the correct dosage of anesthetic can be used. Anesthetic agents can also be injected intramuscularly (IM), intravenously (IV) or intraperitoneally (IP), which is intracelomically in fish.

Oral (per os, PO) medication can be given via stomach tube, or by injecting the anesthetic (diazepam, ketamine) into a suitable food fish that is fed to the patient. Onset of sedation may be variable when anesthetics are given orally. Some anesthetic solutions, such as benzocaine or tricaine at 1 g/l solution, can be topically applied to gills with a spray bottle or bulb syringe for faster induction in larger species, such as elasmobranchs.

6.7.3 Anesthetic Agents Used in Fish

Many commonly used veterinary anesthetics for small animals can also be used with fish (Tables 6.1, 6.2). Not all anesthetics may be available for use in fish in some countries. Check the appropriate drug enforcement agency for applicable regulations on using anesthetics in aquatic animals. Start with a lower dosage if using an unfamiliar drug or inducing anesthesia on a species not usually seen in your practice (Brown, 1993; Ross, 2001; Saint-Erne, 2010; Loh, 2012).

6.7.4 Induction of Anesthesia

Use a container of good quality water with aeration provided by an aquarium air pump connected to an air stone. Add the anesthesia induction solution and mix thoroughly. It is helpful to inject liquid anesthetic through a fine-gauge needle underwater for uniform dispersal in the induction container. Add the fish to the container with the anesthetic solution until the desired level of sedation or anesthesia is reached. At this point, the fish can be removed from the water and placed on a wet surface (plastic sheet, towel, chamois) for treatment, biopsy, or surgery.

If the fish is being maintained in the anesthetic solution, it is important to add untreated water to lower the anesthetic concentration in the water after induction. Monitoring the respiration (opercular movements) and heartbeat (with electrocardiogram, ECG) or blood oxygen saturation (pulse oximeter) can indicate whether the anesthesia is too deep and the anesthetic concentration in the water needs to be reduced. Be sure to maintain aeration in the anesthetic solution with an air pump and air stone, or even by using an oxygen canister with a hose to bubble oxygen into the water.

Table 6.1 Anesthetic agents used in fish.

Agent	Chemical name	Delivery method	Sedative dosage	Anesthetic dosage	Induction time (minutes)	Recovery time (minutes)	Euthanasia	Notes
Alfaxalone	3-alpha-hydroxy-5-alpha-pregnane 11,20-dione	Immersion	1–2 mg/l	1.5–4.0 mg/l; koi 2.5 mg/l	5	3–10	–	–
Benzocaine	ethyl p-aminobenzoate	Immersion	12.5 mg/l	25–500 mg/l	1–3	3–15		May need to be dissolved in ethanol first; fat soluble so prolonged exposure will produce longer recovery times
Carbon Dioxide	CO_2	Immersion		100–400 mg/l	1–2	5–10	Leave fish 60 minutes after respiration stops	A canister of CO_2 is used with an air hose and air stone to bubble gas through the water. Use with caution, under constant observation, and in a well-ventilated area. Avoid breathing CO_2 released from the water
Valium	diazepam	IM/PO	0.1–0.5 mg/kg IM or 1–4 mg/kg PO	–	–	–	–	Sedative and muscle relaxant, used as a pre-anesthetic agent
Ethyl alcohol	ethanol	Immersion	1%	–	–	–	–	20 ml of 100 proof (50%) grain alcohol in 1 l water will produce a 1% solution
Clove oil	eugenol (1 drop = 28.6 mg)	Immersion	3–5 mg/l	30–60 mg/l	2–3	–	114 mg/l for 60 minutes	Mix vigorously with water. Excellent for short duration physical examinations. Not recommended for use in invasive surgeries due to low analgesic effect

Aqui-S	isoeugenol (50% in water solution)	Immersion	3–5 mg/l	15–20 mg/l	12–15			Approved in Australia, Chile, New Zealand and Vietnam
Isoflurane	1-chloro-2,2,2-trifluoroethyl difluoromethyl ether	Immersion		0.25–1 ml/l	2–8	3–30	4 ml/l	Forcefully spray the required dose through a 25-gauge needle under the water while mixing
Ketalar	ketamine hydrochloride	IM injection or immersion	66–100 mg/kg or 1 g/l	–	–	–	–	Provides sedation and immobilization for handling or transportation. Dose can be given orally by injecting into a food fish fed to larger fish needing sedation. Hyperactivity and ataxia can occur during recovery
Xylocaine	lidocaine	IM, IV		0.1–2 mg/kg IM total dose, injected into/ around tisue	–	–	–	Only provides local analgesia
Hypnodil	metomidate hydrochloride	Immersion	0.06–5 mg/l (see notes)	1–10 mg/l	–	–	100 mg/l for 60 minutes after respiration stops for most tropical fish	Doses for tropical marine fish for tranquilization during transportation are 0.06–0.20 mg/l. Dosages for tranquilization used in freshwater fish vary from 2.5 to 5 mg/l. Anesthesia: 1.0–10.0 mg/l of water. The dosage should be individualized, depending upon the fish species and the degree of anesthesia required. May need buffering if water is at a low pH

(*Continued*)

Table 6.1 (Continued)

Agent	Chemical name	Delivery method	Sedative dosage	Anesthetic dosage	Induction time (minutes)	Recovery time (minutes)	Euthanasia	Notes
Nembutal	pentobarbital	IM, IP		20–40 mg/kg		6–24 hours	60–100 mg/kg	Can produce prolonged anesthesia time (6–24 hours) with cardiac and respiratory depression. Secondary method of euthanasia may be used to ensure death once anesthetized
Propofol	2,6-diisopropylphenol	IV		1.5–2.5 mg/kg	5	60–75		Use parentally only
Quinaldine sulfate	2-methylquinoline sulfate	Immersion	5–10 mg/l	25–200 mg/l	2–6	5–20		Acidifies low alkaline water; use sodium bicarbonate buffer in water, as necessary
Tricaine methane sulfonate (MS222)	3-aminobenzoic acid ethyl ester	Immersion	10–40 mg/l	50–400 mg/l induction; 50–100 mg/l for maintenance	1–5	3–15 (in untreated water)		Acidifies water – buffer with equal volume of sodium bicarbonate (baking soda), or use in hard water. Has 21-day withdrawal time when used with food fish in the United States

Table 6.2 Stages of Anesthesia in Fishes.

Stage	Plane	Description	Signs
0	0	Normal	Swimming actively, equilibrium normal
I	1	Light sedation	Reduced motion, ventilation decreased
I	2	Deeper sedation	Motionless unless stimulated
II	1	Light anesthesia	Partial loss of equilibrium
II	2	Deep anesthesia	Total loss of equilibrium
III	1	Surgical anesthesia	Total loss of reactivity when stimulated
III	2	Deep surgical anesthesia	Decrease in respiratory and heart rates
IV	1	Medullary collapse	Cessation of respiratory movements
IV	2	Cardiac arrest	Death

Source: Saint-Erne (2019); adapted from Brown (1993) and Ross (2001).

When aquatic animals are removed from the water after being anesthetized, apply ophthalmic ointment (natural tears) to both eyes to prevent drying and damage to the cornea. Keep the skin moist by covering with wet gauze or cloth and spray with water as needed. Always use wet gloves when handling fish to avoid removing the mucus layer on their skin.

If the fish remains out of the water for more than a few minutes, pump a lower dose of anesthetic solution over the gills to maintain anesthesia (use a syringe, IV bag and drip line, water pump, or aquarium power head). Make sure there is an even flow out both opercula, and the solution is not going down the esophagus. If it is practical, the fish can be periodically returned to the anesthesia solution to maintain sedation or anesthesia.

Methods of monitoring the fish during anesthesia will vary according to the species and the complexity of the procedure, but should include a pre-anesthetic assessment for general health, and adequate monitoring of anesthetic depth (Table 6.2):

- Response to touch, noise, righting reflex.
- Heart rate change is important: take a pre-anesthetic rate reading. In ectotherms, the heart can continue to beat even after death. Use ECG attached to needles inserted into pectoral muscles to monitor the heartbeat.
- Measure the respiratory rate prior to anesthesia, and keep track of the rate during anesthesia and use caution if breathing is slowing.
- A pulse oximetry blood oxygen saturation monitor can be clamped onto caudal fin.
- Maintain proper water quality (aeration, pH, temperature).
- Monitoring and support during anesthetic recovery should include observation of gill membrane color and operculum movements.

6.7.5 Recovery from Anesthesia

Move fish to clean water without anesthetic solution for recovery. The longer the fish is under anesthesia, and the colder the water, the longer the fish will take to recover. Use dim lighting and keep recovery area quiet. Cover the recovery tank if possible. Watch for jumping! Once the fish has recovered from anesthesia and returned to normal swimming, it can be returned to the pond or aquarium.

6.7.6 Decontamination

Effective cleaning is responsible for more than 90% of the success of a decontamination program. Accumulations of soil, dirt, or organic matter provide an effective barrier, protecting pathogens from disinfecting agents. Organic matter rapidly inactivates a number of chemical disinfectants. Some cleaning agents are incompatible with specific types of chemical disinfectants. The effectiveness of certain cleaning compounds and disinfectants depends on the quality and hardness of the water used, the concentration, contact time, temperature and pH. Many disinfectants are corrosive to equipment, and most are irritant to people and toxic to aquatic life. Washwater may still contain viable pathogenic organisms or polluting chemicals which must be disposed of appropriately. Many disinfectants are not effective against spores, and some are only mildly effective against *Mycobacteria* and non-enveloped viruses (Australian Department of Agriculture, Fisheries and Forestry 2008).

Several chemicals successfully kill a wide variety of pathogens. The most widely used and readily available is sodium hypochlorite, but iodophors, hydrogen peroxide and peracetic acid in hydrogen peroxide can also be used (Lilley and Inglis, 1997). Gross contamination such as mud on boots and equipment must always be removed prior to disinfection.

- Chlorination: Sodium hypochlorite and many of the solid chemicals used to provide freely available chlorine in swimming pools and spas, such as calcium hypochlorite, are suitable sources of chlorine. Chlorination of water used to clean equipment, as well as effluent from infected premises or processing facilities, should occur prior to release into the environment. 100 ppm of free available chlorine for 30 seconds is required for this purpose (Alderman and Polglase, 1985). Liquid chlorine sources rapidly lose their strength hence the need to measure free chlorine prior to use.
- Iodine: 100 ppm available iodine supplied as iodophors for up to 32 minutes is an effective disinfectant for crayfish plague. The time necessary is dependent on the iodophor used (Alderman and Polglase, 1985). Iodophors are less corrosive than chlorine-based disinfectants but are not suitable for all items as they leave residual stains (Alderman and Polglase, 1985).
- Treating surfaces with 100 ppm of 5% peracetic acid in hydrogen peroxide for five minutes, a commonly used disinfectant in the food industry, was an effective disinfectant (Lilley and Inglis, 1997).

There can be serious environmental consequences as a result of exposure of unintended targets to waste water containing drugs used to treat fish and aquatic invertebrates. These negative consequences include contributions to the proliferation of antimicrobial resistance, death of desirable organisms, growth of toxic or undesirable algae, and other ecological concerns. The concern of environmental contamination from waste water resulting from treatment of large bodies of water, especially with pharmaceuticals or chemicals such as copper sulfate should not be ignored.

Waste water from infected bodies of water must be contained and disinfected to reduce the likelihood of spread of disease. The potential negative environmental impact of water treatment during an outbreak must be considered and strategies implemented to reduce their impact. Chlorine and iodine-based disinfectants can be rendered harmless prior to discharge by the addition of sodium thiosulphate. Other medicines can be inactivated by carbon filtration, or wait for natural decomposition to occur prior to discharge.

6.8 Vector Controls

Controlling the spread of pathogens between aquaria and ponds are difficult because some agents can be carried to new locations on translocated asymptomatic/carrier hosts, on equipment, motor vehicles, water or by other animals such as water birds or rats. Understanding possible vectors of infection is important in selecting appropriate policies and restrictions during an outbreak.

6.8.1 Rehabilitation Plan

Before a treatment plan has begun, it is vital to consider the rehabilitation and eventual release of stranded, ill or injured wildlife.

6.8.2 End of Life Care (Euthanasia protocols and Agents)

Anesthetic solutions can be used for euthanasia of ornamental fish (Figures 6.16, 6.17), with a recommended euthanasia dose being 10 times that used for anesthesia, leaving the fish in the solution long enough for all opercular motion (respiration) to stop, and then waiting another hour to ensure their death from anoxia while anesthetized and not respiring. The most common method

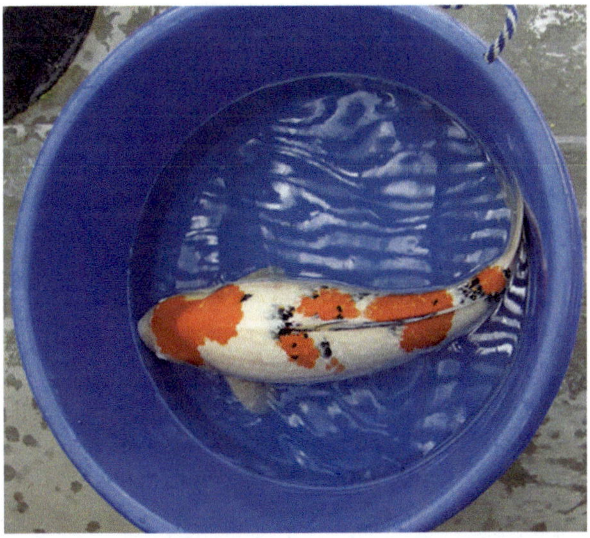

Figure 6.16 Koi fish in anesthetic solution This protocol can also be used for euthanasia. *Source:* Photo by N. Saint-Erne.

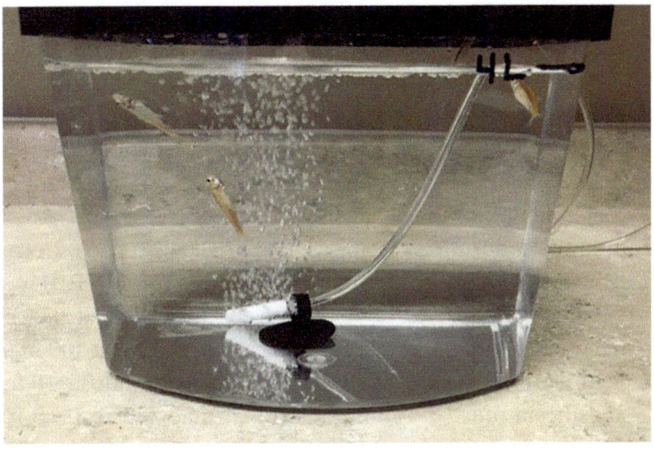

Figure 6.17 Anesthetizing then euthanizing fish in an aerated aquarium. *Source:* Photo by N. Saint-Erne.

of administering anesthetics for euthanasia to fish is by adding the drug directly to the water. Fish rapidly absorb many chemicals through the gill membranes into the blood stream. With this method, it is important to accurately measure the volume of water that is being medicated so that the correct dosage of anesthetic can be used.

Use higher drug doses (10 times the normal anesthetic dose) to rapidly cause unconsciousness. After the fish is unconscious, it will eventually stop respiring, which causes death by hypoxia. Keep the fish in the euthanasia solution for more than 60 minutes after respiration stops. Some fish species (anabantids, catfish, lungfish) are highly tolerant to anoxic conditions and may need longer times in anesthetic solutions for euthanasia, or may need secondary methods of euthanasia once anesthetized.

According to the *AVMA Guidelines for Euthanasia of Animals* (American Veterinary Medical Association, 2020), the following methods are acceptable for euthanasia in fish not intended for consumption:

- Immersion in solutions of buffered tricaine methanesulfonate (MS222), buffered benzocaine, isoflurane and sevoflurane, quinaldine sulfate, 2-phenoxyethanol, and eugenol or clove oil. Fish should be left in the solution for a minimum of 60 minutes after cessation of opercular movement.
- Injections of pentobarbital, ketamine followed by pentobarbital, a combination of ketamine and medetomidine followed by pentobarbital, and propofol followed by pentobarbital. Owners should be advised about the possibility of ketamine-induced muscle spasms during induction when using that agent.

Death must be confirmed before disposal of any animal remains. A combination of criteria is most reliable in confirming death, including lack of heartbeat, lack of breathing (gill movements), lack of response to painful stimuli, gills becoming pale, and rigor mortis. None of these signs alone, except rigor mortis, confirms death. Death can be ensured by physical intervention (pithing, decapitation) after anesthesia.

6.8.2.1 Commonly Used Euthanasia Drug Dosages

- Carbon dioxide (CO_2): A dose of 100–400 mg/l will cause unconsciousness; long exposure will cause death. A canister of CO_2 is used with an air hose and air stone to bubble gas through the water. Use with caution, under constant observation, and in a well-ventilated area. Avoid breathing CO_2 released from the water. Induction is in 1–2 minutes and recovery in 5–10 minutes in fresh water. For euthanasia, leave fish in water after breathing stops for 60 minutes or more.
- Ethanol (ethyl alcohol): 1% added to the water will produce sedation; 3% or more will result in euthanasia; 20 ml of 100 proof (50%) grain alcohol in one liter of water will produce a 1% solution.
- Eugenol/isoeugenol (clove oil): 1 drop = 0.029 ml = 28.6 mg. For sedation during transport, use 3–5 mg/l (1–2 drops/10 l) in shipping water. For anesthesia, use 30–60 mg/l (1–2 drops/l) of water. Mix vigorously with water. Induction occurs in two to three minutes. This preparation is excellent for short-duration physical examinations. It is not recommended for use in invasive surgeries due to low analgesic effect. A dose of 4 drops/l (114 mg/l) induces euthanasia in 60 minutes.
- Metomidate: Sedation concentration is 0.1–1.0 mg/l of water. Doses for tropical marine fish for tranquilization during transportation are 0.06–0.20 mg/l. Dosages for tranquilization used in tropical fish vary from 2.5 to 5 mg/l. For anesthesia use 1.0–10.0 mg/l of water. The dosage should be individualized, depending upon the fish species and the degree of anesthesia required. May need buffering if water is at a low pH. Euthanasia is effective at 100 mg/l in 60 minutes for most tropical fish.
- Pentobarbital: 20–40 mg/kg IM or IP; 60–100 mg/kg IP for euthanasia. Can produce prolonged anesthesia time (6–24 hours) with cardiac and respiratory depression. A secondary method of euthanasia may be used to ensure death once anesthetized.

- Quinaldine sulfate (2-methylquinoline sulfate): Dose at 5–10 mg/l for sedation during transport, 25–200 mg/l for anesthesia. Induction in 2–6 minutes, recovery in fresh water in 5–20 minutes. Acidifies low alkaline water, use sodium bicarbonate buffer in water as necessary.
- Tricaine methane sulfonate, MS222 (3-aminobenzoic acid ethyl ester): Dose at 10–40 mg/l for sedation (handling/ shipping). Dose at 50–400 mg/l for anesthesia induction, and 50–100 mg/l for maintenance. Induction in 1–5 minutes, recovery in 3–15 minutes in clean water. Acidifies water – buffer with equal volume of sodium bicarbonate, or use in hard water. Has 21-day withdrawal time when used with food fish in the United States.

The following methods of euthanasia are not recommended for use when owners of the fish are present and may be disturbed by the fish's response to euthanasia solution (Saint-Erne, 2019):

- Immersion in CO_2-saturated water is not recommended because some finfish exposed to this method may become hyperactive, which can be disconcerting for staff and owners.
- Manually applied blunt force trauma to the head, decapitation, and pithing are not recommended because their application can be distressing for owners and staff.

The following are unacceptable methods of euthanasia in any situation (American Veterinary Medical Association, 2020):

- Flushing of finfish into sewer, septic, or other types of outflow systems is unacceptable for many reasons. Water chemistry and quality may delay time to death and result in exposure to noxious compounds. For systems in close proximity to and/or connected to natural waterways, pathogen release or transmission may occur from diseased or carrier animals.
- Slow chilling or freezing of unanesthetized animals, including placing finfish into a freezer without prior anesthesia, is also an unacceptable method.
- Similarly, death by anoxia and desiccation after removal from the water or by anoxia in water; any death due to exposure to caustic chemicals; and death including prolonged traumatic injury prior to unconsciousness are unacceptable.

Supplementary materials available online

- Imaging methods used in the examination of fish.
- Molecular diagnosis.
- Further reading.

References

Alderman, D.J. and Polglase, J.L. (1985). Disinfection for crayfish plague. *Aquaculture Research* 16: 203–205.

American Veterinary Medical Association. (2020). *AVMA Guidelines for the Euthanasia of Animals: 2020 edition*. Schaumburg, IL: AMVA.

Australian Department of Agriculture, Fisheries and Forestry. (2008). *AQUAVETPLAN: Operational Procedures Manual Decontamination*. Canberra: Department of Agriculture, Fisheries and Forestry.

Barco, S.G., Walton, W.J., Harms, C.A. *et al.* (2016). *Collaborative Development of Recommendations for Euthanasia of Stranded Cetaceans*. NOAA Technical Memorandum NMFS-OPR-56. Silver Spring, MD: US Department of Commerce, National Oceanic and Atmospheric Administration, National Marine Fisheries Service.

Brown, L. (1993.). Anesthesia and Restraint. In: *Fish Medicine* (ed. M.K. Stoskopf), 81. Philadelphia, PA: WB Saunders.

Cannizzo, S.A., Roe, S.C., Harms, C.A. and Stoskopf, M. (2016). Effect of water temperature on the hydrolysis of two absorbable sutures used in fish surgery. *FACETS* 1(1): 44–54.

Chai, N. (2015). Endoscopy in amphibians. *Veterinary Clinics of North America: Exotic Animal Practice.* 18: 479–441.

Lilley, J.H. and Inglis, V. (1997). Comparative effects of various antibiotics, fungicides and disinfectants on *Aphanomyces invaderis* and other saprolegniaceous fungi. *Aquaculture Research* 28: 461–469.

Loh, R. (2012). *Fish Vetting Medicines.* Perth, Australia: Richmond Loh Publishing.

Martínez-Silvestre, A., Bargalló, F. and Grífols, J. (2015). Gender identification by cloacoscopy and cystoscopy in juvenile chelonians. *Veterinary Clinics: Exotic Animal Practice* 18: 527–539.

Novelo, N.D. and Tiersch, T.R. (2012). A review of the use of ultrasonography in fish reproduction. *North American Journal of Aquaculture* 74: 169–181.

Ross, L.G. (2001). Restraint, anesthesia, and euthanasia. In: *BSAVA Manual of Ornamental Fish*, 2nd ed. (W.H. Wildgoose, ed.), 76. Gloucester: BSAVA.

Saint-Erne, N. (2019). Anesthesia Induction and Monitoring in Fish; Lecture notes for WSAVA Convention, Toronto, Canada.

Saint-Erne, N. (2016). Tranquilization, Anesthesia, Analgesia and Euthanasia of Common Exotic Pets; Lecture notes: Midwestern University College of Veterinary Medicine, Glendale, AZ.

Saint-Erne, N. (2010). *Advanced Koi Care*, 2e. Glendale, AZ: Erne Enterprises.

Sande, R.D. and Poppe, T.T. (1995). Diagnostic ultrasound examination and ecocardiography in atlantic salmon. *Veterinary Radiology and Ultrasound* 36: 551–558.

7

Clinical Veterinary Experience and Client Communication

Richmond Loh, Laura Urdes, and Vasile Vulpe

Learning Objectives
The student should be aware of case management concepts and should gain experience in the different aspects of aquatic veterinary medicine. The student should develop the necessary skills to participate in communications with all stakeholders, such as aquarists, aquaculture producers, farmers, wild animal collectors, facility managers.

7.1 Introduction

Historically, aquatic veterinary medicine has focused on farmed species (aquaculture, population medicine), which may not be applicable for the individual patient. Only within the past few decades has the learning base expanded dramatically and become scientifically standardized. Students need to understand how to practice evidence-based veterinary medicine to provide effective services to their clients and to overcome the inertia of historical management or treatments, which are often based on anecdote.

Some brief sources of information relating specifically to aquatic veterinary medicine are listed. As aquatic veterinary medicine may be new to the student, the listed sources will help them develop a network of colleagues who can direct them to a deeper understanding of the differences between aquatic and classical (terrestrial) veterinary medicine. An introductory text on how to assess sources of knowledge, as well as the relevance and quality of these sources, is included.

7.2 Clinical Veterinary Experience

There are many varied and very different specific areas of aquatic animal veterinary practice: pet fish (clinical practice, mobile clinic); ornamental production (retail, wholesale, import, export, farm); research and educational institutes (universities); government (policy, pathology laboratory, field veterinarians, extension, residues); food production (private consultant, employed veterinarian): finfish (e.g., salmonid, tuna, kingfish, grouper, sea bass, tilapia, carp), mollusks (e.g., abalone, oysters, mussels), crustacea (e.g., crabs, shrimp), amphibia, reptiles (e.g., crocodiles, turtles); public/display aquaria (aquariums, zoos, conservation societies).

Fundamentals of Aquatic Veterinary Medicine, First Edition. Edited by Laura Urdes, Chris Walster, and Julius Tepper.

Companion website: www.wiley.com/go/urdes/aquatic-veterinary-medicine

7.2.1 Veterinary Professionalism

A list of some sources of professional development is available in the website materials accompanying this text.

See also 'Assessing Sources in the Context of Clinical Decision Making' below.

7.2.2 How to Identify Diagnostic Laboratories

Usually, diagnostic facilities can be found in government or university laboratories located in geographic areas where aquaculture production is important. Bacteriology and histopathology expertise are pivotal. Check, for example, the availability of specialist bacteriology media, low temperature incubation of plates, veterinary pathologist experience, and whether they are part of a quality assurance program for aquatic animal pathology.

7.2.3 How to Develop and Maintain Appropriate Medical Records

Some important considerations are that records should have traceability, especially the drug volumes used, confidentiality and back-ups. They may contain photographs of patients, site and handwritten notes. Veterinary software is now usually employed for maintaining medical records.

7.2.4 How to Manage an Aquatic Veterinary Practice: Budgeting, Finance and Legal Aspects

Although very low volumes of drugs used in companion fish, some medicines need to be purchased in bulk (many are used for large animal medicine) and most expire before being dispensed. Fees charged to the client should take this into consideration.

Almost all drugs used for companion fish are off-label/unlicensed, so clients need to be made aware of the potential risks. The client should sign a form to confirm the potential risks have been explained to them. This document should be added to the clinical record.

There are a limited number of licensed drugs for use in farmed fish. In some jurisdictions, the availability of drugs may be increased through mechanisms such as the cascade, a risk-based decision-making tree, which is used in European Union countries (UK Veterinary Medicines Directorate, 2021).

Medicines can only be prescribed or dispensed after a valid veterinarian–client–patient–relationship has been established. Depending on the jurisdiction, it may require a clinical check-up ranging from once every three months to once every one to three years.

The serviceable area is only limited by the cost involved in traveling. It is practical to charge by travel time plus mileage and overnight fees if applicable. Reasonable charge-out rates for travel can be calculated using ride-sharing apps or taxi/cab apps for comparison.

Some useful sources of aquatic animal health information are provided in the website materials accompanying this text.

7.2.5 Assessing Sources in the Context of Clinical Decision Making

The best answer to the question, "Why do I need to assess sources of data?" is, "To make the best clinical decisions for my patients". Clinical decisions, such as the best medical treatment for your koi patient with lice (*Argulus* spp.), must be based on strong, up-to-date scientific evidence. In practice, we often rely exclusively on anecdotal experiences, expert opinion, web documents and so on, which are misleading and not always accurate. This approach should be avoided as much as possible. Practicing aquatic veterinary medicine based on evidence may prove challenging sometimes, as you may find that there may not be any science-based evidence available to consider. This is due to the existing gaps in the knowledge of the field and to numerous limitations in the practice of aquatic animal medicine. If this is the case, any source relevant to the topic of interest, including reports, theses, conference proceedings, bibliographies, technical and commercial documentation, and other so-called gray literature sources, should be taken into consideration.

By assessing sources of information correctly, you will be able to increase your overall clinical success by avoiding mistakes and errors in practice (Figure 7.1; RCVS Knowledge, 2021). Holding regular clinical reviews ensure you are practicing evidence-based (aquatic) veterinary medicine. This will improve your diagnostic, prognostic, control and treatment schemes and protocols, allowing you to provide informed choices for your patients and owners.

7.2.6 What is Evidence?

Evidence is data serving as proof to support or refute a fact. Evidence can be weak or strong (sound; Figure 7.1).

In searching for scientifical evidence, one should always aim at searching for the primary (significant) and secondary branches, which usually provide for further enquiry, as depicted in the Diderot and d'Alembert's Tree of Knowledge (1772). Searching the literature should primarily target articles published in reputable peer-reviewed journals. Primary research is original scientific work carried out to collect new evidence to answer a specific research problem. Although assessing the quality of a journal may prove difficult, one way to do that is to check for the journal's impact factor. The Institute for Scientific Information measures the frequency with which an article in a given journal has been cited in other journals in a particular year. Other journals may be assessed by their popularity(i.e., by immediacy factor or citation half-life). However, these two factors do not reflect the journal's quality.

Secondary research or review articles, which are syntheses and interpretations of existing knowledge arising from previously conducted (primary) research studies, are often valuable sources of information, provided that they are up to date. If you are looking for an unfamiliar topic, it is advisable to start by reading a good review article. This type of article usually provides search terms that can be used for further literature surveys.

Books and textbooks are seen as less reliable sources of material by those interested in research and scientific writing. One of the reasons is that, in general, these draw, with scant acknowledgment, on other books previously published.

"Gray literature" is a mass of heterogenous, non-peer-reviewed material, produced by various institutions and organizations, which is not controlled by commercial publishers. These are

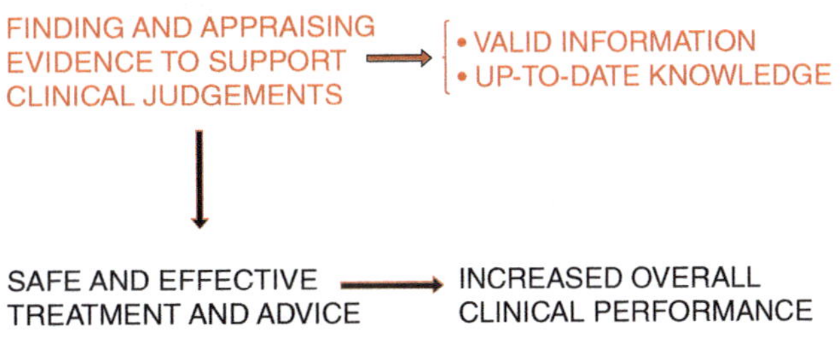

Figure 7.1 Increasing clinical performance by using evidence to support clinical judgment Source: L. Urdes.

commonly produced by (non)governmental organizations, academics, businesses and industries, as reports, theses, conference proceedings, official documents, and so on. Although non-conventional and rather ephemeral, gray literature should not be excluded from a literature survey if it is relevant to the topic of interest. Where there is insufficient knowledge, gray literature may also be the only source available to look into.

Web documents are regarded as the most doubtful resources of knowledge, as these are not usually peer reviewed. Authors can post, modify and withdraw a document without restrictions. In most cases, journal editors would not allow citation of web documents in the reference list of articles.

7.2.7 Questions to Ask when Reading a Paper

A good scientific paper must accomplish two objectives. First, it will clearly and completely describe procedures followed and results obtained. Second, it must provide an interpretation of the outputs of the study in relation to the existing state of knowledge and its significance for future study.

The questions to ask when reading a paper are:

- Is the paper of interest?
- Why was the research done?
- How was the research done?
- What has been found?
- What else is of interest?
- Who wrote the paper?
- In what type of journal was the paper published?
- Who and what is acknowledged?

These questions correspond roughly to the standard structure of a scientific paper: title, abstract, introduction, materials and methods, results, discussion, acknowledgment, literature cited. Answering these questions requires a framework for critical appraisal.

7.2.8 Framework for Critical Appraisal

Critical appraisal involves a structured approach to identify and assess all key aspects of a paper. It also requires an objective assessment of the strengths and weaknesses of the paper. There are four steps in appraising evidence:

1) Identification of information needs. In other words, what information do I need to resolve my patient's medical problem?
2) Transforming the information into a series of questions. This translates a clinical problem (e.g., "Is this a good therapy for my patient's disease?") into an answerable clinical question for which evidence is sought.
3) Searching for the best available evidence to answer your questions. You have to use the most efficient search strategy to identify the evidence that you look for. If there are more questions to answer, in the interest of time, you may have to prioritize them, preferably according to the following considerations, in this order: the patient's welfare; the question you can answer quickly and most efficiently; the question of most interest to you, or which is most rewarding to you in terms of, for instance, cost or clinical benefit.

4) Appraisal of the evidence. The most reliable evidence derives from scientific research based on valid methodologies. This requires you to make a selection of the articles that may yield the most valuable evidence and to look for the statistical strength of the study.

7.3 Client Communication

7.3.1 Work Ethics and Principles of Ethical Practice

Through their activity, veterinarians have to maintain the public trust that the profession has invested in them to avoid any conflicts of interest. The ethics of the veterinarian's actions must be strengthened by the principles noted below.

- The veterinarian should never be influenced by anything other than the patient's welfare, the client's needs and the safety of the public (and maintaining the health of the latter).
- The veterinarian should provide competent medical care according to a relationship between themselves, the client, and the patient, and they should do so with compassion and respect toward animal welfare.
- The veterinarian should respect the rights of their clients and colleagues and should have respectful behavior toward their coworkers.
- The veterinarian needs to abide by professional standards and be truthful in all their professional activities and interactions.
- The veterinarian should be accountable for their actions, should always respect the law and should make an effort in the direction of amending the regulations that work against the superior interest of the patient and public health.
- The veterinarian should continue to study and apply their scientific knowledge while also keeping up to date with their veterinary education.

With the exception of emergencies, the veterinarian is free to choose their clients, the people they associate with, and the medium where they provide veterinary services. On the other hand, the veterinarian must consult and treat all the patients whose guardians seek their help, regardless of the environment they come from or other professional circumstances.

7.3.2 Effective Communication

In current veterinary practice, the client can seek out professional assistance in several situations. The veterinarian can be called to consult on both privately owned and commercial fish populations. There can be different aspects to communicating with these various clients.

The conversation should always be initiated from a place of trust and truth. Keeping client confidentiality is the main objective. On the other hand, the client should be immediately informed about the obligation to notify state veterinary authorities, such as when consumers' interests are at risk or when epizootic, contagious diseases are discovered.

The anamnesis (collecting data regarding the disease and its context) is done using a common language with the client where the excessive use of medical terms is avoided. The tone must be calm (never accusatory) even when the veterinarian was able to tell that the person is at fault in terms of keeping the fish healthy. If a farm is involved, the veterinarian should communicate with its owner, but also with the worker that cares for the aquasystem as the latter can often provide direct and clear information. The vet's questions should always focus on discovering the history of the disease (clinical signs and their evolution over time), including data regarding the fish farming aquasystem, the used technology, and the fish feed.

In cases where aquatic animals are ill, the veterinarian should seek information from the person in charge of the hygiene of the tanks or ponds (including the toxicity of the substances used for cleaning purposes). As for home aquariums, the information should be obtained from different members of the family, including children, who may have interacted with the patients.

The veterinarian may or may not have an office. Depending on the staffing he has, there can be a colleague who only deals with clients, appointments and communications. The communication between the veterinarian and the client could be classic (face to face), or by phone, or can be achieved via a computer and the internet. Fish pathologists can schedule visits (for consultation or collecting samples) to farms or other private locations. Communication with the clients can be done via email, text message, or social networks; test results can be transmitted to clients electronically as long as the communication is secure (confidentiality). Veterinarians can receive messages from their clients via the same channels.

The veterinarian can communicate with the client in several ways. With the help of the internet, the veterinarian can have a website, which although primarily used for public relations and marketing purposes, can also be a place where clients can write and ask questions (to which the vet should respond promptly). This part of the communication process can be a platform where only the truly interested clients can create accounts and to whom the vet can reply with specific information. Here, pictures of the clinical signs or lesions found on the fish can be sent and once the veterinarian analyzes them, they can ask for additional information, offer advice, or indicate the steps for solving a specific situation. Furthermore, applications that allow real-time communication (such as video calls) can be used so that the veterinarian sees a situation that takes place at present or directly solves or explains complex issues to the client (some of which might be harder to understand). Thus, the vet has the possibility to analyze, work, and respond even when they are located in different parts of the world, at great distances from the client.

Supplementary materials

- Sources of professional development.
- Sources of aquatic animal health information.
- Further reading.

References

RCVS Knowledge. (2021). EBVM learning. https://learn.rcvsknowledge.org/course/view.php?id=2 (accessed 29 April 2021).

UK Veterinary Medicine Directorate. (2021). The cascade: prescribing unauthorised medicines. https://www.gov.uk/guidance/the-cascade-prescribing-unauthorised-medicines (accessed 29 April 2021).

8

Public Health, Zoonoses, and Seafood Safety

Olanike K. Adeyemo and Leo Foyle

Learning Objectives
The student should understand the interaction between animal health and human health through the principles of seafood safety, and recognize the public health risks of zoonotic diseases, intoxications and allergies associated with the consumption of seafood. The student must be aware of the veterinarian's role in protecting the environment, as reflected in One Health.

8.1 Introduction

Fisheries and aquaculture products are globally important sources of much-needed high-quality animal proteins, and invaluable providers of employment, income, and foreign exchange. Fishery products are the world's most widely traded foods, with commerce dominated by the developing countries. Approximately three billion people in the world rely on both wild-caught and farmed seafood as their primary source of protein. Fish is a highly perishable animal product; it deteriorates in quality soon after death unless treated properly after harvest, and it can soon become unfit to eat and possibly dangerous to health through microbial growth, chemical change and breakdown by endogenous enzymes. Proper handling, processing, preservation, packaging and storage measures are essential to improve its shelf life, ensure its safety, maintain its quality and nutritional attributes, and avoid waste and losses. The accurate incidence of diseases transmitted by foods is not known in most countries because there is no obligation to report on food-borne diseases to public health authorities. Where there are reporting systems, it is severely underreported, especially because the food item is not usually available for confirmatory analysis.

8.2 Seafood Quality

8.2.1 Sensory Quality of Fish

Freshness is a property of fish that has a considerable influence on its quality. It is the single most important criterion for judging the quality of the majority of fish products. Sensory properties such

Fundamentals of Aquatic Veterinary Medicine, First Edition. Edited by Laura Urdes, Chris Walster, and Julius Tepper.

Companion website: www.wiley.com/go/urdes/aquatic-veterinary-medicine

as appearance, odor, taste, and texture of fish are not only important for quality assessment but they also influence the consumers' choice (Grunert *et al.*, 2004).

Loss of freshness followed by spoilage is a complex combination of microbiological, chemical, and physical processes (Pedrosa-Menabrito and Regenstein, 1990). Changes occur in composition and structure caused by biochemical, physical, enzymatic, and bacterial reactions, negatively affecting the sensory quality of the product (Martinsdóttir, 2002).

Sensory evaluation is a scientific discipline used to measure, analyze, and interpret reactions to characteristics of food as perceived through the senses of sight, smell, taste, touch, and hearing by trained personnel who, with their senses, are able to judge or form an opinion on some aspect of quality in comparison to the normal (Huss, 1994). This requires employing trained and experienced personnel to obtain accurate and reproducible result in sensory evaluation (Connell, 2001; Munoz *et al.*, 1992). Ólafsdóttir *et al.* (1997) reported various techniques to evaluate fish freshness in terms of volatile compounds, microbial methods, and predictive modeling, protein, lipids, adenosine triphosphate (ATP), sensory analysis, and physical measurement using instruments. The instrumental measurement method measures spoilage based on electrical properties, pH and vision properties of fish muscle. Presence of parasites and blood clots in fish fillets are determined by computer-aided vision techniques using commercial pH and texturometers, moisture and fat analyzers (Pau and Olafsson, 1997).

Nucleotide catabolites are degradation products of ATP and can be reliable quality indices of several fish/shellfish, based on K-value. High-performance liquid chromatography is used in measuring this factor (Venugopal, 2002). Total volatile basic nitrogen, ammonia, trimethylamine, and volatile acids can be measured by titration and used as spoilage indicators (Wong and Gill, 1987; Venugopal, 2002). Total volatile basic nitrogen can be used as an indicator of fitness for consumption rather than as an index of freshness during storage of fish, since it is mainly produced during bacterial decomposition (Rezaei and Hosseini, 2008; Popelka *et al.*, 2014).

Factors that affect the sensory quality of fish from its living stage include the water quality of its habitat, its feed, fish species, the age sex, sexual maturation, the season, genetics and more (Green-Petersen, 2010). Postmortem and processing chain factors that affect sensory quality include packing method, quality of the gutting, filleting or other types of ennobling (Hyldig *et al.*, 2007), microbial contamination, or by physical damage (Green-Petersen, 2010), storage temperature and duration (Ólafsdóttir *et al.*, 1997), packaging atmosphere (Hong *et al.*, 1996), chemical composition (Robb *et al.*, 2002) and lipid content (Katikou *et al.*, 2001).

Several sensory grading schemes have been developed over the years for use in assessing fish freshness. Some examples are the European Union (EU) grading scheme for whole fish, the Torry Sensory Assessment scheme and the Quality Index Method.

8.2.1.1 The EU Grading Scheme for Whole Fish

The EU grading scheme for whole fish was developed and introduced by European Council Decision No. 103/76 in 1976 and is commonly acceptable in EU countries. This scheme assesses the skin color, flesh texture, shape of the eyes, color and odor of the gills using the senses of sight, smell and touch, the parameters are graded as follows:

- E high quality
- A good quality
- B low quality
- C fish are not fit human consumption.

8.2.1.2 Torry Sensory Assessment Scheme

The Torry scheme for both whole raw and cooked fish was developed by Torry Research station (Shewan *et al.*, 1953). The Torry freshness scoring uses freshness parameters such as texture, odor, and flavor to determine the sensory response of cooked fish samples (Martinsdóttir *et al.*, 2001).

8.2.1.3 Quality Index Method

The Quality Index Method (QIM) adds up demerit points from 0 to 3 to give an index; it was developed by Bremner in 1985. The QIM has been described by several authors as being precise, objective, non-destructive, rapid, simple to apply. It is a species-specific sensory method for an independent description of outer appearance attributes of postmortem raw fish that is being inspected (Olafsdottir *et al.*, 1997; Huidobro *et al.*, 2001; Martinsdóttir *et al.*, 2009). It is reliable, systematic and practical. QIM employs a score system ranging from 0-1, 0-2, 0-3, 0-4 or more demerit points (Jonsdottir, 1992). In estimating the quality attributes of the fish in an objective way based on the significant parameters for raw fish, the total sum of all points gives an overall sensory score referred to as the quality index (Martinsdóttir, 2002). A quality index closer to zero is indicative of fresher fish; larger totals indicate higher levels of fish deterioration (Huss, 1995; Martinsdóttir *et al.*, 2001) The index points are recorded and can be used in making possible predictions for the remaining shelf life of the product in ice if a straight line theoretical index format is followed (Hyldig and Neilsen, 1998; Luten *et al.*, 1997).

8.2.2 Biochemical and Chemical Quality of Fish

Biochemical and chemical evaluation of seafood quality is used to set quantitative standards. The establishment of tolerance levels of chemical spoilage indicators would eliminate the basing of decisions regarding fish product quality on subjective perception associated with sensory evaluation. Some of the useful procedures for the objective measurement of biochemical and chemical seafood quality are amines (total volatile basic amines), ammonia, trimethylamine (TMA), dimethylamine (DMA), biogenic amines, nucleotide catabolites, ethanol, and measurements of oxidative rancidity.

8.2.2.1 Total Volatile Basic Amines

Total volatile basic amines are one of the most widely used measurements of seafood quality. It is a general term which includes the measurement of TMA (produced by spoilage bacteria), DMA (produced by autolytic enzymes during frozen storage), ammonia (produced by the deamination of amino acids and nucleotide catabolites) and other volatile basic nitrogenous compounds associated with seafood spoilage. These measurements generally reflect only the later stages of advanced spoilage and are generally considered unreliable for the measurement of spoilage during the first ten days of chilled storage.

8.2.2.2 Ammonia

Ammonia is formed by the bacterial degradation/deamination of proteins, peptides and amino acids. It is also produced in the autolytic breakdown of adenosine monophosphate in chilled seafood products.

8.2.2.3 Trimethylamine

TMA is a pungent volatile amine often associated with the typical "fishy" odor of spoiling seafood. Its presence in spoiling fish is cause by the bacterial reduction of TMA oxide (TMAO), which is naturally present in the living tissue of many marine fish species.

8.2.2.4 Dimethylamine

DMA is produced together with formaldehyde in frozen storage with accompanying formaldehyde-induced toughening of the proteins. The amount of protein denaturation is roughly proportional to the amount of formaldehyde and DMA produced. Because it is associated with membranes in the muscle, its production is enhanced with rough handling and with temperature fluctuations in cold storage facility.

8.2.2.5 Biogenic Amines

Fish muscle has the ability to support the bacterial formation of a wide variety of amine compounds that result from the direct decarboxylation of amino acids. Histamine, putrescine, cadaverine, and tyramine are produced from the decarboxylation of histidine, ornithine, lysine, and tyrosine, respectively. Histamine has received most of the attention since it has been associated with incidents of scombroid poisoning in conjunction with the ingestion of tuna, mackerel, and mahi-mahi. Most biogenic amines are stable to thermal processing, so their presence in finished canned products is a good indication that the raw material was spoiled prior to heating.

8.2.2.6 Nucleotide Catabolites

The analysis of the complete nucleotide catabolite profile is always recommended. Since the levels of each of the catabolic intermediates rise and fall within the tissue as spoilage progresses, quality assessment must never be based upon levels of a single catabolite. Examples of catabolites are adenosine monophosphate (AMP), inosine monophosphate (IMP), inosine (Ino), hypoxanthine (Hx).

8.2.2.7 Ethanol

Ethanol has been used for many years as an objective indicator for seafood quality, although it is not nearly as common as the analysis of TMA. Since ethanol can be derived from carbohydrates via anaerobic fermentation (glycolysis) and/or deamination and decarboxylation of amino acids such as alanine, it is a common metabolite of a variety of bacteria.

8.2.2.8 Measurements of Oxidative Rancidity

The highly unsaturated fatty acids found in fish lipids are very susceptible to oxidation. The primary oxidation products are the lipid hydroperoxides. These compounds can be detected by chemical methods, generally by making use of their oxidation potential to oxidize iodide to iodine or to oxidize iron (II) to iron (III). The concentration of the hydroperoxides may be determined by titrimetry or spectrophotometry.

8.2.3 Microbiological Quality of Fish

The microbiological risk associated with seafood other than raw molluskan shellfish is much lower and appears to result from recontamination or cross-contamination of cooked with raw products, or from contamination during preparation followed by time/temperature abuse (e.g., holding at a warm temperature long enough for microbial growth or toxin production to occur). This occurs mainly at the food service (post-processing) level, which is common to all foods and not specific to seafood products. Microbial quality of seafood and seafood products is therefore an essential criterion for evaluation of its safety. Countries in the EU have laid down rules and directive that live bivalves must contain fewer than 300 fecal coliforms or fewer than 230 *E. coli* per 100 g shellfish flesh and must contain no *Salmonella* species. Vessels exporting fish and fisheries products to EU countries must carry a veterinary certificate and the processing factories must be inspected and passed by a national competent authority accredited by the EU. Additionally, the following microbiological tests are required for fresh frozen raw fish (Huss, 1994):

- Aerobic plate count (total viable count) must not exceed 100 000/g.
- Coliforms (zero level of fecal coliforms, while *E. coli* should be <10/g tissue).
- *Salmonella* (not to be detected in 25 g of animal tissue),
- *Staphylococcus aureus* (<1000/g). For Japan, marine products imported into the country must not contain *V. cholerae*, fecal coliform or *Staphylococcus* species (Venugopal, 2002).

8.2.3.1 Parasitic Infection

Seafood-related parasitic infections are even less common than bacterial and viral infections. Anisakids and cestodes have the greatest public health significance in the United States. In general, parasitic infections are concentrated in certain ethnic groups that favor the consumption of raw or partially cooked seafoods.

8.2.3.2 Viral Infection

Norwalk virus of the genus *Norovirus* is incriminated in most non-bacteria gastroenteritis epidemic outbreaks worldwide (Lindesmith *et al.*, 2003) and probably up to 50% of all food-borne outbreaks of gastroenteritis in the United States (Widdowson *et al.*, 2005).

8.2.3.3 Natural Toxins

Most seafood outbreaks are related to biotoxins (ciguatoxin), scombrotoxin, or the consumption of raw molluscan shellfish (Huss *et al.*, 2000).

8.2.4 Fish Spoilage

Fish spoilage has been attributed to three main factors by Wogu and Maduakor (2010): microbial activities, enzymatic autolysis, and chemical oxidation. Of these, microbial action is considered the main cause of deterioration. Fish spoilage is indicated by deterioration which is a loss of fish quality, the effect of which is reflected in the characteristics of the fish such as the color, flavor, odor, or texture (Huss, 1988, 1994, 1995). The process of spoilage begins as soon as the fish dies, and occurs in a sequential order resulting from chemical reactions of the fish lipids, autolytic and microbiological activity (Gram and Huss, 1996).

The poikilothermic nature of fish, their moist environment, and pH after death (neutral or slightly acidic) favors the growth of a wide range of microorganisms (Chebet, 2010). The presence of non-protein nitrogen components, such as TMAO, creatine, methionine, free amino acids, cystine, histamine, carnosine, volatile nitrogen bases such as urea, especially in cartilaginous fishes, support microbial growth and the production of their related metabolites that are responsible for fish spoilage during storage (Huss, 1994). Pathogenic bacterial growth and activities of organisms like *Vibrio* species, *Salmonella* species, Coliforms, *Pseudomonas*, *Shigella* species, *Listeria* species, streptococci, staphylococci and *Clostridium* species have been incriminated in spoilage of fish (Rahman and Noor, 2012). The microflora associated with a particular fish is directly related to the surrounding aquatic environment (Clucas and Ward, 1996; Eze *et al.*, 2011), while the bacterial flora in the gastrointestinal tract corresponds to the condition of the fish (Liston, 1980). The consumption of spoiled seafood has been reported to be one of the possible factors responsible for food-borne diseases.

8.3 Nature and Extent of Public Health Risks from Aquatic Animals and Seafood

Seafood is recognized as being a highly nutritious food source, but it can be associated with potential hazards, both infectious and non-infectious. Working with marine animals and keeping them as pets and exhibits also carries the risk of exposing people to potentially harmful infectious agents and toxins. Choice of diet, such as fresh and live seafood, and seasonality, namely higher *Vibrio* spp. during warmer summer months, are consistent risk factors for seafood-related illness in humans

(Weir, 2012). The term "hazard" as related to seafood refers to "a biological, chemical, or physical agent in or condition of, food with the potential to cause an adverse health effect" (Codex Alimentarius Commission, 2009).

8.3.1 Biological Hazards

Biological hazards are most commonly reported because they often present acute cases of illness that may be sudden and spread over a large population. Causes of biological hazards are most often one or more disease-causing bacteria, viruses, parasites, molds, yeasts, and naturally occurring toxins. They sometimes affect the taste and sensory qualities of the fish, making it relatively easily detectable. Bacteria organisms like *Clostridium botulinum*, *Listeria monocytogenes*, *Staphylococcus aureus*, *Salmonella* species, *Shigella* species, and *E. coli* are considered as non-indigenous pathogens (Kvenberg, 1991) because their presence in fish and other seafoods is usually due to contamination from an external source, while *Vibrio* and *Aeromonas* are described as indigenous bacterial pathogens, as they are naturally found in fish's habitat (Eze *et al.*, 2011).

Bacterial pathogens commonly incriminated with seafoods include: *Bacillus cereus*, *Campylobacter jejuni*, *C. botulinum*, *C. perfringens*, *E. coli*, *L. monocytogenes*, *Salmonella* spp., *Shigella* spp., *S. aureus*, *Vibrio cholera*, *V. parahaemolyticus*, *V. vulnificus*, *Yersinia enterocolitica*. *Salmonella* species have been described as the leading cause of food-borne illness during the past few years, followed by *Campylobacter*, *Shigella* species, and staphylococcus intoxication (World Health Organization, 1999; Centers for Disease Control and Prevention, 2021). Håstein *et al.* (2006) found that while *Salmonella* spp. may be harbored and survive in fish, seafood seldom harbors salmonella. They observed that fish may be exposed to salmonella through consumption of contaminated feed or living in contaminated water. For a long time, salmonella in feed has been well-recognized problem in multiple species (including terrestrial animal systems). The same authors found that the level of salmonella contamination in the feed must be extremely high if the bacteria are to persist in the fish for more than a few days. Fecal contamination is usually responsible for the presence of *Salmonella* spp. in freshwater or marine fish species. Iwamoto *et al.* (2010) reported that, in the United States between 1973 and 2006, infection and intoxication by bacteria agents was responsible for approximately three fourth of the total outbreaks; Viral agents (norovirus and hepatitis A) were incriminated for one fifth of the outbreaks and less than 5% were linked to parasites.

8.3.2 Physical Hazards

Physical hazards are easily detected and cleaned up in the course of fish handling and preparations.

8.3.2.1 Chemical Hazards

Chemical hazards are a resultant effect of chemicals like heavy metals, pesticides, and other environmental chemicals that on their own are not necessarily harmful, but can accumulate to the level of becoming dangerous to the health of living tissues. Fish and other aquatic animals become contaminated with these chemical toxicants when their habitat is polluted. Pollution could be from several man-made sources, including discharge from ships, atmospheric deposition, river run-off, industrial waste discharge, run-off from agricultural treatment chemicals, and untreated sewage (Heberer, 2002; Adeyemo *et al.*, 2010). In seafood, chemical hazards are not physically visible and may not affect the taste and appearance of the fish; chemical contaminants are often not biodegradable or destroyed by preparation methods, rather they tend to bioaccumulate and magnify with increase intake causing chronic diseases. Chemical hazards or pollutants can be categorized according to their source, natural or anthropogenic, and according to the nature of the chemical, organic, inorganic and production/processing chemicals.

8.4 Zoonoses of Aquatic Animal Origin

The term "zoonoses" refers to a disease that can be transferred from animals, whether wild or domesticated, to humans. With the global growth of aquaculture and the increasing volume of international trade in live aquatic animals and their products (Food and Agriculture Organization, 2020), zoonoses require special attention. The increasing interface between humans and aquatic animals that may harbor infectious agents is a potential public health concern. Despite an increased awareness of zoonotic disease agents, their diagnosis in humans by clinicians and medical practitioners is often hampered by a poor knowledge of the zoonotic potential of disease agents in aquatic species and the associated clinical signs (Evans *et al.*, 2009). Pathogens associated with fish and amphibians are transmitted to humans through accidental ingestion of organisms found in fecal material or direct contact of these organisms with broken, abraded, or chapped skin. People who are immunocompromised, including those who have a medical condition or are taking medications that affect the immune system, such as steroids, immunosuppressive drugs or chemotherapy, are at greater risk of developing disease after exposure to these pathogens. Aside from food poisoning, the overall incidence of transmission of disease-producing agents from fish to humans is low. However, there are a number of agents found in fish and aquarium water with potential to be transmitted to humans.

8.4.1 Bacterial Zoonoses

Many bacteria associated with fishes are linked with human disease but their true role as zoonotic agents is often not that clear, and in many cases the fish act as vectors of infectious agents rather than as a true zoonotic source. The World Health Organization defines a zoonosis as any disease or infection that is naturally transmissible from vertebrate animals to humans (World Health Organization, 2020). Bacterial diseases supported as true fish-borne zoonoses include *Mycobacterium* spp., *Clostridium botulinum*, *Streptococcus iniae* and *Vibrio vulnificus* (Gauthier, 2015) while other agents have also been considered zoonotic, including *Aeromonas hydrophila*, *Edwardsiella tarda*, *Vibrio damsela* and *Erysipelothrix rhusiopathiae* (Haenen *et al.*, 2013; Boylan, 2011). Outbreaks of disease are often related to management and husbandry issues, such as the organic loading of the water and high stocking densities, both of which can increase bacterial loads on the external surface of the fish potentially increasing transmission of infectious agents to humans (Haenen *et al.*, 2013). Probably the most important fish-borne zoonotic bacterial agents are the mycobacteria. These Gram-positive, aerobic, non-spore-forming, acid-fast positive, non-motile rods are found throughout marine and freshwater environments.

8.4.1.1 Mycobacteria

Mycobacteria are non-motile, acid-fast rods. Many of these mycobacteria are described as being atypical, being different from the more familiar species, *M. tuberculosis*, *M. bovis* and *M. avium*. These *Mycobacterium* spp. are slow-growing, mildly psychrophilic to mesophilic environmental organisms that typically cause infections in the extremities of humans where temperatures are cooler than 33°C (91°F). Others are described as non-tuberculous mycobacteria and exclude *M. tuberculosis* complex and *M. leprae*. There are approximately 150 species of non-tuberculous mycobacteria (Bi *et al.*, 2015), with *M. marinum*, *M. fortuitum*, and *M. ulcerans* discussed most commonly as fish-borne zoonoses (Boylan, 2011). Two species, *M. fortuitum* and *M. marinum*, are recognized as pathogens of tropical fish.

Humans are typically infected by contamination of lacerated or abraded skin with aquarium water or fish contact. Other sources of infection are spine punctures, cleaning fish, shrimp, or crabs, getting scratched on fish tanks, mouth-siphoning fish tanks, dolphin bites, diving around reefs, splinters from fish net handles. A localized granulomatous nodule (hard bump) may form at the site of infection, most commonly on hands or fingers approximately six to eight weeks after exposure to the organism. All these aquatic *Mycobacterium* spp. can cause acute to chronic disease in fish, which may be associated with multiple and varied clinical signs, most commonly the chronic form with signs such as exophthalmia, lethargy, scale loss, abdominal distention, pigment changes, poor body condition, and superficial ulcers. Many fish undergo subclinical (inapparent) mycobacteriosis, and shed bacteria without overt disease manifesting. Other fish may undergo acute infections, shedding the bacteria prior to the onset of the clinical symptoms. The fecal–oral route is the most likely route of transmission among fish or via ingestion of infected tissues. However, release of infectious organisms from infected gill tissue or ulcerated skin lesions may also be a route through which *Mycobacterium* spp. spread within water.

Mycobacterium spp. often affect people who handle or work with fish, and the resultant infections have been called fish handlers' disease or fish tank granuloma. In affected humans, lesions typically develop on the extremities and are either ulcerative or raised granulomatous nodules. Most infections in humans are limited to the extremities, possibly because of the preference of aquatic *Mycobacterium* spp. for lower temperatures (<30°C/<86°F) or because these sites represent the points of contact with infective material. In a few rare cases in humans, systemic mycobacteriosis has been described; these infections generally develop in immunocompromised individuals and result in symptoms of respiratory tract disease or osteomyelitis. Non-tuberculous mycobacteria can be found in freshwater fish and their products, requiring appropriate handling and treatment before consumption of such products (Lorencova *et al.*, 2013). Disinfection following exposure to atypical mycobacteria is difficult. Thick cell walls and biofilms make atypical mycobacteria resistant to frequently used aquatic disinfectants, such as quaternary ammonia compounds and dilute sodium hypochlorite (bleach; Boylan, 2011). Removing biofilms by mechanical scrubbing will allow glutaraldehydes and oxidants to effectively kill atypical mycobacteria. Phenols, high concentrations of alcohol, and strong sodium chlorite solutions are also effective disinfectants. Disposal of contaminated aquarium water varies by location. Therefore, relevant local authorities should be contacted regarding specific regulations.

8.4.1.2 Streptococcus iniae

S. iniae is another bacterium of major concern because of the serious clinical signs that develop in infected humans. First isolated from Amazon freshwater dolphins (*Inia geoffrensis*) with subcutaneous abscesses at aquaria in San Francisco and New York in 1976, *S. iniae* is a Gram-positive, non-motile coccus that causes multiple clinical signs in freshwater and marine fish including abdominal distention, epidermal and dermal petechiation, exophthalmia, and death. Tilapia (*Oreochromis* spp., *Sarotherodon* spp., and *Tilapia* spp.), striped bass (*Morone saxatilis*), and their respective hybrids are reported to be predisposed to infection with *S. iniae* and may be chronic carriers of the bacterium, although many other food and tropical species can also harbor the pathogen. Humans infected with *S. iniae* can develop cellulitis, systemic arthritis, endocarditis, and meningitis which can be fatal (Weinstein *et al.*, 1997). Most humans have been infected via an existing wound or a fresh puncture wound during handling of live or dead fish.

8.4.1.3 Vibrio Species

Vibrio spp. are Gram-negative, motile, facultative anaerobic rods of the family Vibrionaceae. Most commonly, V. *vulnificus*, *V. parahemolyticus*, and *V. cholera* are identified in aquatic environments. While *Vibrio* spp. can occasionally be isolated from freshwater fish, they are more often associated with marine and brackish environments because of their preference for high salinity waters. *Vibrio* spp. typically proliferate in warm water and are usually more abundant during the warmer months. The degree of *V. parahaemolyticus* contamination in raw shellfish is also known to relate to the water temperatures. Therefore, it is more likely to detect *V. parahaemolyticus* in oysters harvested in the spring and the summer than in the winter (Su and Liu, 2007). *Vibrio* spp. can also be cultured from the skin and gastrointestinal tracts of fish that appear clinically normal; however, in fish subject to stressful conditions, these bacteria can cause disease. Clinical signs in fish infected with *Vibrio* spp. are similar to those of other bacterial infections and cannot be relied on for diagnostic purposes, and include anorexia, lethargy, skin ulcers, exophthalmia, and erythema around the anus and base of the fins. In humans, *V. vulnificus* infection is the most common fish-derived *Vibrio* infection, and the major route of exposure has been reported to be through puncture wounds and ingestion (Lehane and Rawlln, 2000). Biotype 2 of *V. vulnificus*, considered an obligate pathogen of eels (*Anguilla* spp.), may also be an opportunistic pathogen in humans. Skin-penetrating scratches received while handling fish have been reported to cause necrotizing dermohypodermatitis in fish workers, as well as local cellulitis and even life-threatening disease due to fish-spine injuries (Håstein *et al.*, 2006). As a consequence, appropriate care must be taken by consumers at risk, as well as by fish farmers handling diseased eels. Both the infected fish and the water may be sources of infection. An Israeli case demonstrated how changes in packaging of pond-reared fish resulted in human infections (Bisharat and Raz, 1996). In many cases, the infections were initiated by exposure to the fins of the fish. A change in trade patterns meant that fish were no longer packed in ice but were sent live in containers. When producers changed back to selling the fish on ice, no further infections were recorded.

8.4.1.4 Septicemia

Septicemia after ingestion of *V. vulnificus* (typically in shellfish) results in death in 50% to 60% of clinically affected humans (Oliver, 2005). *V. parahaemolyticus* is frequently isolated from a variety of seafoods including cod, sardine, mackerel, flounder, clam, octopus, shrimp, crab, lobster, crawfish, scallop, and oyster (Su and Liu, 2007), and consumption of raw or undercooked seafood, particularly shellfish, contaminated with *V. parahaemolyticus* can lead to development of acute gastroenteritis characterized by diarrhea, headache, vomiting, nausea, abdominal cramps, and low-grade fever. *V. parahaemolyticus* is recognized as the leading cause of human gastroenteritis associated with seafood consumption in the United States and is an important seafood-borne pathogen throughout the world. A key risk factor for ready-to-eat cooked prawns and shrimp is microbiological contamination following the cooking process. Poor post-cooking handling processes, such as the use of contaminated sea or drinking water to cool cooked prawns and shrimp, can lead to contamination with pathogenic bacteria. Cross-contamination with uncooked products can also reintroduce pathogens such as *V. parahaemolyticus* (Food Standards Australia New Zealand, 2005; International Commission on Microbiological Specifications for Foods, 2005). Moderate temperature abuse post-harvest during handling, transport and/or storage can allow the growth of *V. parahaemolyticus* (Food Standards Australia New Zealand, 2005).

8.4.1.5 Aeromonads

Aeromonads are non-spore-forming, Gram-negative, rod-shaped, facultative anaerobic bacteria, autochthonous and widely distributed in aquatic and terrestrial environments. These bacteria were thought to be members of the family Vibrionaceae but have now been allocated to their own family Aeromonadaceae (Igbinosa *et al.*, 2012). *Aeromonas* species are known as causative agents of a wide spectrum of diseases in humans and animals, and studies have shown that some motile *Aeromonas* spp. are becoming food- and water-borne pathogens of increasing importance, capable of causing human infection by ingestion of contaminated vegetables, meat, chicken, and seafood (Ansari *et al.*, 2011). *Aeromonas* spp. have been associated with several food-borne outbreaks and are progressively being isolated from patients with traveler's diarrhea. As putatively emerging enteric pathogens, *Aeromonas* spp. appear to have the inherent capability to grow in water distribution systems, especially in biofilms, where they may be resistant to chlorination (Igbinosa *et al.*, 2012). Aeromonads make up a large portion of the bacterial flora among freshwater aquatic organisms that are maintained in a wide range of water temperatures. *A. hydrophila*, *A. caviae*, *A. sobria*, and *A. schubertii* have all been implicated in human disease and are found in association with finfish and crustaceans. These aeromonads frequently cause disease in cultured and pet fish.

Clinical signs of aeromonas infections in fish are rarely specific and include ulcerative lesions of the skin around the base of the fins and anus, raised scales, abdominal distension, and exophthalmia, all of which are signs that are commonly seen with other bacterial infections. Depending on the severity of infection, anemia, hepatomegaly, and ascites may develop in affected fish. Aeromonad infections in fish are often secondary to other stressors such as a suboptimal environment, poor water quality, parasitism, and nutritional deficiencies. The primary route for transmission to humans is from handling fish and contact with mucus and tissues from infected or carrier fish. Cuts and abrasions already present on the hands of the handler, as well as wounds caused by handling fish directly, are likely routes of infection. Aeromonads can cause life-threatening septicemia related to underlying diseases such as leukemia, cancer, cirrhosis, and various infections such as urinary tract infections, surgical wound infections, meningitis, peritonitis, and endocarditis.

Some predisposing factors for aeromonas infection include hepatic diseases, diabetes, hematologic malignancies, hepatobiliary, and renal diseases. In healthy individuals, the most common signs of an *Aeromonas* spp. infection include localized wound swelling and gastroenteritis. *A. salmonicida* is another important member of this group and is responsible for large economic losses in cultured salmonid populations through what is commonly called furunculosis. An atypical strain of *A. salmonicida* can also cause the so-called goldfish ulcer disease in goldfish and erythrodermatitis in carp. However, *A. salmonicida* does not grow at 35°C (Igbinosa *et al.*, 2012), and to our knowledge, there are no reported zoonotic cases despite the widespread prevalence and severity of disease among salmonids and cyprinids.

8.4.1.6 Enterobacteriaceae

Enterobacteriaceae includes several genera of bacteria that have zoonotic potential, including *Edwardsiella*, *Escherichia*, *Salmonella*, and *Klebsiella* spp. and indeed, most of the bacterial causes of diarrhea are zoonotic (Weir *et al.*, 2012). The Enterobacteriaceae contain Gram-negative, facultative anaerobic rods that are directly associated with fish species or freshwater aquatic environments. *E. ictaluri* and *E. tarda* are the only important primary fish pathogens and both cause major losses in the commercial food-fish industry. *E. ictaluri* is the etiologic agent of enteric septicemia of catfish.

The main route of infection to humans is inoculation through a wound received while handling or examining fish, followed by contamination of existing cuts and abrasions. *E. tarda* infection in catfish has been termed emphysematous putrefactive disease, and humans infected with *E. tarda* via a wound or ingestion may develop necrotic skin lesions and gastroenteritis. Infections with any of these bacteria can remain localized at the point of entry or can become systemic, potentially resulting in severe meningitis.

8.4.2 Parasitic Zoonoses

Very often, snails or crustaceans are involved as first intermediate host and fish as second intermediate host, while the sexually mature parasite is found in birds or mammals as the final host. In between these hosts, one or more free living stages may occur. More than half a billion people are at risk from helminth parasites transmitted by shellfish and fish with some of these parasites being highly pathogenic (Lima dos Santos and Howgate, 2011). Not only do parasites affect humans by direct ingestion, but ingestion of parasites can also cause allergic reactions against parasite antigens with *Anisakis simplex* being the main organism implicated to date (Ivanovic *et al.*, 2015). Fish-borne parasites come from three main groups: digenetic trematodes, especially species of the families Opisthorchiidae and Heterophyidae; nematodes, especially species of the families Anisakidae and Gnathostomatidae; and cestodes, especially species of the family Diphyllobothriidae. Trematodes are the most important of these based on the morbidities of the associated diseases. Keiser and Utzinger (2005) reported that 601 million people are at risk of infection with *Clonorchis sinensis*, 292.8 million with *Paragonimus* spp., 91.1 million with *Fasciola* spp., and 79.8 million with *Opisthorchis* spp.

Human infection is through consumption of poorly cooked or raw fish products infested with these parasites. The incidence of development of human disease has increased in the past few years for a number of reasons. There is now better diagnostic capability, with increased consumption of raw fish where traditionally it is eaten, increased consumption of dishes like sushi, sashimi, ceviche, carpaccio based on raw or minimally processed fish in areas where raw fish was not traditionally eaten. The international market in fish and fish products has grown, and there is continuing development of aquaculture (Lima dos Santos and Howgate, 2011). Because of the worldwide consumption of Japanese cuisine in particular, the traditional Japanese fish dishes sushi and sashimi that are served in Japanese restaurants and sushi bars have been suspected of causing fish-borne parasitic zoonoses, especially anisakiasis (Nawa *et al.*, 2005).

Since around 2000, much evidence has been published linking not only wild-caught fish but also aquaculture products with fish-borne parasites. The important trematodes are the liver flukes, especially *C. sinensis*, *O. viverrini* and *O. felineus*. The former two flukes, in particular, are capable of initiating cholangiocarcinomas in humans and are as a consequence, listed as group 1 biological agents (carcinogens) by the International Agency for Research on Cancer (Kim *et al.*, 2016). The life cycle can be completed by humans through the consumption of raw, undercooked, or otherwise underprocessed fish containing the infective stage of the parasite (World Health Organization, 1995; Tran *et al.*, 2009).

The life cycle of *C. sinensis* is characterized by an alternation of sexual and asexual reproduction in three different hosts, such as snails, fish, and mammals. The definitive host is a human or other piscivorous animal such as cats, mink, badgers, rats and dogs, followed by two intermediate hosts, snail and fish. The parasite matures in the definitive host and eggs are shed in the feces of the host. Highlighting the importance of human hygiene and the exclusion of vermin, if the eggs reach water (human or animal feces) they develop into miracidia, which are ingested by a snail, the first intermediate host. There, they develop asexually and are ultimately shed into the water as motile cercariae which penetrate into the mucus and skin before encysting in subcutaneous tissues or muscle of the second intermediate (fish) host.

If contaminated fish is consumed undercooked, raw salted, pickled, dried, or smoked, this allows liberation of the metacercariae from the flesh through gastric juice digestion and excystation of the larvae in the duodenum, by a combined action of trypsin and cysteine proteases. Subsequently, the excysted flukes migrate to intrahepatic bile ducts through the ampulla of Vater, develop into adult flukes, and can survive for up to 30 years. One worm in a human host can produce approximately 4000 eggs a day by sexual reproduction (Kim *et al.*, 2016).

Fish source and farming system is influential in the final parasite burden in fish flesh. Within reason all wild-caught fish should be assumed to have parasites (e.g. Anisakids) and processed accordingly (Panel on Biological Hazards, 2010). Fish exposed to human activities can also be potentially affected. Fish raised in periurban wastewater-fed aquaculture systems in Vietnam have been found to be a risk of infection with trematode parasites (Nguyen *et al.*, 2007); the infected fish included the non-native tilapia (*Oreochromis niloticus*) and three species of carp, including silver carp (*Hypophthalmichthys molitrix*), which is commonly used in raw fish dishes. Many parasites are associated with the organs and the quick removal of the viscera post-harvest can reduce parasite transfer into the flesh (Codex Alimentarius Commission, 2016). In a separate study, high densities of metacercariae were found encysted in fish viscera compared with flesh (2.3–72.9 metacercariae/50 g). These parasites pose a threat for cross-contamination during dish preparation: it is not just about the flesh, which may have low levels of metacercariae but also about cross-contamination (Tran *et al.*, 2009).

Anisakis simplex is a nematode which uses sea mammals as the definitive host. Various species of fish act as intermediate hosts for the larvae, which are approximately 2 cm in length. Certain regions, particularly Japan and Spain (45% of hake in Spain), are notable for high rates of infestation (AAITO-IFIACI Anisakis Consortium, 2011). The larvae are susceptible to heating (>60°C for 10 minutes) or freezing (20°C for 48 hours), but their allergens are resistant to cooking, freezing, and partially to digestion. In one study, allergen release during freezing and after freezing was higher than in controls, which was attributed to rupture of the cuticle and active liberation of excretion/secretion allergens during freezing (Sánchez-Alonso *et al.*, 2018). The authors concluded that the pathogenic potential of frozen and thawed larvae could not be ignored. There is no effective anti-Anisakis drug. In humans, live larvae in raw or undercooked seafood are usually ejected by vomiting and diarrhea or destroyed by digestion. Larvae not killed or ejected can attach to gastric mucosa, forming granulomas and a self-limiting gastroenteritis. Systemic reactions may occasionally occur. Anisakis infection should be considered in patients highly suspected of having had an adverse reaction to seafood but who have tested negative to allergy tests. Skin testing and specific immunoglobulin E to the parasite itself have proved inconsistent. Diagnosis and treatment are made by endoscopic confirmation and surgical removal of the granulomas (Bahna, 2016).

8.4.3 Viral Zoonoses

Shellfish including oysters, mussels and clams are filter feeding mollusks which can bioaccumulate human pathogens at levels higher than those in surrounding waters. Shellfish-borne enteric viral illnesses have resulted in human disease outbreaks worldwide. The consumption of contaminated shellfish has resulted in illness due to hepatitis A and Norwalk-like viruses. Bioconcentration and accumulation in shellfish may increase the concentration of viruses 10- to 100-fold compared with the water column. Enteroviruses may remain infectious for 9 days in marine waters and 19 days in sediment and up to 30 days in shellfish.

These viruses may cause a wide range of diseases in different individuals, such as aseptic meningitis, respiratory illness, myocarditis, fever, diarrhea, rash, nephritis. Small round viruses such as Norwalk virus, Snow mountain agent, astroviruses, caliciviruses, and others have been implicated in adult gastroenteritis incidental to shellfish association. These viruses are heat stable and are resistant to chlorine. Rotavirus and adenovirus have not been documented as shellfish associated disease. This may be due to low survival in marine environment or incorrect diagnoses. The public impact of these viruses is probably not fully appreciated.

8.4.3.1 Norwalk Virus

Norwalk virus is shed in the feces of infected people, making handwashing extremely important. People who have contracted the virus can still spread it days after their symptoms cease, making cleanliness very important when preparing food. Immunity to this virus is not permanent and reinfection can occur. There is no specific treatment available for Norwalk-like virus infection; however, fluid replacement therapy may be needed for severely dehydrated individuals.

8.4.3.2 Hepatitis A

Hepatitis A is a highly contagious virus affecting the liver and spreading by the fecal–oral route through close person-to-person contact or through contaminated food or water. Signs of jaundice, fatigue, abdominal pain, loss of appetite, nausea, diarrhea, dark urine, and fever characterize hepatitis A. This virus typically has no long-term effects, and once a person is infected with the disease, they cannot acquire it again. However, 15% of people who were infected with hepatitis A will have prolonged relapsing symptoms over a six- to nine-month period.

8.5 Intoxication

8.5.1 Botulism

The anaerobic bacterium *Clostridium botulinum* is a commensal in both fresh and seawater fish and it has been reported as causing intoxication in farmed fish, terrestrial animals, and humans. *C. botulinum* types B, E and F are frequently found in the sea and in mud, and type E (and occasionally some varieties of B and F) may be found in fish intestines and gills, and can grow in fish products under 5°C, unlike other types. In anaerobic conditions, a potent neurotoxin may be produced, resulting in food-borne botulism and human death, typically 12–36 hours after consumption. The onset of symptoms is dose dependent and results in symptoms of flaccid paralysis, including difficulty swallowing or speaking, dry mouth, facial weakness on both sides of the face, blurred or double vision, drooping eyelids, trouble breathing, nausea, vomiting and abdominal cramps, and eventually paralysis. The toxin is destroyed by cooking since it does not survive exposure to 70°C for two minutes.

Botulism in fish products has been associated with dried and vacuum-packed products, including hot-smoked fish. The modern flavor and health preference for hot-smoked fish is with much less smoke and salt, and much more moisture, with the result that any *C. botulinum* present can more readily form toxin when the fish are kept warm for some length of time. Botulism is also more likely to occur with certain preparations that reflect different cultures and geographic locations, such as the whale meat mukluk in the Alaskan and Canadian Arctic, rakish in Norway, salted gray mullet fesikh in Egypt, salted eviscerated whitefish kapchunka in Israel and New York City, uncooked salmon ashbal in Iran, fermented fish preserved in rice izushi in Japan, and imported vacuum-packed whitefish in Europe (Horowitz, 2010).

Several factors must be present before *C. botulinum* toxin can develop in seafood. The organism must be present in the fish, the time and temperature of storage must be favorable for toxin production (time and temperature abuse), and the chemical composition of the product must be such that it supports the growth of the organism. Elimination of one or more of these risk factors will control the product. Cann (2001) states that, realistically, it is not possible to rid a contaminated fish of the bacteria but rapid evisceration and removal of gills, followed by thorough washing of the gutted cavity with tap water, can reduce contamination by as much as 90%. Implementing a dry curfew (withholding food) in farmed trout (*Oncorhynchus mykiss*) for one to three days before harvesting is beneficial, as fish with empty guts cause less contamination during processing. For this procedure to be effective, however, the starved fish should be held in concrete or plastic ponds; hungry trout in dirt ponds will feed off the contaminated mud. In some fish products, *C. botulinum* types B, E and F can grow and produce toxin in temperatures typically used in refrigeration; the lowest recorded temperature for growth in any food is 3.3°C; the product took 31 days to become toxic. Control of cold chain by ensuring fish are adequately slush-iced immediately after catching/harvesting and kept below 4°C at all stages of processing until eaten, will contribute significantly to food safety.

The UK Ministry for Agriculture, Fisheries and Food, based on work by the Food and Agriculture Office of the United Nations, recommends that:

> *caterers and retailers receiving deliveries of fresh fish inspect and where necessary re-ice them to maintain the temperature of the fish below 4°C. Where the amount of ice on receipt is insufficient, the supplier should be notified. A chillroom operating at 4°C can be used to conserve ice around fish but cannot be used satisfactorily to cool uniced fish or keep them cool. Packaged fish should carry a "Sell by" date according to the type of product, clearly marked "Store below 4°C" and carry a recommendation that the contents be eaten within 24 hours if kept at room temperature and within 3 days if kept in a refrigerator. Fish presented for sale without refrigeration should be discarded if unsold at the end of a day's trading (Cann, 2001).*

Changing the chemical and microbiological composition of fish by adding sufficient salt or acetic acid can make fish safe but the high concentration required is not acceptable to most consumers. A pH of 4.5 in marinated products, however, or a salt concentration of 3% in smoked fish products, is usually acceptable and affords added protection and extension of refrigerated shelf life.

8.5.2 Histamine Poisoning

Scombroid poisoning, also known as scombrotoxic fish poisoning, scombroid ichthyotoxicosis, Mahi-Mahi flush, or histamine fish poisoning, is caused by bacterial spoilage of a limited number (Håstein *et al.*, 2006) of fish species: mackerel (*Scomber scombrus*), bonito (*Sarda* spp.), various tuna species (*Thunnus* spp.), swordfish (*Xiphias gladius*), common dolphinfish (mahi-mahi; *Coryphaena* spp.). It has been reported as the most common fish food-borne chemical agent in the United States (Traylor and Goldstein, 2020). Scombroid toxicity closely mimics the pathophysiology of histamine release, including face and neck flushing, diarrhea, urticaria, and headache. Rarely, patients can have severe bronchospasm or cardiac effects, usually in those patients with predisposing medical conditions such as asthma or significant cardiac disease. Scombroid poisoning is entirely preventable and results from temperature abuse (improper storage) following catch or harvesting. The primary toxic agent implicated in scombroid poisoning is histidine (normally found in dark fish meat), which breaks down to histamine.

In temperatures warmer than 4°C, the fish undergo bacterial overgrowth and subsequently convert histidine to histamine. In properly stored and iced fish, histamine is normally less than 0.1 mg/100 g flesh, but histamine levels in contaminated fish are at least 20–50 mg/100 g fish; human tolerance for histamine is reported as 10 mg/100 g flesh (Håstein *et al.*, 2006). The responsible bacteria are most commonly *E. coli*, *Vibrio*, *Proteus*, *Klebsiella*, *Clostridium*, *Salmonella*, and *Shigella*. Affected fish do not have a distinct odor or appearance, although after cooking the skin may appear honeycombed, which makes detection prior to eating difficult. Occasionally, patients report a "peppery" taste to the fish while eating (Traylor and Goldstein, 2020). Classically, histamine toxicity is associated with eating the dark-meat fish, especially the Scombridae and Scomberesocidae families (tuna, mackerel, bonito, skipjack), hence the name scombroid poisoning. Scombroid poisoning occurs mostly in recreationally caught fish more so than commercial harvests, because of the strict regulation of commercial fishing vessels. Non-scombroid species, such as amberjack, bluefish, mahi-mahi, sardine, yellowtail, and herring are also commonly responsible. Rarely, contaminated Swiss cheese may cause a reaction after bacterial contamination of the raw milk prior to processing.

8.5.3 Ciguatera Fish Poisoning

Ciguatera fish poisoning causes substantial human health, social, and economic impacts, and is the most frequently reported natural marine seafood toxin illness in the world (Friedman *et al.*, 2017). Symptoms usually appear one to three hours after consuming contaminated fish. Poisoning is characterized by abdominal pain, nausea, vomiting, and diarrhea, followed by neurological complications 3–72 hours later.

A complex array of gastrointestinal, neurologic and neuropsychological, and cardiovascular symptoms, which may last days, weeks, or months, have been described. There have been reports of fatalities from the Pacific, Caribbean, and Indian Ocean regions (Chan, 2016). Several contributory factors have been identified, including consumption of ciguatoxin-rich fish parts (ciguatoxins are lipid soluble and heat stable and are concentrated in the fish head, liver, intestines, roe, and other viscera), consuming the more ciguatoxic fish species (e.g., moray eel, *Gymnothorax flavimarginatus*) and reef fish collected after storms, as well as individual susceptibility.

Clinical features are generally dominated by convulsions and coma, with various focal neurological signs. Among other symptoms such as paresthesias (i.e., numbness or tingling) in the hands and feet, or oral region, metallic taste, generalized pruritus, myalgia (muscle pain), arthralgia (joint pain), headache, and dizziness, patients have described a sensation of loose teeth, and have reported cold allodynia (not being able to distinguish between hot and cold by either taste or touch), also called "hot–cold reverse", and a symptom some consider pathognomonic, although not all patients experience it. Cold allodynia can also be experienced with other seafood toxicities (e.g. neurotoxic shellfish poisoning). Friedman *et al.* (2017) reported that rarely, severe central nervous system symptoms, such as coma or hallucinations, have been described. Neuropsychological symptoms, may become apparent in the days or weeks after the initial or acute illness, including subjectively reported cognitive complaints such as confusion, reduced memory, and difficulty concentrating, depression or irritability, and anxiety. Fatigue or malaise have been reported and may be debilitating. Cardiac symptoms and signs often include hypotension and bradycardia which may necessitate emergency medical care, and may manifest, generally in the early stage of the illness.

With many variable symptoms described, agreeing on a case definition has proved challenging but Friedman *et al.* (2017) have proposed a case definition based on other those of other bodies including the Centers for Disease Control and Prevention's Yellow Book (2019), the US Food and

Drug Administration's Bad Bug Book (2012), and the European Food Safety Authority's Framework Agreement. Geographical variation of symptoms, presumably due to the presence of different ciguatoxin congeners (i.e. chemical structure variants) has also been described with neurological symptoms often becoming more prominent after gastrointestinal symptoms following consumption of fish from the Caribbean. In the Pacific, neurological symptoms and signs may predominate acutely and there have been a few reports of more severe acute neurologic effects including coma, while in the Indian Ocean, ciguatera fish poisoning has been associated with neurological, neuropsychiatric, and mental status alterations, with reports of hallucinations, giddiness, incoordination, and loss of equilibrium.

Humans are poisoned by consuming fish containing ciguatoxins, the naturally occurring toxins. Unlike other fish-borne natural toxins, ciguatera fish poisoning is not due to the mishandling of fish and is not prevented by any particular storage, preparation, or cooking methods. The ciguatoxins are tasteless, colorless and odorless, and significantly, cannot be destroyed by cooking, smoking, freezing (at least six months at commercial freezing temperatures), salting or any other method of food preparation. Outbreaks can occur seasonally or sporadically, particularly after storms. Not all fish of a given species or from a given area will be toxic. Ciguatoxins and their precursors are produced by dinoflagellates, in the genus *Gambierdiscus*. These bottom-dwelling dinoflagellates are typically found attached to seaweeds, living and dead corals, and other surfaces in shallow tropical and subtropical waters. *Gambierdiscus* requires light and a substrate, which limits ciguatoxin production to shallow coastal habitats (e.g., reefs, atolls). Oceanic fish whose nutrition is derived from pelagic (i.e., in open sea waters and away from the shore) food webs rather than shallow water and coastal food webs are less susceptible to the accumulation of ciguatoxins.

Examples of common ciguatoxic fish species, and further details about ciguatera fish poisoning are available in the website materials accompanying this text.

8.6 Seafood Allergies

Seafood is one of the top eight allergens attributable to immunoglobulin E-mediated reactions and is a common cause of food-induced anaphylaxis, a major global public health issue. Fin fish and shellfish have multiple allergens that are distinct from one another. Cross-reactivity between fin fish and shellfish is exceedingly rare (Bahna, 2016). There are multiple types of the major allergens parvalbumin in fish and of tropomyosin in shellfish as well as other allergens: aldolase, enolase and vitellogenin in fish, and arginine kinase, myosin light chain and sarcoplasmic binding protein in shell fish. The effect of the allergens is affected by processing and usually increases by heating and decreases with canning, gastric acidity and enzymes.

Twenty-one allergens from 15 fish species are officially recognized by the World Health Organization/International Union of Immunological Societies at present, and the range of allergens in crustacea is even more diverse. Fish and shellfish are among the most common culprits of food allergies. A cross-sectional study in the United States found the lifetime prevalence rate for reported fish allergy was 0.4%, while 0.2% of population experienced both fish and shellfish allergy (Tong *et al.*, 2018). Worldwide prevalence of shellfish allergy was found to be 0.6% with higher incidence reported in the Asia Pacific region. In the United States, the lifetime prevalence rate for reported shellfish allergy was 2%. Shellfish allergy is highly prevalent among teenagers in the Philippines (5.12%) and Singapore (5.23%), and is the leading cause of food anaphylaxis in

Hong Kong and Taiwan. Bahna (2016) reported a telephone survey in the United States which revealed that 2–3% of participants self-reported the presence of seafood allergy (2.2% to shellfish and 0.6% to fish). In this survey, shellfish allergy was reported to be much less prevalent in children than in adults (0.5% vs. 2.5%). In a decreasing frequency, the causative triggers of reported allergy to shellfish were shrimp, crab, lobster, clam, oyster, and mussel. In an international survey administered to 17 280 adults from 15 countries, symptoms attributed to seafood ingestion were reported to be caused by shrimp in 2.3%, oyster in 2.3%, and fish in 2.2% with a general food allergy/intolerance range of 4.6% in Spain to 19.1% in Australia (Woods *et al.*, 2001). The variation may reflect differences in regional consumption and reporting patterns. Growing consumption of seafood globally may explain the increasing incidence of fish and shellfish allergies. Most hypersensitivity reactions to seafood are usually more severe than the reactions to most other food allergens, and are associated with rapid onset of symptoms, including gastrointestinal, cutaneous, respiratory, or multiple organ system symptoms, consistent with anaphylaxis (Bahna, 2016). Exposure occurs by ingestion, skin contact, or inhalation. Airborne allergen exposures are particularly abundant in the vicinity of cooking seafood by boiling, steaming, or frying. Skin exposure can occur more in occupational settings, and the manifestations are commonly cutaneous in the form of urticaria or allergic contact dermatitis but can also be respiratory or systemic. Occupational asthma in seafood processers (e.g., the snow crab, *Chionoecetes* spp.) has also been described.

8.7 The Veterinarian's Role in Protecting Public Health and Seafood Safety

Food safety is best assured by an integrated, multidisciplinary approach which considers the entire food chain. A food safety system should take into account the complexity of food production and the globalization of the food supply, and should be risk-based. It should consider hazards and potential associated risks at each stage of the food chain (i.e. primary production, transport, processing, storage and distribution), and should integrate risk management responses to such risks at the most appropriate points along the food chain. Veterinarians are trained in both animal health (including food-borne zoonoses) and food hygiene, which makes them uniquely equipped to play a central role in ensuring food safety, especially the safety of food of animal origin. The prevention, detection, and control of food-borne hazards throughout the food chain are generally more effective in reducing or eliminating the risk of unwanted health effects than relying on controls of the final product.

8.7.1 Monitoring and Control of Seafood Safety

The responsibility for monitoring and control of seafood safety is usually divided among various agencies of the government. In the United States, the oversight on seafood safety is carried out by the Food and Drug Administration, the Environmental Protection Agency, the National Marine Fisheries Service, and the state administrations. Potential health hazards are ascribed to chemical, microbial, and parasitic contaminants of seafood (e.g., natural toxins, toxic metals, synthetic substances, microorganisms, and parasites). These agents are acquired from three sources: Fecal pollution of the aquatic environment, the natural aquatic environment and the industry, retail, restaurant, or home processing and preparation.

The most well-known methods of managing quality and safety are:

- Good hygiene and manufacturing practices and sanitation.
- Sanitary standard operating procedures.
- Hazard analysis critical control point.
- Quality control.
- Quality assurance and management – ISO standards
- Quality systems
- Total quality management.

An "ideal" portion of fish may include attributes of taste, texture, color, but also an absence of anything harmful. Anything contributing to this ideal consistently, can be considered as a good manufacturing practice. The Food and Agriculture Organization of the United Nations (2001) describes good manufacturing practices as those procedures for a particular manufacturing operation that practitioners of, and experts in, that operation consider to be the best available, using current knowledge. This can include describing the requirements for facility design and construction, storage conditions, and harvesting and processing procedures. Some of these procedures will relate specifically to sanitation and health. Good hygiene practices refer to all practices regarding the conditions and measures necessary to ensure the safety and suitability of food at all stages of the food chain. It is clear that a whole-of-chain approach is integral to these concepts, and everyone, at each stage of the food chain, must be fully involved. All of these best practices must be identified, documented and implemented. When fully thought out, a food safety plan that includes all best practices, and applied daily as standard operating procedures, should control all product, personnel and environment. Sanitary standard operating procedures describe how good hygiene practice is to be achieved (i.e., minimizing microbial, chemical and physical contamination). For example, how could a food-producing company say they will produce food free of significant levels of coliforms and salmonellae if no one is ensuring that staff wash their hands after going to the toilet, or use footbaths after the toilet, and no one is disinfecting the tables and equipment?

8.7.1.1 Hazard Analysis Critical Control Point

The hazard analysis critical control point (HACCP) concept is based on the recognition of microbiological hazards that exist at various points in food processing, and measures that can be taken to control these hazards. That is, the anticipation of hazards and the identification of control points.

The HACCP system therefore offers a rational and logical approach to control food hazards. The HACCP system is a tool that can be applied, where this is possible, in addition to good hygiene practices. In other words, good hygiene practices constitute the foundation for ensuring that food hygiene is implemented in the first place, and the HACCP system is a potential add-on. Because the good hygiene practices are applied first, the international standard ISO 22000 names them prerequisite programs: "basic conditions and activities that are necessary to maintain a hygienic environment throughout the food chain suitable for the production, handling and provision of safe end products and safe food for human consumption", although there are other definitions of prerequisite programs (Wallace and Williams, 2001).

Best practices may vary between countries and operations but certain ones are core, including the safety of water and ice, the condition and cleanliness of food contact surfaces, prevention of cross-contamination from unsanitary objects to food, maintenance of facilities for personal hygiene, protection of food and food contact surfaces from adulteration, proper labelling, storage and use of toxic compounds, control of employee health conditions, waste management, transportation, traceability, and exclusion of pests.

When best practices are fully implemented, they should control the product. They impart generic control (e.g., bacteria rather than a particular bacterium). Once the food system is fully controlled, attention can turn to controlling specific hazards of concern with a HACCP approach.

To obtain fresh and frozen fish products, live fish are taken from the sea or from aquaculture systems and further handled and processed without any chemical additive or preservatives and distributed to sales points under frozen condition. Contamination with pathogenic bacteria can be from humans or animal reservoirs and can occur when the landing place is unhygienic. Washing and cleaning before packaging can also be a point of contamination if the fish are washed with contaminated water. Usually, fish are cooked before eating and this helps to eliminate the risk of pathogenic bacteria, although a few countries have a tradition of eating raw or partially cooked fish.

In identifying the critical control points (CCP) for fish and fish product processing, it is essential to first consider the temperature condition at all times, from capture to the point of sales and distribution (CCP-1) to prevent the growth of pathogenic and spoilage bacteria, and this works with time. There should be a specified maximum time at which products can be allowed at temperatures over 5°C, as most pathogenic bacteria do not grow at temperatures below 1°C. A sensory assessment (appearance, odor) of the fish at the port of landing is CCP-2 for ensuring that until this point the fish product has been maintained under adequate temperature control. Hygiene and cleanliness of handlers and fish harbor are CCPs for preventing contamination of products with microorganisms; water quality is a CCP-1 in preventing contamination from this source. The seriousness of the hazard varies, depending on the intended end use of the product.

HACCP is a worldwide-recognized systematic and preventive approach that addresses biological, chemical and physical hazards through anticipation and prevention, rather than through end-product inspection and testing. End-product testing can still be used, but as a verification that the HACCP plan is working.

Since the establishment of the World Trade Organization (WTO) in April 1995, the Codex Alimentarius Commission is recognized as the reference for international food safety requirement. Recognizing the importance of HACCP to food control, in June 1997, the Commission incorporated HACCP principles into their international code of practice *General Principles of Food Hygiene* (Codex Alimentarius Commission, 2020). Given this recommendation, HACCP has become the international reference system for food safety assurance for all WTO signatory governments. The Codex *General Principles of Food Hygiene* lay a firm foundation for ensuring food hygiene. They follow the food chain from primary production through to the consumer, highlighting the key hygiene controls at each stage and recommending a HACCP approach wherever possible to enhance food safety. Guidelines for the application of the HACCP system were presented by the Commission in 1997, and recommended that prerequisite programs (good manufacturing and health practices delivered through standard operating procedures and individual work instructions) be functional prior to the application of HACCP principles.

The seven principles of HACCP system are:

1) Identify potential hazards and assess the risk of occurrence.
2) Determine the Critical Control Points (CCPs).
3) Establish criteria to be met to ensure that each CCP is under control.
4) Establish a monitoring system.
5) Establish corrective action when CCP is not under control.
6) Establish procedures for verification.
7) Establish documentation and record keeping.

The 12 steps of HACCP food system consist of assembling a HACCP team, description of the product, identification of the intended use, constructing a flow diagram, on-site confirmation of flow diagram, listing all potential hazards with each step on the flow diagram and considering any measure to control the hazard at that step, and describing the CCPs. Additionally, the system involves the CCP, establishing critical limits, a monitoring system for each CCP, corrective actions, verification procedures, and a record keeping system.

More details about the setting up a HACCP food system are available in the website materials accompanying this text.

8.7.1.2 Operational Prerequisite Programs

The outcome of good manufacturing and health practices is the global reduction of the contaminant load (i.e., facility-wide), whether they compromise food safety or food suitability. Yet, in some cases, the level of hazards can still remain too high and unacceptable. This is why the food operator conducts a hazard analysis after the good manufacturing and health practices have been put in place and implemented. When a hazard is still identified for which there is no CCP, the ISO 22000 standard recommends establishing operational prerequisite programs: "identified by the hazard analysis as essential in order to control the likelihood of introducing food safety hazards to and/or the contamination or proliferation of food safety hazards in the product(s) or in the processing environment" (International Organization for Standardization, 2018). The elements of an operational prerequisite program are those of a CCP except that no critical limit is required for the control measures. Food safety is thus achieved thanks to good manufacturing and health practices and operational prerequisite programs determined through the application of HACCP principles, and where possible through the establishment of CCPs.

8.7.1.3 Weaknesses of HACCP

Despite rigorous CCPs in place in food production processes, there are often food safety issues, such as glass contamination or bacterial contamination after a controlling step (e.g., *Listeria monocytogenes* on hot-smoked salmon because a worker or the environment was unhygienic and recontaminated the product after smoking), poor storage conditions, or rat infestation. These are all issues that are controlled by good manufacturing and health practices. The HACCP system is implemented under the working assumption that good manufacturing practices are in place and that hazards associated with poor practices (peripheral hazards) have already been addressed and controlled; however, this assumption may be wrong. When a decision as to what size sieve to use to remove foreign material or what temperature to apply to eliminate harmful bacteria, HACCP provides an excellent decision making tool. However, hundreds of food safety decisions with no less of an impact on food safety are made without any real decision-making tool. It is crucial for the processor to acknowledge that HACCP is not designed to compensate for shortcomings in manufacturing and health practice, and that hazards controlled by good practices can be as significant as those being controlled by CCPs. Usually, larger companies will have quality assurance programs and quality-control teams that manage and deliver the HACCP plant efficiently; small companies may struggle to devote the required amount of time and personnel. Correct hazard analysis may not be performed, meaning that the entire HACCP plant may have fundamental flaws and despite the effort, may not be functional. Similarly, assessing the severity of risk differs between operators and this may render the HACCP plan ineffective. As with all plans, the HACCP system may deteriorate over time, even if originally well-constructed. Small changes going unnoticed will soon accrue to the point that large mistakes can occur. The better designed the HACCP plan the more likely it is to withstand change, but only constant monitoring and verification will keep it in shape.

8.7.2 The Role of Aquatic Animals and Seafood in the Emergence, Maintenance and Transmission of Antimicrobial Resistance to Humans

The emergence of drug resistance in microorganisms has become a serious problem both in the medical and agricultural fields. Antibiotic-resistant strains of bacteria are an increasing threat to animals and human health, with resistance mechanism having been identified and described for all known antimicrobials currently available for clinical use (McDermott *et al.*, 2002). Scientific data have revealed an increasing connection between the overuse of antimicrobial drugs in medicine, agriculture, the food industry, and the emergence and spread of antibiotic resistant bacteria. Antibiotic use has been largely responsible for the development of resistance in the bacterial pathogens. Extensive use in humans and indiscriminate use in veterinary practice, especially for the purpose of preventing (prophylaxis) or treating microbial infections. International use of antibiotics is also not coordinated, and they are prohibited in some countries while being permitted in others.

8.7.2.1 Antimicrobial Use and Antimicrobial Resistance in Aquaculture

In recent time, aquaculture has intensified due to its potential to provide sustainable, safe, and reliable alternative food production systems. To enhance fish survival and market value, a number of key strategies are regularly employed: extensive aquaculture, where predators are removed and competitors are controlled; semi-intensive, where food is supplemented and enhanced; and intensive, where all food needs are supplied. Because of the growing demands for finfish and shellfish, there has been a shift from extensive to semi-intensive and intensive systems, as they can produce greater yields (Dawood and Koshio, 2016). However, this intensification increases stocking density and nutrient pollution, often leading to poor water quality issues.

The combination of high density and poor water quality increases the likelihood of pathogen outbreaks. One outcome of higher disease rates in intensive farming is a reliance on antibiotics and other supplements, especially in countries where regulatory limits may not be clearly defined or closely monitored (Cabello, 2006; Santos and Ramos, 2016). Data on the amounts of antibiotics used in aquaculture are scarce, as few countries monitor the quantity of antibiotics used (Smith, 2008). However, in general, the use of antibiotics in aquaculture depends on local regulations, which vary widely. In some countries (specifically Europe, North America, and Japan), regulations on the use of antibiotics are strict and only a few antibiotics are licenced for use in aquaculture. In Europe, for example, the practice of non-therapeutic prophylactic use of antibiotics was banned in 2001 by the European Union Veterinary Medicinal Products Directive, as amended and codified in Directive 2001/82/EC (European Council, 2001 a,b,c). However, 90% of the world aquaculture production is carried out in developing countries that lack regulations and enforcement on the use of antibiotics (Chual *et al.*, 2016). This leads to high variability in antibiotic use. The prophylactic use of antibiotics in aquaculture has been commonplace in the past, particularly in shrimp (Holmström *et al.*, 2003) and salmon aquaculture (Buschmann *et al.*, 2012), and the difficulty in treating individual affected finfish and shellfish means that metaphylactic use of antimicrobials to treat entire populations is still commonplace (Cabello, 2006; Cabello *et al.*, 2013; Chual *et al.*, 2016; Economou and Gousia, 2013).

Antimicrobials and other medicaments are usually prescribed by veterinarians to food animal producers, including aquaculture. Residues of veterinary drugs include the parent compounds and/or their metabolites in any edible portion of the animal product, and include residues of associated impurities of the veterinary drug concerned. Some drugs used in food animals include topical antiseptics, bactericides, fungicides, ionophores, steroid anabolic growth promoters and other production enhancers, anti-parasitic drugs, and antibiotics. Other food animal drugs are those that modify the gastrointestinal environment to reduce the likelihood of rumen foaming and bloat in cattle, organic and inorganic water treatments that reduce the chances for water or fish infection in aquaculture, miscellaneous drugs and compounds used with the advice of veterinarians to treat specific conditions. The risk to human health include drug residue allergy, cancer, reproductive, and developmental effects, development of antibiotic resistant microbes, and so on.

Further information on pesticides, hormones, and growth promoters is available in the website materials accompanying this text.

8.8 The Veterinarian's Role in Preventing Environmental Contamination

8.8.1 Legal Disposal of Aquatic Animal Remains and Other Biohazards

Strategies for the disposal of dead animals (entire animals or parts thereof) should be prepared well in advance of any emergency. Major issues related to the disposal of dead animals include the number of animals involved, biosecurity concerns over the movement of infected or exposed animals, people and equipment, environmental concerns, and the psychological distress experienced by farmers and animal handlers. Disposal methods for aquatic animal remains should take into consideration a range of factors, including the cause of mortality. It may be appropriate to carry out a risk assessment on the disposal options. In the case of euthanizing animals for disease control purposes or unusually large mortalities, this may require approval from, or supervision by, the competent authority. In the event of aquatic animal mortalities of a significant nature in aquaculture or in the wild, the competent authority should be notified so that necessary steps can be taken to dispose of the dead aquatic animals, to minimize the risk of possible spread of aquatic animal disease. Cooperation among all relevant agencies and stakeholders involved in aquatic animal health is necessary to ensure safe handling and disposal. In this context, the following aspects should be addressed:

- Physical, logistical and data access by relevant personnel, in cooperation with stakeholders, including access of the competent authority to the aquatic animal waste.
- Movement controls and the authority to make exemptions under certain biosecurity conditions, for example for transport of aquatic animal waste to another location for disposal.
- The determination of the method and location of disposal, and the necessary equipment and facilities by the competent authority, in consultation with other authorities including government organizations responsible for the protection of human health and the environment.

Following collection, aquatic animal waste should be stored for the minimum time practical; the storage area should be separated from aquaculture sites and bodies of water to minimize the risk of spread of pathogenic agents. The disposal plant should operate using procedures that minimize the risk of spread of pathogenic agents. Disposal plants should maintain records related to quantity and type of raw material received, supplier, quantity and type of finished product, receivers, critical check points, and deviations from provisions stipulated in relevant regulations. These should be made available to the competent authority on request.

Further information on the disposal of high- and low-risk waste is available in the website materials accompanying this text.

8.9 Effluent Treatment Protocols

Intensive farming uses significant inputs to maximize production. In aquaculture, the accumulated byproducts (e.g., fish feces, excretions, uneaten feed) must be removed continuously to maintain health and welfare of the fish and to achieve optimal growth. Suspended solids and dissolved nutrients in the effluents have potential negative impacts on the environment. The amount of these materials in the effluent depends on a wide range of factors. Their environmental impact can be decreased either by improved farm management, or by physical and/or biological treatment of the effluent. Modern intensive land-based aquaculture systems can be divided in two types: open and closed systems.

In open systems, water used to rear fish, from whatever source, is discharged to the environment with its content of solids and nutrients, after passing through the farm. In closed systems, at least part of the water is recycled after specific treatments to reduce the content of solids and dissolved nutrients. Innovative methods and technologies for farm effluent water treatment, water reuse and byproducts recycling will reduce the quantity of clean water used in fish farming and the amount of materials discharged to the environment.

8.9.1 Effluent Water Treatment

Water quality regulations developed by governmental agencies usually have effluent standards and rules for issuing and enforcing permits for individual effluent outflows (Tesley, 2016). Water quality standards are designed to prevent effluents from causing negative impacts on receiving waters (Gallagher and Miller, 1996; Boyd, 2000). Standards normally specify limits for selected water quality variables and may contain other restrictions. A water quality standard might contain the following restrictions: pH 6–9; dissolved oxygen 5 mg/l or more; five-day biochemical oxygen demand 30 mg/l or less; total suspended solids 50 mg/l or less. Sometimes, the standard also may place a restriction on discharge volume or restrict discharge volume indirectly by specifying a maximum daily load for a variable. Effluent water treatment involves characterization of effluent, followed by solids removal, which is considered as the first important part of any treatment system. There are two methods for reducing suspended solids in fish farm effluent, each of which removes suspended solids from suspension: sedimentation and mechanical filtration.

8.9.1.1 Sedimentation

Sedimentation uses gravitational settlement systems of differing complexity. The sedimentation rate is measured in centimeters per second. In aquaculture, a favorable settlement speed is considered to be 1 cm/s. Most unused feed and feces are separable by sedimentation. Simple sedimentation is achieved by structures, variously called sedimentation, or settling, ponds and basins, which make use of the settlement characteristics of the solids.

Channels, with or without physical barriers, are often designed with frequent changes of water flow direction to reduce the energy of the solids and accumulate the waste at specific points. The channels can be built in concrete to facilitate cleaning. Alternatively, where space is available, channels can be excavated in water meadows providing sufficient transit time for the solids to settle.

Quiescent zones and in-raceway solids collection (cones) are where sections of raceways, usually located before the outlet, can be screened to exclude the fish, thus providing an area with reduced turbulence where solids can settle. A further improvement on this is the installation of collection cones within the floor of the raceway.

Lamellar settlement tanks achieve settlement of solids in a restricted land area, by more sophisticated parallel and inclined barriers. They are complicated, expensive to construct and difficult to clean. They are rarely used for fish farm effluent treatment.

Centrifugal concentrators (hydrocyclones) make use of centrifugal force to separate solids from water. Incoming water is directed tangentially at the top of the cylindrical uppermost part of the hydrocyclone vessel and the velocity of the inflow water is converted to rotary motion, thus creating centrifugal force. Heavy solids are thrown outwards and settle into the lower, conical, part of the vessel for subsequent removal. Hydrocyclone tanks are effective for high-density solids such as sand and mud but are difficult to use with large flows or with solids having a specific gravity close to that of water, such as fish feces.

8.9.1.2 Mechanical filtration

Mechanical filtration uses energy and filtration meshes with the dimension fashioned to trap solids. The meshes remove solids from water using physical barriers through which the solid particles cannot pass. This is usually achieved with a packed medium such as sand or with a mesh. Mechanical filters will remove both settling solids and those that will not settle due to their small particle size or low density.

8.9.2 Algal Ponds

Algae use solar energy to turn nutrients (in effluents) into usable resources, by the process of photosynthesis. The treatment must be well adjusted to balance the quantity of O_2, CO_2 and nutrient exchanges between the heterotrophic and autotrophic compartments. Where this is so, the fish wastes are considered to be a resource for the algae, which restore the water quality for the fish culture. Accordingly, algal growth is related to fish-effluent parameters (particularly nitrogen, phosphorus, dissolved oxygen) but it is also affected by temperature and light in outdoor systems.

8.9.3 Constructed Wetlands

Natural wetland systems can have a dramatic effect upon the quality of water as it passes through them. Particulate matter suspended in the inflow water, together with dissolved organic nutrients, coliform bacteria and even industrial and agricultural chemical pollutants, can be significantly reduced. Their subsequent impact in the downstream receiving waters is ameliorated by passage through a wetland system. Constructed wetlands do successfully clean waste water. Polluted water enters the system and the water that leaves it is significantly cleaner.

The success of any particular system depends on a number of design features which work together to create the optimum conditions for the physiochemical and biological processes to occur, and to enable a practicable level of their active management.

Supplementary materials
Ciguatera fish poisoning. Setting up a hazard analysis critical control point food system. Pesticides, hormones and growth promoters. Methods for waste. Further reading.

References

AAITO-IFIACI Anisakis Consortium (2011). Anisakis hypersensitivity in Italy: prevalence and clinical features: a multicenter study. *Allergy* 66: 1563–1569.

Adeyemo, O.K, Adedeji, O.B and Offor, C.C (2010). Blood lead level as biomarker of environmental lead pollution in feral and cultured catfish (*Clarias gariepinus*). *Nigerian Veterinary Journal* 31(2).

Ansari, M., Rahimi, E. and Raissy, M. (2011). Antibiotic susceptibility and resistance of *Aeromonas* spp. isolated from fish. *African Journal of Microbiology Research.* 5: 5772–5775.

Bahna, S.L. (2016). Not every seafood "allergy" is allergy! *Annals of Allergy, Asthma and Immunology* 117: 458–461.

Bi, S., Hu, F.S., Yu, H.Y. *et al.* (2015). Nontuberculous mycobacterial osteomyelitis. *Infectious Diseases* 47: 673–685.

Bisharat, N. and Raz, R. (1996). Vibrio infection in Israel due to changes in fish marketing. *Lancet* 348: 1585–1586.

Boyd, C.E. (2000). *Water Quality, An Introduction.* Boston, MA: Kluwer Academic.

Boylan, S. (2011). Zoonoses Associated with Fish. *Veterinary Clinics: Exotic Animal Practice,* 14: 427–438.

Bremner, H.A. (1985). A convenient easy to use system for estimating the quality of chilled seafood. Proceedings of the fish processing conference, Nelson, New Zealand, 23–25 April 1985. *Fish Processing Bulletin* 7: 59–70.

Buschmann, A.H., Tomova, A., Lopez, A. *et al.* (2012). Salmon aquaculture and antimicrobial resistance in the marine environment. *PLoS ONE* 7: e42724.

Cabello, F.C. (2006). Heavy use of prophylactic antibiotics in aquaculture: a growing problem for human and animal health and for the environment. *Environmental Microbiology* 8: 1137–1144.

Cabello, F.C., Godfrey, H.P., Tomova, A. *et al.* (2013). Antimicrobial use in aquaculture re-examined: its relevance to antimicrobial resistance and to animal and human health. *Environmental Microbiology* 15: 1917–1942.

Cann, D.C. (2001). *Botulism and Fishery Products.* Torry Advisory Note No 22 (revised). London: Ministry of Agriculture, Fisheries and Food, Torry Research Station.

Centers for Disease Control and Prevention. (2021). Division of Bacterial and Mycotic Diseases, Disease Information. Salmonella. https://www.cdc.gov/salmonella/index.html (accessed 27 May 2021).

Centers for Disease Control and Prevention. (2019) *CDC Yellow Book 2020.* New York, NY: Oxford University Press.

Chan, T.Y.K. (2016). characteristic features and contributory factors in fatal ciguatera fish poisoning--implications for prevention and public education. *American Journal of Tropical Medicine and Hygiene* 94: 704–709.

Chebet, L. (2010). "Rapid" (Alternative) Methods for Evaluation of Fish Freshness and Quality. Master thesis. University of Akureyri. https://skemman.is/handle/1946/5682?locale=en (accessed 2 May 2021).

Chuah, L., Effarizah, M.E., Goni, A.M. and Rusul G. (2016). Antibiotic application and emergence of multiple antibiotic resistance (MAR) in global catfish aquaculture. *Current Environmental Health Reports* 3: 118–127.

Clucas, I.J and Ward, A.R. (1996). *Post-Harvest Fisheries Development: A guide to handling, preservation, processing and quality*. Chatham, UK: Natural Resources Institute.

Codex Alimentarius Commission. (2020). *General Principles of Food Hygiene*. CXC 1-1969. Rome: Codex Secretariat, Joint FAO/WHO Food Standards Programme.

Codex Alimentarius Commission. (2016). *Guidelines on the Application of General Principles of Food Hygiene to the Control of Foodborne Parasites*. CAC/GL 88-2016. Rome: Food and Agricultural Organization of the United Nations and world Health Organization.

Codex Alimentarius Commission. (2009). *Food Hygiene Basic Texts, 4e*. Rome: Food and Agricultural Organization of the United Nations and world Health Organization.

Connell, J.J. (2001). *Quality Control in the Fish Industry*. Torry Advisory Note no. 58. London: Ministry of Agriculture, Fisheries and Food, Torry Research Station.

Dawood, M.A.O. and Koshio, S. (2016). Recent advances in the role of probiotics and prebiotics in carp aquaculture: a review. *Aquaculture* 454: 243–251.

Economou, V., Gousia, P., Kansouzidou, A. *et al*. (2013). Prevalence, antimicrobial resistance and relation to indicator and pathogenic microorganisms of *Salmonella enterica* isolated from surface waters within an agricultural landscape. *International Journal of Hygiene and Environmental Health* 216: 435–444.

European Council. (2001a). Directive 2001/82/EC of the European Parliament and of the Council of 6th November 2001 on the Community code relating to veterinary medicinal products. OJ L 311, 28.11.2001, p.1. *Eur-Lex* https://eur-lex.europa.eu/legal-content/EN/TXT/?uri=CELEX%3A02001L0082-20090807 (accessed 2 May 2021).

European Council. (2001b). *EC Enterprise Directorate General. Notice to Applicants: Vol 6B Presentation and Content of the Dossier Part II G and H: Guidance on Data Relating to the Environmental Risk Assessment for Products Containing or Consisting of Genetically Modified Organisms*. Brussels, Belgium: European Council.

European Council. (2001c). *EC Health and Consumer Protection Directorate General. Guidelines on the Assessment of Additives in Animal Nutrition: Additives other than Micro-Organisms and Enzymes*. Brussels, Belgium: European Council.

Evans, J.J., Klesius, P.H., Haenen, O. *et al*. (2009). Overview of zoonotic infections from fish and shellfish. Zoonotic infections from fish and shellfish. Program, abstracts and report of European Association of Fish Pathologists (EAFP) Workshop. EAFP International Conference, 14–19 September, Prague, Czech Republic.

Eze, E.L., Echezona, B.C., Uzodinma, E.C. (2011). Isolation and identification of pathogenic bacteria associated with frozen mackerel fish (*Scomber scombrus*) in a humid tropical environment. *African Journal of Agricultural Research* 6: 1918–1922.

Food and Agriculture Organization. (2020). *The State of World Fisheries and Aquaculture: Sustainability in action*. Rome: Food and Agriculture Organization of the United Nations..

Food and Agriculture Organization. (2001). *Manual on the Application of the HACCP System in Mycotoxin Prevention and Control*. FAO Food and Nutrition Paper 73. Rome: Food and Agriculture Organization of the United Nations.

Food and Agriculture Organization. (1998). *Food Quality and Safety Systems: A training manual on food hygiene and the hazard analysis and critical control point (HACCP) system*. Rome; Food and Agriculture Organization of the United Nations.

Food Standards Australia New Zealand. (2005). *Proposal P265: Primary Production and Processing Standard for Seafood: Final assessment report*. Canberra.

Friedman, M.A., Fernandez, M., Backer, L. C., *et al.* (2017). An updated review of ciguatera fish poisoning: clinical, epidemiological, environmental, and public health management. *Marine Drugs* 15: 72.

Gallagher, L.M. and Miller, L.A. (1996). *Clean Water Handbook. 2e*. Rockville, MD: Government Institutes.

Gauthier, D.T. (2015). Bacterial zoonoses of fishes: a review and appraisal of evidence for linkages between fish and human infections. *Veterinary Journal* 203: 27–35.

Gram, L. and Huss, H.H. (1996). Microbiological spoilage of fish and fish products. *International Journal of Food Microbiology* 33: 121–137.

Green-Petersen, D.M.B. (2010). *Sensory Quality of Seafood – in the chain from catch to consumption*. PhD Thesis. National Food Institute, Technical University of Denmark.

Grunert, K.G., Bredahl, L. and Brunso, K. (2004). Consumer perception of meat quality and implications for product development in the meat sector: review. *Meat Science* 66: 259–272.

Haenen, O.L., Evans, J.J. and Berthe, F. (2013). Bacterial infections from aquatic species: potential for and prevention of contact zoonoses. *Revue Scientifique et Technique* 32: 497–507.

Håstein, T.H.B., Lillehaug, A., Utne Skåre, J. *et al.* (2006). Food safety hazards that occur during the production stage: challenges for fish farming and the fishing industry. *Revue Scientifique et Technique* 25: 607–625.

Heberer, T. (2002). Occurrence, fate, and removal of pharmaceutical residues in the aquatic environment: a review of recent research data. *Toxicology Letters* 131: 5–17.

Holmström, K., Graslund. S., Wahlstrom. A. *et al.* (2003). Antibiotic use in shrimp farming and implications for environmental impacts and human health. *International Journal of Food Science and Technology* 38: 255–266.

Hong, L.C., Leblanc, E.L., Hawrysh, Z.J. *et al.* (1996). Quality of Atlantic mackerel (*Scomber scombrus* L) fillets during modified atmosphere storage. *Journal of Food Science* 61: 646–651.

Horowitz, B.Z. (2010). Type E botulism. *Clinical Toxicology* 48: 880–895.

Huidobro, A., Pastor, A., López-Caballero, M.E. *et al.* (2001). Washing effect on the Quality Index Method (QIM) developed for raw gilthead seabream (*Sparus aurata*). *European Food Research and Technology 2001*; 212: 408–412.

Huss, H.H. (1995). *Quality and Quality Changes in Fresh Fish*. FAO Fisheries Technical Paper no. 348. Rome: Food and Agriculture Organisation of the United Nations.

Huss H.H. (1994). *Assurance of Seafood Quality*. FAO Fisheries Technical Paper no. 334. Rome: Food and Agriculture Organization of the United Nations.

Huss, H.H. (1988). *Fresh Fish – Quality and Quality Changes: A training manual prepared for the FAO/DANIDA Training Programme on Fish Technology and Quality Control*. FAO Fisheries Series no. 29. Rome: Food and Agriculture Organisation of the United Nations; Danish International Development Agency.

Huss, H.H., Reilly, A. and Embarek, P.K.B. (2000). Prevention and control of hazards in seafood. *Food Control* 11: 149–156.

Hyldig, G. and Nielsen, J. (1998). A rapid sensory method for quality management. In: *Methods to Determine the Freshness of Fish in Research and Industry* (ed. G. Olafsdóttir, J. Luten, P. Dalgaard *et al.*), 297–305. Paris: International Institute of Refridgeration.

Hyldig, G., Larsen, E. and Green-Petersen, D. (2007). Fish and sensory analysis in the fish chain. In: *Handbook of Meat, Poultry and Seafood Quality* (ed. L.M.L. Nollet), 499–510. Oxford: Blackwell Publishing.

Igbinosa, I.H., Igumbor, E.U., Aghdasi, F. *et al.* (2012). Emerging *Aeromonas* species infections and their significance in public health. *Scientific World Journal* 2012: 625023.

International Commission on Microbiological Specifications for Foods. (2005). *Microorganisms in Foods 6: Microbial Ecology of Food Commodities*. 2e. ed. New York, NY: Springer.

International Organization for Standardization. (2018). *Food Safety Management Systems: Requirements for any organization in the food chain*. ISO22000:2018. Geneva: ISO.

Ivanovic, J., Baltic, M.Z., Boskovic, M. *et al.* (2015). Anisakis infection and allergy in humans. *Procedia Food Science* 5: 101–104.

Iwamoto, M., Ayers, T., Mahon, B. E. *et al.* (2010). Epidemiology of seafood-associated infections in the United States. *Clinical Microbiology Reviews* 23: 399–411.

Jonsdottir, S. (1992). Quality index method and TQM system. In: *Quality Issues in the Fish Industry* (ed. R. Olafsson and A.H. Ingthorsson), 81–94. Reykjavik: Research Liaison Office, University of Iceland.

Katikou, P., Hughes, S.I. and Robb, D.H.F. (2001). Lipid distribution within Atlantic salmon (*Salmo salar*) fillets. *Aquaculture* 202: 89–99.

Keiser, J. and Utzinger, J. (2005). Emerging foodborne trematodiasis. *Emerging Infectious Diseases* 11: 1507–1514.

Kim, T.-S., Pak, J.H., Kim, J.-B. *et al.* (2016). Clonorchis sinensis, an oriental liver fluke, as a human biological agent of cholangiocarcinoma: a brief review. *BMB Reports* 49: 590–597.

Kvenberg, E.J. (1991). Non-indigenous bacterial pathogens, In: *Microbiology of Marine Food Products*. (ed. R.W. Donn And H. Cameron), 263–291. New York, NY: H. Van Nostrand Reinhold.

Lehane, L. and Rawlln, G.T. (2000). Topically acquired bacterial zoonoses from fish: a review. *Medical Journal of Australia* 173: 256–259.

Lima dos Santos, C.A.M. and Howgate, P. (2011). Fishborne zoonotic parasites and aquaculture: a review. *Aquaculture* 318: 253–261.

Lindesmith, L., Moe, C., Marionneau, S. *et al.* (2003). Human susceptibility and resistance to Norwalk virus infection. *Nature Medicine* 9: 548–553.

Liston, J. (1980). Microbiology in fishery science. In: *Advances in Fish Science and Technology. Jubilee Conference of Torry Research 23–27 July*. (ed. J.J. Connell). Farnham, UK: Fishing New Books.

Lorencova, A., Klanicova, B., Makovcova, J. *et al.* (2013). Nontuberculous mycobacteria in freshwater fish and fish products intended for human consumption. *Foodborne Pathogens and Disease* 10: 573–576.

Luten, J.B., Børresen, T. and Oehlenschläger, J. (1997). *Seafood from Producer to Consumer, Integrated Approach to Quality*. Developments in Food Science 38. Amsterdam: Elsevier.

McDermott, P.F., Zhao, S., Wagner, D.D. *et al.* (2002). The food safety perspective of antibiotic resistance. *Animal Biotechnology* 13: 71–84.

Martinsdóttir, E. (2002). Quality management of stored fish. In: *Safety and Quality Issues in Fish Processing* (ed. H.A. Bremner), 360–378. Cambridge: Woodhead Publishing.

Martinsdóttir, E., Schelvis-Smit, R., Hyldig, G. *et al.* (2009). Measuring sensory evaluation of seafood: methods. In: *Fishery Products: Quality, safety and authenticity*. (ed. H. Rehbein and J. Oehlenschlager), 425–443. Chichester: Wiley-Blackwell.

Martinsdóttir, E., Sveinsdottir, K., Luten, J. *et al.* (eds.). (2001). *Sensory Evaluation of Fish Freshness: Reference manual for the fish sector*. Ijmuiden, Netherlands: QIM Eurofish.

Munoz, A.M., Civille, G.V. and Carr, B.T. (1992). *Sensory Evaluation in Quality Control*. New York, NY: Springer.

Nawa, Y., Hatz, C. and Blum, J. (2005). Sushi delights and parasites: the risk of fishborne and foodborne parasitic zoonoses in Asia. *Clinical Infectious Diseases* 41: 1297–1303.

Nguyen, T.H., Nguyen, V.D., Murrell, D. *et al.* (2007). Occurrence and species distribution of fishborne zoonotic trematodes in wastewater-fed aquaculture in northern Vietnam. *Tropical Medical and International Health* 12(Suppl 2): 66–72.

Ólafsdóttir, G., Martinsdóttir, E., Oehlenschläger, J. *et al.* (1997). Methods to evaluate fish freshness in research and industry. *Trends in Food Science and Technology* 8(8): 258–265

Oliver, J.D. (2005). Wound infections caused by *Vibrio vulnificus* and other marine bacteria. *Epidemiology and Infection* 133: 383–391.

Panel on Biological Hazards. (2010). Scientific opinion on risk assessment of parasites in fishery products. *EFSA Journal* 8: 1543.

Pau, L.F. and Olafsson, R. (eds.). (1997). *Fish Quality Control by Computer Vision*. New York, NY: Marcel Dekker.

Pedrosa-Menabrito, A. and Regenstein, J.M. (1990). Shelf-life extension of fresh fish: a review. Part III. Fish quality and methods of assessment. *Journal of Food Quality* 13: 209–223.

Popelka, P., Nagy, J., Pipová Monika, *et al.* (2014). Comparison of chemical, microbiological and histological changes in fresh, frozen and double frozen rainbow trout (*Oncorhynchus mykiss*). *Acta Veterinaria Brno* 83: 157–161.

Rahman, F. and Noor, R. (2012). Prevalence of pathogenic bacteria in common salad vegetables of Dhaka Metropolis. *Bangladesh Journal of Botany* 41: 159–162.

Rezaei, M. and Hosseini, S.F. (2008). Quality assessment of farmed rainbow trout (*Oncorhynchus mykiss*) during chilled storage. *Journal of Food Science* 73: H93–H96.

Robb, D.H.F., Kestin, S.C., Warriss, P.D. *et al.* (2002). Muscle lipid content determines the eating quality of smoked and cooked Atlantic salmon (*Salmo salar*). *Aquaculture* 205: 345–358.

Sánchez-Alonso, I., Carballeda-Sangiao, N., Gonzalez-Munoz, M. *et al.* (2018). Pathogenic potential of Anisakis L3 after freezing in domestic freezers. *Food Control* 84: 61–69.

Santos, L. and Ramos, F. (2016). Analytical strategies for the detection and quantification of antibiotic residues in aquaculture fishes: a review. *Trends in Food Science and Technology* 52: 16–30.

Shewan, J.M., Macintosh, R.G., Tucker, C.G. *et al.* (1953). The development of a numerical scoring system for the sensory assessment of the spoilage of wet white fish stored in ice. *Journal of the Science of Food and Agriculture* 4: 283–298.

Smith, P. (2008). Antimicrobial resistance in aquaculture. *Revue Scientifique et Technique (International Office of Epizootics)* 27: 243–264.

Su, Y.C. and Liu, C. (2007). *Vibrio parahaemolyticus*: a concern of seafood safety. *Food Microbiology* 24: 549–558.

Tesley, A.E. (2016). *The ABCs of Environmental Regulations*. 3e. Lanham, MD: Bernan Press.

Tong, W.S., Yuen, A.W., Wai, C.Y. *et al.* (2018). Diagnosis of fish and shellfish allergies. *Journal of Asthma and Allergy* 11: 247–260.

Traylor, J.M.A. and Goldstein, S. (2020). *Histamine Toxicity*. StatPearls. Treasure Island, FL: StatPearls Publishing.

Tran, T.K., Murrell, K.D., Madsen, H. *et al.* (2009). Fishborne zoonotic trematodes in raw fish dishes served in restaurants in Nam Dinh Province and Hanoi, Vietnam. *Journal of Food Protection* 72: 2394–2399.

US Food and Drug Administration. (2012). *Bad Bug Book: Handbook of foodborne pathogenic microorganisms and natural toxins*. Silver Spring, MD: FDA.

Venugopal, V. (2002). Biosensors in fish production and quality control. *Biosensors and Bioelectronics* 17: 147–157.

Wallace, C. and Williams, T. (2001). Pre-requisites: a help or a hindrance to HACCP? *Food Control* 12: 235–240.

Weinstein, M.R., Litt, M., Kertesz, D.A. *et al.* (1997). Invasive infections due to a fish pathogen, *Streptococcus iniae*. *New England Journal of Medicine* 337: 589–594.

Weir, M., Rajić, A., Dutil, L. *et al.* (2012). Zoonotic bacteria and antimicrobial resistance in aquaculture: opportunities for surveillance in Canada. *Canadian Veterinary Journal* 53: 619–622.

Widdowson, M.A., Sulka, A., Bulens, S.N. *et al.* (2005). Norovirus and foodborne disease, United States, 1991–2000. *Emerging Infectious Diseases* 11: 95–102.

Wogu, M.D. and Maduakor, C.C. (2010). Evaluation of microbial spoilage of some aquacultured fresh fish in Benin City Nigeria. *Ethiopian Journal of Environmental Studies and Management* 3(3). doi: 10.4314/ejesm.v3i3.63960.

Wong, K. and Gill, T.A., (1987). Enzymatic determination of trimethylamine and its relationship to fish quality. *Journal of Food Science* 52: 1–3.

Woods, R.K., Abramson, M., Bailey, M. *et al.* (2001). International prevalence of reported food allergies and intolerances. Comparisons arising from the European Community Respiratory Health Survey (ECRHS) 1991–1994. *European Journal of Clinical Nutrition* 55: 298–304.

World Health Organization. (2020). Zoonoses. Fact Sheet. www.who.int/topics/zoonoses/en (accessed 2 May 2021).

World Health Organization. (1999). Joint FAO/NACA/WHO *Study Group on Food Safety Issues Associated with Products from Aquaculture*. WHO Technical Report Series 883. Geneva: WHO.

World Health Organization. (1995). *Control of Foodborne Trematode Infections: Report of a WHO Study Group*. WHO Technical Report Series 849. Geneva: WHO.

9

Legislation, Regulations, and Policies

Myron Kebus and Chris Walster

Learning Objectives
Students should be familiar with the various areas of legislation that affects practicing aquatic veterinarians.

9.1 Introduction

To practice veterinary medicine and deliver services to clients, every veterinarian will be required to have a good understanding of regulations pertaining to aquatic veterinary medicine. Although veterinary jurisprudence is included in veterinary curricula, it is important that every practicing veterinarian understands the laws and regulations which might have an impact on them and their clients.

Most legal requirements fall into three categories: legislation, regulations, and policy. All are formulated or promulgated by government agencies. Most frequently, legislation is developed by a legislative body in a country, state or province, and provides general intent of a law to be enacted. Once enacted, this allows the appropriate governmental body overseeing the topic of the legislation to address or promulgate specific regulations or policies, always fulfilling the general intent of the legislation. In most cases, regulations are "hard" rules of what must or must not be done, while policies usually provide guidance or suggestions on similar issues. Often, the governmental agency with oversight over regulations and policies has responsibility for their enforcement and is given the legal authority to prosecute violations.

Aquatic veterinarians need to follow regulations and policies affecting veterinary practice in their local jurisdiction, but there is greater emphasis and need to understand legislation pertaining to aquatic animals regarding their import/export, welfare, disease reporting and notification, sampling for disease, use of drugs and vaccines, food safety, incoming water, effluent treatment, wild and domestic interactions, zoo and aquaria licensing and premise registration. This requirement comes about due to the largescale movement and international trade in aquatic animals, the lack of licensed medicinal products, environmental restrictions on the use of medicinal products, greater public scrutiny of the environmental impact of farming practices

Fundamentals of Aquatic Veterinary Medicine, First Edition. Edited by Laura Urdes, Chris Walster, and Julius Tepper.

Companion website: www.wiley.com/go/urdes/aquatic-veterinary-medicine

coupled with the interaction and exchanges that occur between wild and "domesticated" animals. Some basic points to consider:

- Legislation varies between jurisdictions and within some jurisdictions, often being dependent on the presence or absence of certain diseases or a desire of a jurisdiction to control a specific disease. Aquatic veterinarians often find that they require knowledge of the legislation and regulations of multiple jurisdictions.
- Aquatic veterinary medicine is not the sole province of veterinarians. Some European Union (EU) countries, for example, allow suitably qualified biologists and others to practice aspects of aquatic veterinary medicine. The same is true of countries in Asia and Africa. In Norway, the title of aquatic medicine biologist is considered equivalent to the title of veterinarian and they have limited prescription rights. This has historically come about due to a perceived lack of interest by veterinarians for aquatic veterinary medicine and a shortage of suitably trained veterinarians.

9.2 Regulations Affecting the Practice of Veterinary Medicine

Regulations are covered in undergraduate veterinary courses. However, practicing aquatic veterinary medicine and complying with the regulations can be difficult. You may work within a larger team of health professionals that includes not only veterinary nurses and technicians but also fisheries biologists, farm managers, and others often termed paraprofessionals. Sites may be remote and impractical to visit, creating difficulties establishing traditional veterinarian–client relationships, ability to prescribe, and how you advise your client. All these issues can be solved by having clear lines of responsibilities and communications within the team, organizing routine visits, or possibly making use through telemedicine or remote diagnosis. If you are uncertain that you can meet all the ethical and legal requirements expected, then it is better to discuss the issues with your regulatory body before accepting the case. Ignorance of legislation is not a legal defense if a veterinarian is accused of malpractice.

The body that regulates the practice of veterinary medicine in your jurisdiction is a good place to start or, alternatively, you can contact your local veterinary association. In the United States, all regulations affecting the practice of veterinary medicine are overseen by state boards. An alphabetical list of veterinary state board websites can be found on the American Veterinary Medicine Association website (avma.org), together with a model Veterinary Practice Act. In the UK, veterinarians need to follow the Royal College of Veterinary Surgeons Code of Professional Conduct for Veterinary Surgeons (rcvs.org.uk).

9.3 Animal Health Regulations

As discussed in the introduction, veterinarians treating aquatic animals need to be aware of multiple areas of legislation covering veterinary practice, veterinary medicines, animal health, welfare, environment, transportation, and slaughter. Generally, regulations, any supplemental legislation and an explanation of their intent can be found by searching the internet.

The Animal Health Regulations for the EU can be found on the Eur-Lex (2020) platform. This platform provides the text of the regulation, the background and intent, together with supplemental legislation. Within the EU, a regulation is binding on all member states and must be adopted on the same day. An EU Directive provides the intended result, but member states are free to determine how it is transposed into national law. This can lead to differing dates of adoption and potentially differences in interpretation.

9.4 International Animal Disease Regulations and Standards

The World Animal Health Organisation (OIE; www.oie.int) is an intergovernmental body dedicated to improving the health of animals. It currently includes 182 member countries and is recognized by the World Trade Organization as the reference body for standards relating to animal health and zoonoses. Two reference codes and manuals (terrestrial and aquatic) are published. "The *Terrestrial Animal Health Code* and *Aquatic Animal Health Code*, respectively, aim to assure the sanitary safety of international trade in terrestrial animals and aquatic animals, and their products." (World Animal Health Organisation, 2021).

"The purpose of the Manual of Diagnostic Tests for Aquatic Animals (the Aquatic Manual) is to provide a standardised approach to the diagnosis of the diseases listed in the Aquatic Code, to facilitate health certification for trade in aquatic animals and aquatic animal products. Although there are many publications on the diagnosis and control of aquatic animal diseases, the Aquatic Manual is a key reference document describing the methods relevant to the OIE-listed diseases and other important diseases for use by aquatic animal health laboratories around the world. Adoption of the specified methods will help to increase efficiency of laboratories and to promote improvements in aquatic animal health world-wide." (World Animal Health Organisation, 2021).

Veterinarians working in aquatic veterinary medicine should be familiar with both the Aquatic Code and Manual. You should not only be aware of the diseases listed but also the meaning of terms used (e.g., competent authority, zones and compartments). As well as containing disease specific chapters, the Code provides information on surveillance, risk analysis, disease prevention and control, trade measures, antimicrobial use, and welfare. The manual provides not just laboratory diagnostic techniques, but information on etiology, prevalence, control and prevention, among other useful information.

9.5 Economic Impact of Disease Regulations

The costs related to aquatic animal diseases are not well tracked. Aquatic animal farmers do not always appreciate the cost of disease losses. In many cases, the costs associated with regulations are considered as a burden on aquaculture. Even less well defined are the economic benefits of prevention of disease introductions. It is a challenge to demonstrate the economic impact of diseases, until a farm experiences disease loss first hand, although one can carry out simple cost–benefit analyses where figures are available. Official figures are unlikely to be farm specific but by jurisdiction. It is feasible to estimate costs of losses versus costs of prevention in discussion with the farmer.

Losses from aquatic animal diseases include mortality, facility closure orders, restriction of movement orders, inability to replace stock, market losses, reduced quality of survivors, reputation diminished, and missed markets.

9.6 Regulated and Non-Regulated Diseases

Part of the challenge is to determine which diseases warrant regulation and which do not. The criteria to answer this question include the degree of economic loss and market disruption it causes, whether it is a new or emerging disease, whether the disease can be detected with a test, whether it can be controlled and its spread limited, and the potential impact on free-living populations.

Regulated disease which may be referred to as listed, controlled, notifiable or reportable, can vary between jurisdictions, although all lists will be based on what is covered in the OIE *Aquatic Animal Health Code* and *Manual of Diagnostic Tests for Aquatic Animals*. Differences are dependent on presence or absence of the pathogen or affected species and whether the jurisdiction wishes to control other pathogens of interest to it locally. There are many examples where countries regulate aquatic diseases not found in the OIE Code.

Some examples of regulations dealing with aquatic animal diseases are available in the website materials accompanying this text.

9.7 Role Of Diagnostic Laboratories and Use of Assays

Diagnostic laboratoriess primarily perform assays to help to confirm the veterinarian's clinical assessment or narrow down their diagnostic suspicions. All countries have access to approved diagnostic laboratories and use assays in the OIE Manual for OIE-listed diseases. Most countries have developed assays for diseases which are not referred to in the OIE Manual and Code. The American Fisheries Society Fish Health Section *Blue Book* (2014) contains examples of non-OIE disease assays. When possible, it is important that veterinarians are always involved in submitting diagnostic samples and interpreting the results obtained.

The laboratory can also be seen as a third-party verifier that a disease organism is present. Selection of samples is based on the purpose for sampling. As an example, for a mandated aquatic animal health inspection you will probably use a specified laboratory; for detection of a listed disease you will probably use a reference laboratory; for in-farm or hobbyist use (e.g., a private client) a commercial or in-house laboratory with experience in aquatic animal health may be suitable. Generally, the number of animals or diagnostic samples required for an aquatic animal health inspection is based on the likelihood of detecting a pathogen based on certain criteria, such as disease prevalence. Details about sampling aquatic animals are provided in Chapter 5.

When reporting specific pathogens to the regulatory authority, it is imperative that the sample collection and the laboratory testing procedures are specified. Veterinarians need to be aware of their obligation to report to the regulatory authority their suspicion or knowledge of the presence of a reportable disease.

Examples of countries providing lists of reportable diseases and the actions required are available in the website materials accompanying this text.

9.8 Import/Export Regulations, Health Certificates and Movement Permits

It is widely accepted that a state or country's aquatic animal health is most at risk from the import of diseased aquatic animals or their products from another state or country. The intent of jurisdictional aquatic animal health regulations has been primarily to protect the health of aquatic animal within that jurisdiction. To accomplish this, import health requirements specify that animals imported to their jurisdiction must be tested for specific pathogens or assessed for signs of animal disease prior to import, to show they are free of specific pathogens. These requirements are typically captured in certificates of veterinary inspection (often called "health certificates"; see also Chapter 8, Microbiological Quality of Fish). Veterinarians need to be aware of which government agency to contact within their jurisdiction or, in the case of export, the receiving jurisdiction.

Creating a working network with colleagues in government agencies is essential to ensure that veterinarians keep abreast of requirements of legislation. Importantly, many issues related to certifying the health of animals moved between jurisdictions are covered in Section 5 of the OIE Aquatic Animal Health Code.

As an example, within the United States, legal authority for state aquatic animal health standards resides in agriculture agencies or resource agencies. Federal health standards applying to international import and export of aquatic animals is administered by the US Department of Agriculture or for salmonids, the US Fish and Wildlife Service. One example where similar programs apply to interstate movement of fish is found in Wisconsin's fish health regulations (Kebus, 2006).

9.8.1 General Considerations

Commerce of live aquatic animals and their products is a major economic activity. The risk of disease spread and pathogen introduction is greatest in facilities that receive aquatic animals from many regions and stock most widely. Importation presents the greatest risk of disease spread and introduction of pathogens. Additionally, many aquatic animals migrate and may travel from infected regions to pathogen/disease-free regions.

Aquaculture can impact free-living aquatic animal populations by disease spread or amplification of pathogens in open waters. Whether a facility is state-supported or private, the aquatic animal health standards must be uniform and science-based. Conversely, pathogen transmission from aquatic animals through open water can adversely affect cultured species. The health status of broodstock and those acquired from the wild and introduced into facilities should be subject to stringent health assessments. Unintentional introduction of pathogens derives from many sources, including diseased or carrier animals or fomites harboring infective material. Facilities should employ appropriate measures to reduce the risk of these pathogens entering the aquatic system.

The risk of introducing disease generally depends on the type of aquaculture facility (recirculating, raceway, pond, net pen), the health management practices, and stocking practices. Animals reared in open water are at greater risk of introducing pathogens to the water or receiving pathogens from open water than self-contained facilities (e.g., indoor recirculating tanks). The greater the level of health assessment and disease testing, the lower the risk of disease. Facilities that stock public and private waters have an increased risk of introducing disease compared with facilities that do not move live aquatic animals off of their facility.

Additionally, chemical control and treatment of potentially pathogenic organisms can impact open water. The decision to use chemicals should be made only after very thorough and careful consideration. Shotgun treatment, treatment with multiple chemicals in an effort to treat a disease that has not been accurately diagnosed, should never be practiced. There is far greater opportunity to damage animals and the environment with this approach rather than benefit animal health. Animal disease treatment should rely heavily on improving management and husbandry, whether chemicals are used or not. Many aquatic animal diseases can be controlled without chemicals. There are some cases where chemical treatment is essential to prevent severe mortality. Farmers should use only legally approved chemicals. Aquaculture veterinarians should be consulted for professional guidance on chemical use on facilities.

Facility practices can impact human health. The major categories are drug residues and other contaminants in edible aquatic animal products, antibiotic resistance, and zoonotic diseases (animal to man). Facility practices directly affect the first two categories and are a concern in the United States and worldwide. Consumers expect the aquatic animals they consume to be safe and wholesome. Seafood producers and facilities that release animals which may be caught and eaten are obliged to ensure that the edible tissues are not tainted with chemicals or other contaminants. As for the zoonotic diseases of aquatic animal origin, these are comparatively rare compared with zoonotic diseases transmitted by other animals.

To determine the requirements for transfer of specified species, it is essential that the veterinarian consult with both the state of origin and the state of destination. The pathogens of interest and the test procedures required will be specified by the importing governmental agency. These agencies constantly update target pathogens. In addition, it is important for the veterinarian to also consider that there may be transfer of exotic or introduced species with a shipment. It is imperative that the shipment be checked for both animal and plant species to prevent introduction of unwanted species. Many jurisdictions require the following information and data:

- Does the facility raise or distribute aquatic animals?
- What species are to be imported (to assist in avoiding the introductions of aquatic plant/animal nuisance species)?
- What is the origin of the source water?
- Is the origin and transport history of specified species traceable?
- Has the species been reared in an environment containing salmonids and/or cyprinids?
- Have pathogens of concern been found on the facility?
- Have chemicals, antibiotics or irradiation been used? (see Chapter 8).
- What is the nature and cause of mortality for the past one to five years?
- Were species obtained as eggs or as live animals?

9.8.2 Role of Producer Best Management Practices

Best management practices can be helpful in directing farmers on the best way to prevent pathogens from entering any aquatic animal farm. Verifying best management practices is best done by a third party. Regulatory agencies often mandate the production of a standard operating procedure, which should reflect best production practices.

General practices to consider:

- Provide the best water quality.
- Avoid overcrowding.
- Avoid over- and underfeeding.
- Minimize stress.
- Remove dead animals immediately.
- Call for professional assistance early.
- Obtain the best animal stock.
- Invest in good facility design and construction.

Strict biosecurity is one of the major components of best management practices on aquatic animal farms and import health standards are one of the most important components of a farm's biosecurity plan. Veterinarians should always be involved in helping producers develop and implement biosecurity best management practices. For more information on biosecurity see Chapter 8. Critical points to consider include:

- Introducing new animals.
- Introducing new water.
- Facility traffic (visitors).
- Vermin control (birds, rats, etc.).

9.9 Veterinary Drug, Biologics, and Pesticide Regulations

Always refer to the legislation and regulations applicable to your local jurisdiction. A discussion on the use of antibiotics and other treatments can be found in Chapters 5 and 7.

Examples of websites covering regulatory aspects of veterinary medicines, and an explanation of the cascade in the UK and investigational new animal drugs in the United States are available in the website materials accompanying this text.

9.10 Other Regulations

Food safety regulations are described in Chapter 8.

It is imperative to be aware of the environmental impact of waste water discharge and to refer to your local environmental protection agency or equivalent (see Chapter 8).

Supplementary Materials

- Some examples of regulations dealing with aquatic animal diseases.
- Examples of bodies with lists of reportable diseases and the actions required.
- Examples of agencies covering regulatory aspects of veterinary medicines.
- Further reading.
- Further resources.

References

American Fisheries Society Fish Health Section. (2020). *Blue Book*. https://units.fisheries.org/fhs/fish-health-section-blue-book-2020

Eur-Lex (2020) The EU's animal health law. https://eur-lex.europa.eu/legal-content/EN/TXT/?uri=LEGISSUM%3A3005_2 (accessed 20 May 2021).

Kebus, M.J., (2006). Wisconsin's Veterinary Approach to Fish Health. In: *Aquaculture Biosecurity: Prevention, Control and Eradication of Aquatic Animal Disease* (ed. A.D. Scarfe, C-S. Lee and P.J. O'Bryen), 69–76. Ames. IA: Blackwell Publishing.

World Animal Health Organisation. (2021). International standards. https://www.oie.int/en/what-we-do/standards (accessed 20 May 2021).

10

Principles of Aquatic Animal Welfare

Laura Urdes and Chris Walster

Learning Objectives
Students should demonstrate knowledge of current issues related to aquatic animal welfare and an ability to assess the welfare status of key aquatic species (e.g. effects of capturing, handling, transportation, specific signs of stress and pain and how to mitigate them). Students should be also familiar with local jurisdiction welfare legislation and aware of international (World Organisation for Animal Health) and supranational (European Union, International Air Transport Association) sources. Additionally, they should be aware of the numerous schemes provisioning increased welfare standards (e.g. RSPCA Assured (UK), Marine Stewardship Council, Responsible Fishing Scheme, Industry Codes of Practice, European Food Safety Authority Opinions on the Welfare of Farmed Fish).

10.1 Introduction

It is fair to say that, despite the fact humans have exploited aquatic animals for thousands of years as sources of food and other commercial products, as well as pets, aquatic animal welfare has never been high on the public agenda. Perhaps a case of out of sight out of mind? From roughly the 1960s or somewhat before, this situation has started to change.

There is increasing recognition that the oceans are not an infinitely exploitable resource, raising concerns over the environment and ecosystems. Greater recognition that changes in production methods for farm animals and lifestyle for pets has impacted the type and frequency of disease seen. Minimizing stress at slaughter has produced better-quality carcasses giving premium prices for the product. There are issues with the availability, speed, and ease of slaughter methods for aquatic animals. The effects of stocking density on both infectious and non-infectious diseases, as well as undesirable behaviors such as territorial aggression or repetitive behaviors.

Rapid movements of live aquatic animals around the world facilitates the hobby of fish keeping, but enhances the spread and impact of new or exotic diseases (Walster, 2008, 2015).

Fundamentals of Aquatic Veterinary Medicine, First Edition. Edited by Laura Urdes, Chris Walster, and Julius Tepper.

Companion website: www.wiley.com/go/urdes/aquatic-veterinary-medicine

The general public expects that the same welfare standards to be applied to aquatic animals as in the case of the more familiar terrestrial animals, but our ability to accurately assess and provide the welfare needs of aquatic animals is hampered and complicated by:

- The alien environment in which they live, which makes it difficult to observe natural behavior.
- The number of taxa and species involved (around 600 species of fish are farmed and up to 6000 species are traded or kept as ornamental or pet fish).
- The debate over pain and sentience in fish, crustacea, and cephalopods.
- The reliability, complexity, cost and practicality of monitoring welfare indicators. Commercial aquaculture facilities are often found in hard to reach places, requiring remote monitoring. Fish will often congregate in schools and vary their depth dependent on environmental cues affecting observed stocking densities. Dissolved oxygen measurements are dependent on where the monitor is placed (e.g., lowest at the end of a raceway or where fish are likely to school).
- New aquaculture species are obtained from the wild and are less adapted to the production process than domesticated species.
- The limited availability of licensed medicines and vaccines, as well as welfare issues connected with administering them (e.g., abdominal adhesions due to intraperitoneal injection of vaccines or the need to sedate ornamental fish prior to injecting).

Management procedures often require keeping animals in confined spaces which can be detrimental to water quality (e.g., grading, transportation, and slaughter). To ensure good water quality, animals are often fasted beforehand.

Welfare is an economic luxury. In Asia and Africa, much aquaculture is carried out by subsistence farmers where putting food on the table is more important to them than animal welfare. What is our ethical and moral responsibility regarding welfare? Bear in mind that we can only influence welfare when we have some sort of control over the animal. In laboratory animals, regulated procedures are done deliberately; in aquaculture, welfare is a consequence of the production process, whereas with ornamental fish welfare issues are often due to a lack of knowledge. The rights of indigenous peoples to carry out traditional hunting (e.g., of whales) also need to be considered.

Many of the above points can be summed up as a lack of knowledge or "more research is needed"; indeed, the number of welfare papers published each year seems to increase exponentially, but improvements in welfare on the ground appear to be slow in coming. A more depressing summation of the above points is that current welfare indicators are often contradictory, depending on the species or system discussed, leaving one with a feeling that applying and assessing good welfare in aquatic animals is a daunting task.

10.2 A Brief Discussion on the Whys and Wherefores of Animal Welfare

As a veterinarian, you have a responsibility not only for the health of an animal under your care but also for its welfare. Fortunately for us, there is a clear link between health, production, and welfare allowing us to use health assessment parameters, in which we are well trained, as a proxy measurement for good or at least acceptable welfare.

A discussion of the multiple concepts that have been proposed to quantify and qualify the welfare of aquatic animals is available in the website materials accompanying this text.

Problems come in deciding what is good welfare. The definition is influenced by your moral and ethical standpoint and that of your clients and the public, the definition of welfare used, the amount of control exercised over the animal, the practicality of implementing welfare procedures and their availability. The following brief discussion is partly based around resources available from the World

Small Animal Veterinary Association (WSAVA) Animal Wellness and Welfare Committee (https://wsava.org/committees/animal-wellness-and-welfare-committee).

Starting with a definition of welfare used by WSAVA, "The physical and psychological, social and environmental well-being of animals", we can see immediately its roots are firmly anchored in the five freedoms (Brambell, 1965) discussed later in this chapter and measurable welfare indicators e.g. obesity and malnutrition.

Welfare consists of inputs and outputs. Inputs are the environment, the animal, management. Outputs are physiology, behavior, health and production. An animal's experience of welfare is shown in Figure 10.1.

Environment/available resources (sensory input)
↓
Brain evaluates (emotions)
↓
Body responds (behavior, physiology)
↓
Animal adapts and survives (homeostasis, allostasis)

Figure 10.1 An animal's experience of welfare.

The four principles of medical ethics (Beauchamp and Childless, 2001) are:

1) Nonmaleficence – do good.
2) Beneficence – avoid harm.
3) Respect for autonomy.
4) Privacy of others or keep your promises.

See Ebsen *et al.* (2012) for further discussion of these four principles.

10.3 Ethical Theories of Welfare

- Deontology – ethics of principle; duty and obligation.
- Utilitarianism – ethics of consequence; what produces the greatest good.
- Teleology – ethics of purpose; the purpose they serve rather than the means by which they arise.

10.3.1 What drives welfare?

- Moral concern – an animal may be harmed.
- Public opinion (that looks bad).
- Commercial concerns (potential loss of sales).
- Science (objective).

10.3.2 Assessment Welfare Frameworks

10.3.2.1 The Five Freedoms (Brambell, 1965)

1) Freedom from thirst, hunger, and malnutrition.
2) Freedom from discomfort.
3) Freedom from pain, injury and disease.
4) Freedom to express normal behavior.
5) Freedom from fear and distress

10.3.2.2 The Five Needs (UK Animal Welfare Act 2006)

1) A suitable environment.
2) A suitable diet.
3) To be able to exhibit normal behavior patterns.
4) To be housed with, or apart from, other animals.
5) To be protected from pain, suffering, injury, and disease.

10.3.2.3 The Five Domains (David Mellor, New Zealand)

1) Nutrition
2) Environmental
3) Health
4) Behavior
5) Mental or affective state (produced/affected by the previous four domains).

10.3.2.4 The Five Opportunities (United States)

1) Opportunity for a well-balanced diet (food and water).
2) Opportunity to self-maintain.
3) Opportunity for optimal health.
4) Opportunity to express species-specific behavior.
5) Opportunity for choice and control.

The five domains provide the areas we need to consider when assessing welfare; the five freedoms are certainly aspirational when it comes to aquatic animals, while the five needs and five opportunities are possibly achievable to some extent, dependent on species, given current knowledge.

Given the wide range of taxa included as aquatic animals, it would be a monumental task to discuss the various welfare needs of all taxa, let alone all species. Our knowledge of aquatic animal welfare is far from complete but, where possible, specific information is given, although the focus is on fish, simply because fish are the ones most known about. The student is encouraged to make use of the references and further resources found in this chapter. It is useful to understand where different groups stand on animal welfare, and a simplistic division might be that animal rights groups base their opinion on ethics, while animal welfare groups base their opinion on science.

10.3.3 Life Quality of Aquatic Animals Related to the Five Freedoms

Applying the five freedoms to aquatic animals throws up some differences compared with the more familiar terrestrial animals, and some conundrums. Most aquatic species are ectotherms (cold-blooded) rather than endotherms (warm-blooded), which means that environmental temperature affects things such as the ability to digest food, wound healing and disease burden, where rising spring temperatures often favor pathogen reproduction before the fish can mount an adequate immune response. Stocking density guidance is given in kg/m^3 rather than kg/m^2, even though the full volume of an aquarium or net pen is rarely fully used and the maximum stocking density achievable depends on our ability to maintain good water quality (see Chapter 1). Water is a universal solvent exposing aquatic animals to a range of adverse events which may not be completely under the control of the keeper or the system they are contained in. Examples are pesticides sprayed in adjacent fields entering ponds, hand lotion and touch pools, heavy metals washed down fjords or rivers after storms in adjacent mountains, and higher levels of chlorine/chloramine in tap water at weekends, when most hobbyists do water changes, due to legal requirements to maintain safe drinking water for people, which does not necessarily mean safe water for fish.

Conundrums include the ability of new aquaculture species to thrive in captivity when sourced from the wild. Unlike terrestrial farmed animals most aquaculture species are only a few generations removed from their wild counterparts and have not had time to adjust to the presence of humans or management procedures. While aquaculture operators will clearly select for animals more suited to the farmed environment, and fish generation times are often short, allowing for rapid selection, there is still an issue of when species can be considered domesticated and whether during this period it is detrimental to their welfare? Does human utility surpass any potential detriment to their welfare?

Do migratory species need to migrate, or by swimming in a net pen are they still able to exhibit natural behavior? Salmonids, globally, are one of the successes of aquaculture in terms of production, but they are a migratory species, often migrating thousands of miles. Is this need to migrate innate or simply down to a need to find food? If it is an innate need, can this need be satisfied by swimming within a net pen?

Do aquatic animals suffer from thirst or hunger? At least in the sense of how mammals suffer from thirst and hunger, this is a problematic question. Animals living in freshwater have to excrete excess water continuously to maintain homeostasis, while for saltwater the problem is the need to actively excrete salt. Where this question does become pertinent is in the use of freshwater or saltwater baths (as appropriate) for therapeutic reasons. Do these treatments cause the animal to suffer thirst? Mammals are considered to have suffered hunger when their stomach is empty and/or there is low blood glucose. Carnivorous fish do not use glucose as their main energy source and many species of fish do not have a stomach. So, can they suffer hunger?

Whether fish suffer pain has been debated for several decades and the debate has now moved on to include other aquatic groups such as crustacea. Pain is the conscious experience of a noxious stimulus, together with a psychological element. Nociception is simply recognition of a noxious stimulus which produces a reflex action that an observer might interpret as pain. Currently, the debate seems to revolve around whether some aquatic animals have the brain structure to feel pain, in that they do not possess a neocortex, although studies have shown this is not necessary to feel pain in all species. In human medicine, it is recognized that it can be extremely difficult to quantitatively measure pain in a patient. As such, the precautionary principle can be used by practicing veterinarians, whereby best practice, would be to consider the necessity and/or benefit of providing pain relief with a given procedure.

10.3.3.1 Fear and Distress Connected to Predators

While land-based facilities can mitigate against predators by using fences (e.g., otters) or nets above ponds (e.g., birds) or by being totally enclosed, problems arise for water-based facilities where this can be much harder. Theoretically, you can mitigate by using "predator secure" nets but these are costly and may have an indeterminate lifespan with weaknesses not being spotted before it is too late. Seals and other marine predators (e.g., dolphins) love salmon, and the net issue (which also relates to escapees) is somewhat ameliorated by acoustic deterrents or shooting of animals. There are papers describing the adverse effect on predators of acoustic deterrents and, in some countries, shooting of predators is banned on conservation grounds. The question arises as to how we determine who has the greater welfare need.

Escapees are a problem for salmon aquaculture. If a net pen fails, then tens of thousands of farmed fish may escape and breed with wild salmon. It is considered that farmed species are "genetically weaker" than wild species and may impact detrimentally on wild populations causing decline. Should farms be placed on migratory routes?

New diseases seem to arise frequently and obviously impact the welfare of species under our control and potentially those that are not. Is this due to our expanding knowledge of the aquatic environment, climate change, keeping large numbers of animals in relatively small volumes, or poor husbandry, allowing pathogens to mutate successfully more frequently?

While many of the above questions are currently unanswerable, we can assess welfare and quality of life based on the five freedoms or any of the other welfare frameworks. It is the duty of a veterinarian to ensure the welfare of animals under their care. That does not mean that everything can and should be done perfectly, but that any husbandry or clinical procedures carried out are at a level acceptable to the majority of their peers. Welfare is a continuing debate and, as individuals, we should keep ourselves informed of any developments.

10.3.4 Freedom from Thirst, Hunger and Malnutrition

Thirst can be avoided by providing a suitable environment. If a species is unfamiliar to you, basic environmental requirements can be assessed by consideration of where it is found in the wild or using websites such as FishBase (fishbase.se). Hunger can be avoided by providing a suitable (e.g., is the species carnivorous, herbivorous, or omnivorous) and varied diet, using appropriately sized pellets or flakes that float or sink depending on whether they are surface, mid-water or bottom feeders. Live food can be provided if necessary, which has its own welfare implications such as introduction of disease. Malnutrition is associated with being underweight (underfeeding) but includes obesity (overfeeding) and unavailability of micronutrients (e.g., thiamine deficiency through the feeding of trash fish containing thiaminase). For some species there are body condition score charts allowing assessment of the body condition of a fish (Clark *et al.*, 2018).

For many species, there are commercial diets available which provide an indication of the amount (percentage body weight) you should provide. In commercial aquaculture, where water temperatures and the quantity of feed are known, it is possible to calculate when the fish will be ready for market. Problems arise when there are delays in sending to market such as insufficient market price, movement restrictions, or lack of equipment such as transport. In these conditions, it is considered better to feed one week in three at the normal rate, rather than providing insufficient food on a continuous basis.

Nutrition is more fully covered in Chapter 3, it is worth making the following comments. Fish can be omnivorous, carnivorous, or herbivorous. They can be surface feeders, mid-water, or bottom feeders. Their nutritional requirements vary during life stage and also the environment the fish is in. Carbohydrates are the most abundant and cheapest source of energy for fish, although doubt has been expressed about the usefulness of carbohydrates in fish feed, particularly in carnivorous species, which use protein for energy. However, the amount of carbohydrate affects whether pellets will float or sink.

Proteins are the most expensive source of energy, with requirement being highest in the initial feeding of fry and generally decrease as fish increase in size. For maximum growth, young fish require 40–60% protein in the diet, while for healthy maintenance most species require 1–1.5 g protein/kg bodyweight/day. As water temperature increases, the requirement for protein to maintain optimum growth increases. Like mammals, fish require ten essential amino acids: arginine, histidine, isoleucine, leucine, lysine, methionine, phenylalanine, threonine, tryptophan, and valine.

Lipids consist of fats, phospholipids (part of cell membranes), sphingomyelins (present in brain and nerve tissue), waxes and sterols (components of several hormones, particularly sexual hormones). Fatty acids are the component parts of lipids. They maybe saturated or unsaturated which can be divided into mono, poly- (PUFA) and highly unsaturated fatty acids. While fish are considered a good source of omega 3 and omega 6 for people, these elements must be included in the diet and are essential fatty acids.

Vitamins can be termed a micronutrient as opposed to the above, which are macronutrients. They are required in very small amounts but are critical for the maintenance of normal physiological behavior. They are divided into water-soluble and fat soluble vitamins. The water-soluble vitamins are vitamin B complex (thiamine, riboflavin, pyridoxine, pantothenic acid, niacin, biotin, folic acid) and B12, choline, inositol, and ascorbic acid (vitamin C). The fat soluble vitamins are A, D, vitamin E and K. Water-soluble vitamins leach out of the diet as soon as the pellet hits the water. If natural feeds are available in the pond as in extensive aquaculture, vitamin supplementation may not be necessary. Conversely, if intensive farming is carried out, supplementation of food with vitamins becomes a necessity.

Of the 26 essential minerals described for animals, only 9 are known to be essential for fish. Fish can absorb minerals from their environment, so supplementation may not be necessary except for those that are required in high concentrations, especially in freshwater fish. Calcium can be obtained from food and through the gills and fins in freshwater. Phosphorus can only be obtained from food as both fresh and saltwater are generally deficient. Fishmeal is rich in both, but feedstuffs of plant origin are deficient in calcium and phosphate is unavailable as it is found as phytic acid, which cannot be absorbed. Magnesium is necessary for the structure of cell walls and cobalt increases hemoglobin formation and improves growth in common carp.

10.4 Production

10.4.1 Breeding

- All brood stock require increased nutrition prior to spawning to ensure that they have enough energy to give to the developing gonads. In salmon, which do not feed when spawning naturally, this increased nutrition must be given six to nine months prior to spawning, when it will be laid down as fat reserves. In carp, this extra feeding should be supplied prior to the decrease in water temperatures as winter approaches. Carp naturally spawn with increasing water temperature in the spring, but the gonads were already developed in the previous year. There is no benefit in feeding them in the spring.
- Carp can be prepared with natural feeding and cereals at 2% body weight/day. The ponds need to be fertilized to produce enough natural food.
- When fish have finished spawning, they may have lost between 5–10% of body weight and will be in poor condition. If they are to be used as brood stock again then it is essential that they be fed well. Not only to replace the lost weight but to help prevent disease.

10.4.1.1 Eggs

- Eggs do not require feeding. However, they are very tasty for all manner of creatures. Dead and diseased eggs should be removed. The batch should be treated with malachite green at 5 ppm (malachite is banned in food fish in the EU, and the only licensed product available is Pyceze® (Novartis Animal Vaccines), which is based on bronopol).
- If eggs hatch early and the ponds are not ready to receive them, they can be fed finely minced hardboiled egg yolk for a couple of days.

10.4.1.2 Fry

- After three to four days in the hatchery, the fry are ready to go into the pond.
- The pond should have been prepared a couple of weeks earlier. This can be done by liming, which kills any disease organisms and helps to break down silt, thus liberating nutrients. The pond can also be fertilized.

- The number and type of plankton should be carefully monitored to ensure sufficient number and the right sort of plankton.
- The type of feed that fry can use is dependent on two factors: their size and their high metabolic needs. For the first few days, rotifers will supply their needs but soon they will need to move on to medium sized zooplankton such as *Moina*. *Artemia* as newly hatched or frozen nauplii may be used at this stage. However, rotifers are considered of better nutritional quality.
- *Daphnia* provide the final food source. This whole process will take about three to four weeks.
- Artificial diets can be fed from day one; even if the fry do not eat them, the plankton will. The benefit of supplying an artificial diet early is that it helps wean fry on to it.
- Many facilities will culture their own plankton. This is relatively easy to do. It requires appropriate water, nutrition, oxygen, and a light source. A culture of appropriate algae can be added as required. The advantage is that you have a known food source. In the pond there may be unwelcome additions such as cyclops. The disadvantage is that it is hard to control production of the plankton if you get an algal bloom.

10.4.1.3 Fingerlings

- Prepare the pond. For fingerlings, you would lime the pond in the spring. As well as the benefits already mentioned, liming increases the buffering capacity, provides calcium for invertebrates, and precipitates organic matter in suspension.
- Add fertilizer. Manure may be added or artificial fertilizer. As the fingerlings may be in this pond for much of the summer, if you require maximum natural food then this will need to be done every fortnight.
- The fish should be taking artificial diets well now. The size of the pellets used relates to the size of the fish. Starting with crumbs, as the fish grow the larger the pellet that can be given. Diets can be fed at up to 10% with 40% or higher protein.
- In warm climates, fish may grow to three to four inches in size within two months.

10.4.1.4 Growing On

- The protein requirement decreases in older fish.
- If you feed too much carbohydrate, then it will be laid down as fat.
- In ornamentals where color matters, then it is worth adding spirulina or carotenoids to the diet to enhance color. Most ornamental fish require at least one winter to produce solid colors. In their first season the color is washed out.
- When using color enhancers it is best to use them for three to six weeks prior to sale.

10.4.2 Health Effects of Poor Nutrition

- Starvation causes poor growth, decreased survival, and increased susceptibility to disease. It may be a result of underfeeding, competition between fish due to size, or inappropriate physical characteristics such as size of pellet.
- Retention and trailing of feces indicates that the fish is constipated. This can be a result of feeding too much dried food and is sometimes thought to occur when old, poorly stored food is given.
- Fatty liver occurs due to too much fat in the diet but also due to rancid fat. As fish rarely are exposed to temperatures above 30°C, they store their fats as PUFA. This keeps the fats liquid. Animal fat can block the gut as it goes solid and cannot be digested. PUFAs are very easily oxidized and turn rancid. Vitamin E helps to prevent oxidation but is itself destroyed in the process. This is why food should be kept in sealed containers and used within a couple of weeks of opening.

- Thiamine deficiency can occur when feeding trash fish, which contain thiaminase, an enzyme which breaks down thiamine. Symptoms are of the nervous system and can include swimming erratically or circling and blindness.
- Vitamin C deficiency causes slow wound repair. If treating a sick fish, it is often advantageous to give an injection of vitamin C as well as any other treatment.
- Aflatoxicoses is caused by aflatoxin, which is produced by *Aspergillus* spp. molds (*A. flavus* and *A. parasiticus*). It occurs when food has been stored in damp conditions. Ornamental fish keepers should be advised to buy no more food than the fish eat within four weeks. Another bad practice is using food left over from the autumn in the following spring.

10.4.3 Health Effects of Good Nutrition

- Good nutrition maximizes production and minimizes waste.
- Fish reach their biological potential.
- Spirulina, used as a complementary feed, improves reds in ornamental fish, thus increasing their value.

10.4.4 Immunostimulants

- Many immunostimulants are derived from yeast polysaccharides. They act by directly stimulating white blood cells. Some organic acids are thought to stimulate the immune system.
- There is no point feeding immunostimulants continuously, as they have no effect. The best way to use them is to feed prior to a stressful management procedure. They all vary but generally they should be fed 10–21 days prior to the event. If you do use them long term, then it is better to do two weeks on six weeks off. Immunostimulants have been used to improve the efficacy of vaccines.
- Probiotics are cultures of bacteria that are thought to be beneficial. It is thought that they work two ways: one is to colonize areas so as to remove other more pathogenic bacteria; the other is to bind to sites in the gut, thus blocking entry points for pathogenic bacteria.
- Astaxanthin and canthaxanthin are carotenoids used to provide the pink color to salmon. There is evidence that they have a beneficial effect on the immune system.

10.4.5 Freedom from Discomfort

For terrestrial animals, freedom from discomfort relates to the provision of a suitable environment, including shelter and a suitable resting area. For aquatic animals, this means suitable water quality, including flow rates (current), depth and volume, suitable lighting, both in terms of luminosity and wavelength, suitable substrate and refugia, such as a plant pot in a home aquarium, or the nooks and crannies of an artificial reef in a public aquarium.

Assessing water quality should involve measuring at least the following six parameters routinely: temperature, pH, dissolved oxygen, NH_3, NO_2 and NO3. However, to properly assess water quality requires the measurement of 36 parameters, a costly and time-consuming process. Flow rates need to be suitable depending on whether species live sedentary or active lives. Depth, together with lighting, relate to the normal position of the animal within the water column while volume relates to the spatial needs of the animal.

10.4.6 Environment

- Local to the fish – is it intensive/extensive aquaculture? In a mud pond or the hatchery? In a hobbyist pond or retail outlet? Species and type of production?
- If the environment is intensive, fish require vitamin supplementation. If extensive and in a mud pond, the vitamins are gained from the environment via plankton, rotifers, and clandocerans.
- In a small hobbyist tank, excess feeding may cause an ammonia spike due to waste food. In a mud pond, the natural fauna would use the excess food.
- The lower the digestibility the higher the rate of feeding and the higher the production of feces. Remember that the higher the concentration of organic waste, the lower the oxidation reduction potential, the greater the use of oxygen, more bacteria in the water so greater chance of infection. Marine species need an oxidation reduction potential of 300 mV, a good freshwater pond is above 250 mV, a pond growing blanketweed is below 250 mV and below 100 mV you grow slime algae.
- Different species require different diets, not just in nutrients. A bottom feeder will not take floating pellets!
- To grow fish one can feed 3–10% body weight/day depending on temperature and age. To maintain fish one can feed 1–1.5% body weight/day. However, while being held in a retail facility, one might only feed at a rate of a quarter to a half percent of the body weight/day. First, because the system is heavily stocked, second because the fish may be sold on, and third to keep costs down. It is not advisable to feed below 1%/day unless temperatures are low. It would be preferable to starve for two weeks and feed for one.
- In a small facility you would hand feed. This allows you to examine the fish feeding. It also gives you greater control of the amount you feed as you can see what is wasted.
- Always know the number of fish stocked and the average weight. This tells you how much to feed. For some species if you know your average water temperatures, the number of fish stocked, the size you wish to grow them to and the time you have to reach that weight, then it is possible to work out a daily feeding regime.
- Do not use diets designed for different species. Koi have often been fed trout pellets. In the short term it is no problem. In the long term it is harmful.

10.4.7 Freedom from pain, injury and disease

Although there are insufficient scientific data indicating that all fish can experience pain, from what is currently known, it may seem appropriate to give fish the benefit of scientific doubt. One must always assume that, during surgical and other routine, potentially painful procedures, fish can feel pain, and should take measures to prevent or alleviate the pain (Box 10.1).

Injuries (also termed "lesions") are structural damage of organs, tissues, or body fluids. Injuries can be caused by physical agents, inflicted by the physical environment (fishing nets may cause laceration, hemorrhage; extreme temperatures produce frostbite, burns, and thermic shock; continuous illumination may cause eye damage in those fish requiring periods of darkness), or by other fish (fin damage caused by biting), chemical agents (e.g., above normal water solutes such as chlorine, nitrogenous compounds, dissolved gases, unsettled sand suspensions modify the chemical and microbiological properties of the epidermal mucus, cause necrosis or inflammation of gills, dermis, and mucosa) or biological agents (e.g., sea lice infections in farmed salmon cause physical damage or stress in the fish, adversely affecting their growth and performance).

Disease occurs when there is loss of homeostasis. It involves structural and functional abnormalities of tissues, fluids and/or organs and translates clinically into lesions and symptoms.

Box 10.1 Pain

The world "pain" was originally used to express an emotional negative sensation which, as it was believed before the eighteenth century, only humans were able to experience (Pringle, 1989). According to the International Association for the Study of Pain, pain is an "unpleasant sensory and emotional experience associated with actual or potential tissue damage, or described in terms of such damage" (Merskey *et al.*, 1979). It follows that pain involves physical, perceptual and emotional elements. The cognitive set required to experience pain is composed by nociceptors, nociceptive processing brain components, nerve bundles, and the cognitive capacity to feel pain. Nociceptors, of which presence has been demonstrated in a few fish species (Mettam *et al.*, 2011), play a major role in detection of noxious or injurious stimuli, in that they respond to these stimuli, allowing for nociception similarly to that described in amphibians, birds, and mammals.

In humans, pain is controlled by four nervous structures: the hippocampus, amygdala, cerebral frontal lobes, and neocortex/neopallium. Neocortex is the major association center, which generates consciousness (including perceptual and emotional sensations) and allows for storage and access to accumulated experiences, including pain-related experiences. The neocortex is lacking in fish and is poorly represented in reptiles, amphibians, birds, and primitive mammals, while in superior mammals it is a complex and well-defined structure (Urdes, 2017a). The absence of a structural neocortex in fish suggests that they may lack the perceptual and emotional basis for pain (or any other feelings, for that matter). Nevertheless, in those animals lacking components of the cognitive set required to experience pain, such as fish, pain experience should be inferred from the behavioral responses of the animal, which translate into removing from the site of aversion (Farm Animal Welfare Committee, 2014; Huntingford *et al.*, 2006).

All these cases, when they arise, cause poor welfare. Freedom from pain, injury and disease refers mainly to minimizing suffering caused by these conditions, by good husbandry practices, which include adequate housing, control of disease and avoiding stress-causing factors, such as those caused by removal of fish from water and crowding. This refers to minimizing pain and preventing unnecessary suffering through adequate housing and nutrition, prompt diagnosis and medical treatment to injured and diseased fish. Especially in the case of farmed fish, the concept includes also prevention of disease and measures taken to prevent unnecessary suffering at the time of killing.

Inadequate housing and nutrition take into consideration instances in which poor welfare may arise. While feed deprivation seems to be less harmful in fish than in warm-blooded animals, sudden feed withdrawal, which is applied usually before handling and transport to reduce metabolism in fish (and hence, to reduce ill-effects of stress), reduce welfare due to increased aggression in the fish. Poor water quality, crowding and removal from water cause maximal stress responses from fish. Effects of poor water quality and how to avoid them are shown in Chapter 1. The choice of site and water supply may be essential in preventing fish pathogens from entering a fish population, as well as it dictates on the chemical composition of the water. For instance, water sourced from boreholes may carry fewer fish pathogens than lake water, it is more temperature-stable and free from chlorine. Algal blooms and gelatinous zooplankton may occur sometimes, reducing the water flow, clogging the gills and suffocating fish.

In the case of fish farms, simple systems in design, which allow for fairly uniform conditions, such as ponds, raceways, sea pens and tanks, may not allow sufficient variation for species-specific (in the case of polyculture) or individual preferences of a fish. Diseased fish may seek different places in a temperature gradient than healthy ones, while in polyculture, some fish may prefer different positions in the water column by light levels and food delivery. Mainly in the case of ornamental fish, excessive or inappropriate environmental enrichment may encourage territoriality and aggression, resulting in injuries. Overcrowding and handling cause skin and fins damage, increasing disease susceptibility of the fish. Apart from the negative effects on the water quality, high stocking density can influence also the fish behavior, as they may exhibit aggressive and territorial responses. Other variables leading to poor welfare related to inadequate housing are pollution events, predators (e.g., aquatic birds and mammals feeding on fish), and escapes. Predators are discussed later in this section and also in Chapter 1.

Escapes occur mainly in farmed fish, when rearing units fail, damaged by predators or extreme weather events, or in the case of inadequately designed units. Those escaping fish which survive generally experience poor welfare, as they may have difficulties in adapting to the new environment in the wild, feeding poorly, losing condition and dying of starvation. Other escaping fishes may reside within the water circulation systems in tanks, raceway or ponds, acting as a potential disease reservoir.

10.4.8 Prevention of Disease, Prompt Diagnosis and Treatment of the Injured and Diseased

To assess welfare from the perspective of prevention, monitoring of behavior, morbidity, mortality, and physical injuries, such as fin and skin damage or deformities, is necessary. To reduce the risk of diseases associated with inappropriate husbandry of the fish, at the designing and planning stages of a fish facility, veterinary input is required to develop appropriate healthcare plans aimed at decreasing the risk of husbandry-associated health conditions.

Individual monitoring of fish would be ideal, but it is usually difficult and often limited in practice, because of the three-dimensional environment, which is typically visible only from the water surface. Hence, monitoring is rather conducted at group level and involves assessment of the fish behavior at feeding and at other times, giving consideration to any behavioral changes, such as food rejection or swimming abnormalities. Underwater cameras and remotely operated vehicles can be used to monitor health status of fish in farms, but follow-up of any arising problem in a systematic manner may prove difficult. Other means of monitoring fish health is by regularly sampling fish for the purpose of monitoring or on other occasions, such as when fish are tagged or vaccinated by hand.

Apart from the fish sampling, clinical examination of fish samples and necropsy of priorly euthanized fish should also be performed for fish stock monitoring. However, this method of monitoring is not always reliable, as fish health condition at the time of sampling may dictate which individuals are subjected to examination. Additionally, catching and culling fish can influence the behavior and may have welfare impact on the rest of the population. In fish farms, biosecurity methods, such as the provision of sites for quarantined fish, appropriate cleaning and disinfection of equipment, and all-in-all-out production are among the most reliable ways to prevent disease. Such measures often reduce the risk of outbreak occurrence and minimize the use of therapeutic medication. As in the case of other farm animals, in fish farms, biosecurity measures, including monitoring and control of disease and physical injury, as well as other measures such as strategies to tackle major common diseases and recording of mortalities, should be part of a written health plan agreed between the producer and the veterinarian involved in the health care of the fish.

As less feasible as it may seem, there is currently agreement on the need for individual monitoring and disease control in fish. Applying group therapeutic medication to fish may be detrimental to the healthy fish and lethal to those with incompatibility to the chemicals and/or concentrations used. There are usually deaths recorded during chemical bathing in salmon, aimed at eliminating sea lice. Also, in-feed group medication may create a number of issues. Sick animals may not ingest sufficient medication, so they will not be adequately treated; healthy fish in the group take the medication although they do not require it.

While group medication does still have its own benefits in treating fish efficiently, reducing the level of agents in the water and thus limiting the possibility for a wider disease distribution, there are generally limitations in using such medications due to environmental and pollution concerns. According to environmental legislation, there are a number of restrictions on the amount of medicines and number of treatments allowed, thus making such treatments less effective.

As in other animal industries, diseases resistance is one of the traits genetically selected. The practice is common in farmed fish (e.g., salmon) but breeding for disease resistance is also practiced in the ornamental fish sector. This practice has its own limitations, with further implications on welfare and production of the fish.

Disease involves suffering and, hence, poor welfare. Infestations with the sea lice *Lepeophtheirus salmonis* in Norwegian salmon production, for example, are currently seen as one of the greatest fish welfare problems, where mortalities can reach extremely high numbers. Sub-lethal injuries consist in physical damage and skin erosion, immunosuppression, chronic stress, and secondary infections, such as viral infectious salmon anemia, where the parasite acts as a mechanical transmitting vector (see Chapter 4). In some cases, disease is favored by poor husbandry and environment because these factors cause stress, impairing development and immunity system of the fish. Increasing temperature to hasten growth and development of fish may increase the incidence of spinal deformities in the fish. Crowding at highest density, moving and transporting fish outside water will cause serious injuries and stress to fish.

Prevention and treatment of disease in farmed fish is often constrained by the limited availability of suitable authorized medicines. To avoid fish suffering, veterinarians are allowed to use available medicinal products to alleviate pain and treat health conditions, in accordance with the cascade principle (or similar, such as investigational new animal drugs in the United States). This is a legislative provision of national and EU legislation recognizing the need for veterinary practitioners to use certain medicines off-label not strictly in accordance with the conditions under which the product was authorized. The cascade principle applies only to veterinarians. Such licenses may be granted by the national competent authority when there is a particular health situation or where no authorized veterinary medicinal product is available in the country but one is available in another member state or a third country.

10.4.9 Pain Management in Fish

For fish kept for food, the OIE Aquatic Animal Health Code is the baseline for fish production, covering the welfare of fish during transport, aspects of stunning and killing for human consumption, and for diseases control purposes. For further information on pain management in fish see Box 10.2.

Further information on preventing unnecessary suffering at the time of killing is available in the further reading section in the website materials accompanying this text.

Further information on the legal context is available in the further reading section in the website materials accompanying this text.

Box 10.2 Pain Management in Fish

Analgesics are used to relieve pain and discomfort in fish. Anesthetics are used in fish to produce insensitivity to painful or discomforting procedures, such as surgery, fin clipping, handling, transportation, and to induce unconsciousness and sleep. Anesthetics are used as the first stage of euthanasia in fish, as well (see also Chapter 6). However, both analgesia and anesthesia in fish are areas where relatively little in terms of clinical data is known or formally reported (Urdes, 2017b). The factors acknowledged as impeding pain management practice in fish as successful as in terrestrial vertebrates are the wide range of species, which makes generalization across species very problematic; analgesic agents tested on fish, as well as licensed anesthetic products for fish, are very limited; the ability to monitor depth of fish anesthesia is restricted to a few specialist research groups globally. Additionally, the use of pre-anesthetic (sedation) protocols in fish, in combination with one or more adequate anesthetics, which ensure avoidance of aversive reactions to anesthetics in other species, is not yet available for fish. The choice of the correct methodology of administration of analgesic and anesthetic agents should take into account three groups of variables:

- Species-related characteristics, such as fish species, strain, body weight and physiological stress
- Environmental conditions, such as water temperature and pH
- Agent-related characteristics, such as chemical composition, pharmacological properties, exposure duration and drug concentration.

Generally, in small to medium-sized fish, anesthetics are administered dissolved into the water where fish are held (equivalent to inhalation anesthesia in mammals) or introduced (i.e., immersion of fish into a water tank or bucket containing anesthetic solution). Administration of anesthetics via injection is restricted only to large fish species of over 10 kg. In the case of anesthesia, monitoring depth of the process by visual assessment and interpretation of ventilation rates (opercular ventilation rates), posture (body movement and equilibrium), and reflex response to stimuli (e.g., tail or fin pinch) are standard practice in fish.

There are four groups of analgesics in fish commonly referred to in the literature: opioids, local anesthetics, non-steroidal anti-inflammatory drugs (NSAIDs), and antidepressants; the latter two have been less explored in fish. Experimentally, the opioid morphine (5 mg/kg) has been shown to minimize pain and discomfort in rainbow trout, flounder, and goldfish. It is assumed that, in fish, the pharmacodynamics of morphine is similar to that in mammals, by inhibiting neurotransmitter release, thus blocking nociceptors and central transmission (presynaptic effect). An exception is that, in fish, excretion rates are much slower (total elimination time is 56 hours), suggesting that its use would be suitable to chronic conditions or after major surgery. Other opioids, such as tramadol, dermorphin, butorphanol, and buprenorphine were also tested on farmed and ornamental fish species, such as cod, trout, carp, dogfish, and koi carp, but appeared to have limited effectiveness and poor analgesic properties.

Local anesthetics block nociceptive transmission. The analgesic effects of lidocaine have been tested in rainbow trout and zebrafish where, at 1 mg/kg, no adverse effects were observed, and it was assessed as a very efficient analgesia. Novocaine (procain) is known to reduce reflex responses in cod, but since it has not been tested in vivo in fish, it is not recommended to be used. Very few NSAIDs have been tested in fish for their analgesic effect, but action of these drugs observed in other species decrease inflammatory reactions by decreasing the production of thromboxanes and prostaglandins. Ketoprofen, tested in koi carp and dogfish with doses of

2–4 mg/kg, has been proven not to be effective, whereas carprofen at doses of 1–5 mg/kg has been found to cause deleterious effects in trout (i.e., increased ventilation and depressed activity).

Anesthesia in fish can be achieved by physical and chemical means. Gradual cooling to 10.3°C is effective in adult zebrafish (*Danio rerio*) to a degree where a surgical plane of anesthesia is achieved. However, it is advised that gradual cooling should be used as a last option and when surfaces and instrumentation can be maintained at 10°C.

There are currently over 15 anesthetics in use in veterinary practices, experimental settings and aquaculture. The most common anesthetics are tricaine methanesulfonate (MS222), benzocaine, lidocaine hydrochloride, clove oil, eugenol, isoeugenol, etomidate and metomidate hydrochloride, 2-phenoxyethanol (2-PE), quinaldine and quinaldine sulphonate, 2,2,2 tribromoethanol, propoxate, 4-styrilpyrydine, propofol, and isoflurane. However, only very few of these substances are approved for use in fish destined for human consumption. A summary of the anesthetic agents applied to fish, showing a range of doses, efficiency and adverse effects of the anesthetics in different fish species is discussed in Chapter 6).

If there is no prior experience with the fish, fish strain and/or analgesic or anesthetic substances we want to use, prior to using them, it is recommended to perform a pilot test using the lowest doses and a small number of fish of different strains, to ensure safety and efficacy of the procedure. *Source:* WSAVA Congress 2017.

10.4.10 Freedom to Express Normal Behavior

In some experimental studies, it has been demonstrated that fish can respond to painful stimuli with reflexes, similar to responses seen in amphibians, birds, and mammals. In the facial skin of trout, there are a number of polymodal nociceptors which respond to mechanical, chemical, and thermal extreme variations (Farm Animal Welfare Committee, 2014). A number of studies have also addressed the effect of pain alleviating chemicals, showing that while the fish in the experiments responded aversively to electric shock, fin pinching, CO_2 saturated water, needle prick, their pain responses decreased at increased levels of analgesics and opioids, such as morphine. It is inferred that opioid receptors and endogenous (endorphin-like) opioids are present in the spinal cord and brain of the fish subjected to such experiments. Although repetition of some experiments by other groups had different or inconclusive results, most studies reported changes in fish behavior after the events.

If pain could be inferred from the behavioral responses of an animal only, we could always determine when or if the animal suffers, without the need to demonstrate that they have a perceptual and emotional basis for feeling something. It is inferred that behavioral changes suggesting anticipation and avoidance – the "keep away" behavior of fish when they are netted, hooked, live cut, and so on, relates to the survival, phylogenetically inherited sense, which shows that they are able to learn from positive reinforcement. In the light of current evidence, the Farm Animal Welfare Committee (2014) recommends that "animals should be given the benefit of any reasonable moral or scientific doubt about their welfare", and that all animals, should have "a life worth living".

While it is difficult to define typical or normal behavior of various fish species, mainly because some are semi-wild (e.g., salmon) or even wild (e.g., wrasse), which means that some generations of fish species have been kept in captivity less than others, it is generally agreed that normal behavior in fish should reflect the provision of adequate space (area), facilities (enrichment, hiding areas for cleaner species) and company of their own, to support normal functions, such as nutrition and reproduction, and to keep homeostasis.

In some cases, allowing fish to perform normal behavior in captivity may be quite challenging. A good example is smolting in salmon, which is a physiological process when the young salmon (fingerling or parr) move from freshwater to sea water. In the wild, this process occurs when the young salmon completes maturation in freshwater. In farmed salmon, this process involves the entire population, which is moved as a group, simultaneously. The individuals which are not ready to move are affected by the salt water and can die. Another example is farmed halibut. In the wild, halibut lives at the bottom, but in farms it is kept in nets with a tight base, where they lie in layers, one on the top of others. While it is currently accepted that a certain degree of stress is unavoidable in fish and that, in many cases, welfare may conflict with production priorities, we should always look for ways to minimize stress through, at least, good husbandry practices and appropriate system designs.

10.4.11 Freedom from Fear and Distress

Generally, in fish, fear and distress are caused by environmental and physical stressors such as loud noises and vibration, ultrasonic calls of predators, sudden changes of the environment, competition for food, handling, crowding/harvesting, and culling. Ornamental fish kept in aquariums and tanks at home or in offices, may be distressed by ultrasonic noise (inaudible to humans) and lights produced by computers, telephones and other devices commonly used in these facilities.

Fish species may respond differently to sound frequency and intensity. Man-made intense sounds, such as those produced by explosion, pile driving, and air guns can cause temporary or permanent hearing loss, change of behavior and disorientation in fish. At close range, underwater blasting may cause tissue damage (e.g., stun) in fish. Noise and vibration may also interfere with the acoustic communication in some species. It seems that fish act differently depending on whether vibrations are at low or high frequencies. Low-frequency vibrations of loud sounds, made for example by shipping, underwater dredging, and drilling, would cause fish to swim away from the source. High-frequency vibrations (of over 10 Hz) of softer sounds can instead attract fish. Devices and machines producing ultrasound vibrations may disturb the species able to detect these types of vibrations in the water (e.g., shads).

As shown previously, fear in fish translates to behavioral and physical changes, aimed at preparing them to react to potential danger or threats. Most commonly, fish would express fear by hiding and running away from the potential danger, quickened breathing and muscle stiffness. Long term exposure to fear-causing stressors may lead to poor mental health, as fish may become continuously alert and fearful. However, since most normal fish behaviors have not been well characterized, there are some general features of fish behavior that clearly signal for signs of stress. These include flashing (scratching body surfaces on objects), gasping at the water surface, fin clamping, color changes, social isolation, changes in activities such as feeding behavior and neophobia (Pasnik *et al.*, 2010; Martins *et al.*, 2011).

Physically, stressed fish may experience digestion and eating issues, as well as heart problems. Just like other animals, fish require good treatment and husbandry conditions to prevent fear and distress. Providing a stress-free environment to fish requires prior knowledge about the species-characteristic needs, about what should or should not be used in their environment. The basic features of aquatic environments and life support systems important to the health of fish and other aquatic animals are outlined in Chapter 1.

General requirements consist in prevention, careful monitoring, and the implementation of stress mitigation measures based on good practice to protect fish from environmental and physical stressors, such as predation, escapes, exposure to unpredictable events, during harvest, handling and transport. Some measures applying to fish husbandry are:

- Optimizing the environment by designing installations which allow for response to changing conditions, optimal movement and minimal handling of the fish to avoid discomfort, injuries and escapes in various weather conditions.
- Maintaining stocking densities in facilities within optimal limits, as communicated by evidence-based science.
- Ensuring good water quality, adequate transport conditions, monitoring and shelter to avoid environmental risk factors such as algal blooms and extreme weather events (see Chapter 1).
- Gentle handling at all times, including during harvest and at the time of killing (Farm Animal Welfare Committee, 2014).
- To overcome transport stress, allow for acclimation following transport and when fish are introduced into new environments (e.g., movement of farmed salmon between hatchery and various growing stages may be disruptive, as it generally involves movement of the fish in groups, without providing for differentiated conditions for individuals).
- Avoid as much as possible exposure of fish to continuous light, loud noises and vibrations.

Further information on noise, vibration and ultrasonic calls is available in the website materials accompanying this text.

10.5 Conclusion

Aquatic animal welfare is a continuing debate, with veterinarians often caught between opposing groups, opposing outcomes, and limited scientific evidence. It is up to all veterinarians to try to drive the debate forward based on scientific evidence, sound objectivity, and an awareness that welfare may need to be compromised in certain instances to ensure the overall benefit of the animals under their care.

Because of the diversity of opinion, our ability to measure welfare simply or accurately and the need for a lot more research, that the aim of this chapter has not necessarily been to provide answers to welfare questions, but to provide the student with sufficient background to be able to consider the complexities that arise. By reading this chapter and using the resources in this book, it is hoped that the student can ensure sufficient knowledge to be aware of differing legislation and welfare concerns dependent on the usage of the aquatic animal, as well as, the drivers behind welfare.

Supplementary Materials

- Noise, vibration and ultrasonic calls.
- Bibliographic references.
- Further reading.
- Further resources.

References

Beauchamp, T.L. and Childress J.F. (2001). *The Principles of Biomedical Ethics*. Oxford, UK: Oxford University Press.

Brambell, F.W.R., Chairman. (1967). *Report of the Technical Committee to Enquire into the Welfare of Animals Kept under Intensive Livestock Husbandry Systems*. Cmnd. 2836. London: HMSO. https://edepot.wur.nl/134379.

Clark, T., Pandolfo, L.M., Marshall, C.M. *et al.* (2018). Body condition scoring for adult zebrafish (*Danio rerio*). *Journal of the American Association for Laboratory Animal Science* Ebsen, M., Andersen, S. and Pedersen, B.D. (2012). Further development of Beauchamp and Childress' theory based on empirical ethics. *Journal of Clinical Research and Bioethics* S6: e001. doi:10.4172/2155-9627.S6-e001.

Farm Animal Welfare Committee (2014). *Opinion on the Welfare of Farmed Fish*. London: FAWC.

Huntingford, F.A., Adams, C.E., Braithwaite, V.A. *et al.* (2006). Current understanding on fish welfare: a broad overview. *Journal of Fish Biology* 68: 332–372.

Martins, C.I., Galhardo, L., Noble, C. *et al.* (2012). Behavioural indicators of welfare in farmed fish. *Fish Physiology and Biochemistry* 38: 17–41.

Merskey, H., Albe Fessard, D., Bonica, J.J. *et al.* (1979). Pain terms: a list with definitions and notes on usage recommended by the IASP subcommittee on taxonomy. *Pain* 6: 249–252.

Mettam, J.M., Oulton, L.J., McCrohan, C.R. and Sneddon, L.U. (2011). The efficacy of three types of analgesic drug in reducing pain in the rainbow trout, *Oncorhynchus mykiss*. *Applied Animal Behaviour Science* 133: 265–274.

Pasnik, D.J., Evans, J.J. and Klesius, P.H. (2010). Stress in fish. In: *Fundamentals of Ornamental Fish Health* (ed. H.E. Roberts), 33–38. Ames, IA: Wiley-Blackwell.

Pringle, L. (1989). *The Animal Rights Controversy*. San Diego, CA: Harcourt Brace Jovanovich.

Urdes, L.D. (2017a). The welfare concept – does it apply to fish, too? Proceedings of the World Small Animal Veterinary Association, Copenhagen, Denmark, 25–28 September 2017. https://www.vin.com/apputil/content/defaultadv1.aspx?id=8506476&pid=20539& (accessed 4 May 2021).

Urdes, L.D. (2017b). Pain management in fish. Proceedings of the World Small Animal Veterinary Association, Copenhagen, Denmark, 25–28 September 2017. https://www.vin.com/apputil/content/defaultadv1.aspx?id=8506475&pid=20539& (accessed 4 May 2021).

Walster, C., Rasidi, E., Saint-Erne, N. and Loh, R. (2015). The welfare of ornamental fish in the home aquarium. *Companion Animal* 20: 302–306.

Walster, C. (2008). The welfare of ornamental fish. In: *Fish Welfare* (ed. E.J. Branson), 269–290. Oxford, UK: Blackwell Publishing.

Index

Page numbers in *italics* refer to illustrations; those in **bold** refer to tables

Fundamentals of Aquatic Veterinary Medicine, First Edition. Edited by Laura Urdes, Chris Walster, and Julius Tepper.

Companion website: www.wiley.com/go/urdes/aquatic-veterinary-medicine

Printed in the USA/Agawam, MA
September 16, 2026

910661.234